DOCUMENTATION FOR REHABILITATION:
A Guide to Clinical Decision Making

SECOND EDITION

Lori Quinn, EdD, PT
Honorary Research Fellow
Cardiff University
School of Healthcare Studies
Cardiff, Wales

Senior Lecturer
New York Medical College
Physical Therapy Program
Valhalla, New York

James Gordon, EdD, PT, FAPTA
Associate Dean and Associate Professor
Division of Biokinesiology and Physical Therapy
  at the School of Dentistry
University of Southern California
Los Angeles, California

SAUNDERS

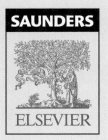

ELSEVIER

SAUNDERS
ELSEVIER

3251 Riverport Lane
Maryland Heights, Missouri 63043

DOCUMENTATION FOR REHABILITATION: ISBN: 978-1-4160-6221-9
A GUIDE TO CLINICAL DECISION MAKING
Copyright © 2010, 2003 by Saunders, an imprint of Elsevier Inc.

Notice

Library of Congress Cataloging-in-Publication Data
Quinn, Lori.
  Documentation for rehabilitation : a guide to clinical decision making / Lori Quinn, James Gordon. – 2nd ed.
     p. ; cm.
  Rev. ed. of: Functional outcomes documentation for rehabilitation. c2003.
  Includes bibliographical references and index.
  ISBN 978-1-4160-6221-9 (pbk. : alk. paper)
  1. Physical therapy. 2. Physical therapy assistants. 3. Medical protocols. 4. Communication in medicine. I. Gordon, James, Ed.D. II. Quinn, Lori. Functional outcomes documentation for rehabilitation. III. Title.
  [DNLM: 1. Medical Records. 2. Physical Therapy Modalities. 3. Disability Evaluation. 4. Documentation. 5. Patient Care Planning. WB 460 Q74d 2010]
  RM700.Q85 2010
  615.8'2--dc22

                                                                                          2009041665

Vice President and Publisher: Linda Duncan
Executive Editor: Kathy Falk
Senior Developmental Editor: Melissa Kuster Deutsch
Publishing Services Manager: Patricia Tannian
Project Manager: Carrie Stetz
Designer: Teresa McBryan

To Ann Gentile, a never-ending source of inspiration to us both.

Contributors

Helene M. Fearon, PT
Partner
Fearon & Levine Consulting
Wilton Manors, Florida
www.fearonlevine.com
Chapter 15

Jody Feld, DPT, MPT, NCS
Manager of Clinical Support and Education
Bioness Inc.
Valencia, California
Case Examples

Janet A. Herbold, PT, MPH
Senior Administrator
Burke Rehabilitation Hospital
White Plains, New York
Chapter 16

Stephen M. Levine, PT, DPT, MSHA
Partner
Fearon & Levine Consulting
Wilton Manors, Florida
www.fearonlevine.com
Chapter 15

Agnes McConlogue, PT, MA
Clinical Assistant Professor
Department of Physical Therapy
Stony Brook University
Stony Brook, New York
Chapter 14

Karen Dauerer Stutman, PT, MS
Physical Therapist
Carlson Physical Therapy
Bethel, Connecticut
Case Examples

Preface

This book was born out of necessity. It began its life, in a rudimentary form, as a teaching manual for students in the physical therapy program at New York Medical College. We needed a textbook that would provide a framework for functional outcomes documentation, and no satisfactory texts existed. So we wrote one.

The main philosophical idea underlying this textbook is simple: not only is the logic of clinical reasoning reflected in documentation, but documentation itself shapes the process of clinical reasoning. Thus, we would argue, one of the best ways to teach clinical reasoning skills is by teaching a careful and systematic approach to documentation. This book is therefore not just a "how-to" book on documentation of physical therapy practice. Rather, it presents a framework for clinical decision making.

In this second edition, we have undertaken some fundamental changes to the structure and organization of this text. Most significantly, we have incorporated the International Classification for Functioning, Disability, and Health (ICF) model. This change has occurred for two reasons: (1) the ICF framework has now been almost universally adopted, including recent adoption by the American Physical Therapy Association; and (2) we believe this framework provides a better structure for understanding the complex relationships between a person's health condition and his or her ability to participate in life skills.

This switch to the ICF model has conceptual implications as well as practical ones for this textbook. The ICF terminology inherently focuses on the positive aspect of a person's health, and we believe this is important to adopt within clinical documentation. The ICF structure in some ways is not too different from that of the Nagi model; therapists can somewhat readily translate information that was previously referred to as "disability" to "participation," from "function" to "activities," and from "pathology" to "health condition" ("impairments" has stayed the same).

The terms *participation, activities, impairments,* and *health condition* are now incorporated into the vocabularies of contemporary physical therapists and certainly of entry-level physical therapy students.

Nevertheless, for physical therapists to "walk the walk" rather than just "talk the talk," the framework exemplified by the ICF model must be incorporated into how they design and implement evaluations and interventions. This process is reflected in the documentation written by physical therapists. The outside world views physical therapy primarily by words that are written—as communicated in a medical record, progress notes given to a patient or physician, or forms completed for an insurance company. We believe that documentation shapes and reflects the advances in the science of physical therapy and therefore requires an updated framework that incorporates current knowledge regarding the disablement and rehabilitation process.

The purpose of this book is to provide a general approach to documentation—not a rigid format. It is, first and foremost, a textbook for entry-level physical therapist and physical therapist assistant students. It is intended to promote a style and philosophy of documentation that can be used throughout an entire physical therapy curriculum. However, it is also a book that we hope will appeal to practicing physical therapists and physical therapist assistants who are searching for a better structure for the note-writing process. We have provided examples and exercises related to wide-ranging areas of physical therapy practice, including pediatrics, rehabilitation, women's health, health and wellness, orthopedics, and acute care. This book was designed to help students and therapists organize their clinical reasoning and establish a framework for documentation that is easily adaptable to different practice settings and patient populations. Although this book has many examples and exercises, it certainly does not include all possible types of documentation or all the details of how to document in different settings. Rather, this book provides a method for learning good documentation skills that can be adapted to different settings.

Although physical therapist assistants and physical therapist assistant students will find this book relevant, their practice is inherently limited to writing treatment notes. A large portion of this book focuses on documentation of the initial evaluation. However, the components listed in each of these chapters, particularly documentation of activities, are important components of the daily note documentation.

The book is divided into three sections. The first section provides the overall theoretical framework. The second section explains in detail each of the specific components of a functional outcomes initial evaluation and provides extensive examples and practice. The third section considers other types of documentation, such as progress notes and letters to third parties. Importantly, we have added three new chapters to this text: "Legal Aspects of Documentation," "Payment Policy and Coding," and "Documentation in Pediatrics," which has allowed us to significantly expand our coverage of these areas.

We believe that a standardized format for documentation should be introduced early in a physical therapy curriculum so that students can practice writing notes in successive clinical courses. Furthermore, we have structured the book so that students should be able to learn the approach on their own without requiring a separate course on documentation. Thus we have provided many opportunities for practice of documentation skills through exercises at the end of most chapters. Nevertheless, the book will work best when an instructor is guiding the learning process and is available to answer questions. The exercises are written primarily for physical therapist students and physical therapist assistant students in entry-level education. However, depending on their level of education and the design of the curriculum, many students may not be able to complete all the exercises. This is particularly true for exercises in which the reader is asked to rewrite problematic documentation. Some students may only have limited knowledge to be able to rewrite the statements accurately.

As much as possible, we have attempted to incorporate the terminology and main ideas of the *Guide to Physical Therapist Practice*. For the most part, they are relevant to and consistent with functional outcomes and documentation. Readers should find this book "*Guide*-friendly," and we have reprinted figures and adapted components of the *Guide* into our documentation framework.

Readers will note that although the *Guide* uses the term "patient/client" to denote individuals served by physical therapists, we have chosen to use only the term "patient." This is solely for ease and consistency, although we recognize the importance of the differentiation of these two terms in physical therapy vocabulary.

This book should be used in conjunction with other resources and references related to functional outcomes and documentation. Many of these resources are listed in the appendixes of this book. In particular, there are important legal aspects of documentation. We have provided a foundation for key elements related to legal aspects of documentation; however, readers should consult state and federal laws to ensure that their documentation is in compliance with current guidelines.

Documentation for third-party payment is an important and often challenging type of physical therapy documentation. We discuss this with more depth than in the first edition and have added an entire chapter devoted to payment policy and documentation (Chapter 15). This chapter has been written with invaluable contributions from Steve Levine and Helene Fearon, who have extensive experience in this area. In addition, we have discussed our framework and suggestions with many therapists and managers who have experience with Medicare payment policy. However, we caution the reader that this framework does not necessarily comply with specific Medicare requirements or standards, which change frequently. We do believe that the principles discussed in this book are applicable to all forms of documentation, including Medicare, as they are currently used in clinical settings.

As this book goes to print, the United States is in the midst of a change in its health care system. Most significantly, what is at stake is the funding of health care and ensuring that most Americans are covered by some form of health care insurance. We believe that these policy changes will have an effect on medical record documentation and payment policy; however, what types of effects at this point are unknown.

Finally, we do not intend that this book should be the last word on documentation in physical therapy. On the contrary, we see it as a beginning. We hope that physical therapists will continue to explore new forms of documentation that will better reflect the changing patterns of practice and that will facilitate improvements in patient care. We invite readers to send comments, suggestions, and criticisms to us and to publish alternative approaches in journals and textbooks. Discussion and debate about the best ways to document will help us to find the true path to best practice.

Lori Quinn
James Gordon

Acknowledgments

The authors would like to acknowledge the contributions by many people who provided examples, ideas, insights and, most importantly, critiques of this book at various stages of its inception. First, we owe a debt of gratitude to current and past students of the Physical Therapy Program at New York Medical College. We have benefited so much from the thoughtful insights of students for whom this material was first designed.

Next, we would like to thank the staff and faculty of the Program in Physical Therapy at New York Medical College, the Department of Biokinesiology and Physical Therapy at the University of Southern California, and the Physiotherapy Program at Cardiff University, Wales. Many of the faculty provided important comments for this book, wrote or reviewed case examples, or helped with editorial components.

We would also like to thank our contributors: Karen Stutman and Jody Feld, for providing some excellent case examples, and Agnes McConlogue, Janet Herbold, Steve Levine, and Helene Fearon for their tireless work writing and editing their respective chapters.

We gratefully acknowledge the following individuals who provided insightful feedback for this second edition:

Monica Busse, PhD, MSc (Med), BSc (Med), Hons BSc (Physio)

Kate Button, PhD, MSc, BSc physiotherapy, MCSP

Stephanie Enright, PhD, MPhil, MSc, MCSP, PG Cert HE

Julie Fritz, PT, PhD, ATC

Barbara Norton, PT, PhD, FAPTA

Patricia Scheets, PT, DPT, NCS

We thank the many reviewers who carefully read and provided insightful comments about the book. We have made every effort to incorporate their suggestions into this second edition.

We also gratefully acknowledge the work of our editors, who provided great support and encouragement during this process. We would like to thank Kathy Falk, Melissa Kuster, and Carrie Stetz, as well as the entire editorial staff, for their expert assistance in completing this project.

Last, we thank our families for their never-ending support. With gratitude:

to Eric, Annabel, and Samantha

to Provi, Jason, Anita, and Maddie

Lori Quinn

James Gordon

Contents

DOCUMENTATION FOR REHABILITATION

Theoretical Foundations and Documentation Essentials

CHAPTER 1

Disablement Models, ICF Framework, and Clinical Decision Making

LEARNING OBJECTIVES

After reading this chapter and completing the exercises, the reader will be able to:

1. Define a functional outcome and discuss its importance in physical therapy documentation.

2. Identify and describe three historical models of disablement.

3. Define the components of the International Classification of Functioning, Disability, and Health (ICF) model.

4. Classify clinical observations and measurements according to the ICF.

This book outlines a method for physical therapy documentation and clinical decision making based on the general principle that documentation should focus on functional outcomes. An *outcome* is a result or consequence of physical therapy intervention. A *functional outcome* is one in which the treatment effect is the individual's ability to accomplish a goal that is meaningful for that individual. Functional outcomes should be the focus of physical therapy documentation:

1. Examination procedures should determine relevant limitations in functional activities and the impairments that cause those limitations.

2. Goals should be explicitly defined in terms of the functional activities that the patient will be able to perform.

3. Specific interventions should be justified in terms of their effects on functional outcomes.

4. Most importantly, the success of interventions should be measured by the degree to which desired functional outcomes are achieved.

Traditional physical therapy documentation formats do not easily adapt to a functional outcomes focus. Therefore several authors have attempted to present documentation formats that are generally referred to as *functional outcomes reports* (FOR) (Stamer, 1995; Stewart, 1993). The FOR format presented in this book is based in part on ideas derived from these published documentation formats and the authors' own clinical and teaching experience.

This book has two main purposes: (1) to provide a framework for clinical decision making that is based on a functional outcomes approach and (2) to provide guided practice in writing functional outcomes documentation.

Clearly there is no single correct way to write physical therapy documentation. Documentation must be adapted to the context in which it is written. The purpose of this book is therefore not to present a rigid format for writing documentation. Instead, the book offers a set of guidelines for writing documentation in a functional outcomes format. This set of guidelines is flexible and should be adaptable to many different practice settings.

The framework for documentation presented herein is based on the now widely accepted International Classification of Functioning, Disability and Health (ICF) model of how pathologic conditions lead to disability. Until 2008, the American Physical Therapy

Association (APTA) endorsed the Nagi framework as a guiding disablement framework (Nagi, 1965, 1991). In fact, the Nagi model is an integral part of the current version of the *Guide to Physical Therapist Practice* (the *Guide*) and the first edition of this textbook. In July 2008, the APTA joined the World Health Organization (WHO), the World Confederation for Physical Therapy, the American Therapeutic Recreation Association, and other international organizations in endorsing the ICF model. Accordingly, we have adapted the documentation format in this textbook to the ICF model.

To the extent possible, we have incorporated the *Guide* into our documentation framework. The main purpose of the *Guide* is to "help physical therapists analyze their patient/client management and describe the scope of their practice" (APTA, 2001, p. 12). Importantly, the *Guide* has helped to establish a common set of definitions and physical therapy terminology. This book attempts to use that terminology in addition to an overall conceptual framework that is consistent with that of the *Guide*.

In this chapter, we discuss the history of disablement models and development of the ICF model. We also consider how this model can be used to understand the role of physical therapists (PTs) in the diagnostic process and planning appropriate interventions. Finally, the importance of the ICF framework to documentation is discussed. The exercises at the end of the chapter provide practice in classifying conditions according to the Nagi model.

Historical Perspective of Disablement Models

The use of disablement models as an organizing framework for physical therapy was one of the key conceptual developments of the 1990s (Jette, 1994). Various models of disablement have been developed and explored, including the original WHO model (1980), the Nagi model (1965), and the National Center for Medical Rehabilitation Research (NCMRR) model (National Advisory Board on Medical Rehabilitation Research, 1991). These models are illustrated in Figure 1-1. Despite differences in terminology, each model provides a framework for analyzing the various effects of acute and chronic conditions on the functioning of specific body systems, basic human performance, and people's functioning in necessary, expected, and personally desired roles in society (Jette, 1994).

The differences among the various disablement models represent more than simple differences in terminology; important theoretical differences also exist (which are beyond the scope of this book).

Nevertheless, these differences are small compared with the overwhelming similarity of the models. All the models are based on the assumption that the process of disablement can be analyzed at multiple levels. In the 1990s the Nagi model gained considerable acceptance in North America, whereas the WHO model has been used more widely in Europe, Australia, and Asia.

Disablement describes the consequences of disease in terms of its effects on body functions, the ability of the individual to perform meaningful tasks, and the ability to fulfill one's roles in life. The arrows in Figure 1-1 imply a causal chain leading from active pathology to disability using the Nagi model as an example. Indeed, the causal links between elements in the models are useful; they help to conceptualize the relationships between findings at different levels. Nevertheless, the arrows often were interpreted as indicating a temporal series of events, which many health professionals found problematic. Furthermore, it was believed that these models did not capture the complexity of the relationships between different levels that were often multidirectional.

INTERNATIONAL CLASSIFICATION OF FUNCTIONING, DISABILITY AND HEALTH

In 2001 the WHO revised its disablement model to address the criticisms of current models. The ICF seeks to use the positive terms *activity* and *participation* to redefine what Nagi refers to as *functional limitation* and *disability*. Thus although the general structure is similar to the original WHO model and the Nagi model, the focus of this new model is on the "positive" ("ability") aspects of disablement.

In this new model, the process of disablement is a combination of (1) losses or abnormalities of **body function and structure**, (2) limitations of **activities**, and (3) restrictions in **participation** (Figure 1-2). Of note, the terms *activity* and *participation* focus on a person's abilities versus inabilities or disabilities. As shown in Figure 1-2, the ICF model relinquishes the notion of simple, unidirectional causal links between levels. The individual's pathologic state (health condition) becomes a broader category that influences all other levels. Furthermore, contextual factors—both extrinsic (environmental) and intrinsic (personal)—are specifically identified as affecting the relationship between body structures and functions and activities, and participation. Personal factors can consist of such things as family support, whereas extrinsic factors might include environmental barriers. These important additions highlight the multiple factors that can be related to any one person's "disability."

WHO Classification

Disease ⟹ Impairment ⟹ Disability ⟹ Handicap

Nagi Model

Active Pathology ⟹ Impairment ⟹ Functional limitation ⟹ Disability

NCMRR Model

Pathophysiology ⟹ Impairment ⟹ Functional limitation ⟹ Disability ⟹ Social limitation

FIGURE 1-1   Different models of the disablement process.

The ICF is endorsed by the WHO as the international standard used to measure health and disability (resolution WHA 54.21). In addition to the overall model presented in Figure 1-2, the ICF provides definitions (Box 1-1) and detailed descriptions of what each "level" encompasses (Figure 1-3). Figure 1-3 provides sample descriptions from the ICF framework that could be used for a patient who has had a stroke and has gait impairments, mobility limitations, and faces environmental barriers in the workplace. Within each of the ICF domains there is a hierarchy of description (Chapter, second, third, and fourth levels as needed). This ultimately leads to a code that can be used to refer to a specific domain. These definitions and codes provide common terminology that can be used by all health professionals, whether describing individual patient characteristics (as in Figure 1-3) or conducting large-scale population-based research.

ICF is part of the WHO family of international classifications, which includes the *International Statistical Classification of Diseases and Related Health Problems* (ICD). ICD-9 is the version currently in use by health professionals in the United States to classify diseases, disorders, or other health conditions. However, a more recent version of these classifications, ICD-10, is set to be adopted by 2013. Each disease or health condition has its own ICD-9 or ICD-10 code. These codes are used most frequently by PTs in the United States for billing purposes (see Chapter 15); however, they are designed to provide a common international language for communication and research. More information on the ICF and the online version are available at *http://www.who.int/classifications/en/*.

REHABILITATION: THE REVERSAL OF DISABLEMENT

The ICF model provides the conceptual framework for a "top-down approach" to understanding a patient's problems. Such an approach represents the natural

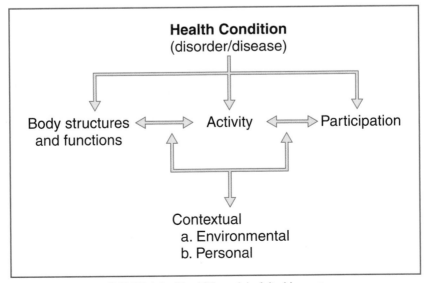

FIGURE 1-2   The ICF model of disablement.

Definitions of the Components of ICF

Body functions are physiologic functions of body systems (including psychological functions).

Body structures are anatomic parts of the body such as organs, limbs, and their components.

Impairments are problems in body function or structure such as a significant deviation or loss.

Activity is the execution of a task or action by an individual.

Participation is involvement in a life situation.

Activity limitations are difficulties an individual may have in executing activities.

Participation restrictions are problems an individual may experience in involvement in life situations.

Environmental factors make up the physical, social, and attitudinal environment in which people live and conduct their lives.

From World Health Organization: *Towards a common language for functioning, disability and health*, Geneva, 2002, World Health Organization. Retrieved January 12, 2009, from *http://www.who.int/classifications/icf/ training/icfbeginnersguide.pdf.*

way in which PTs solve clinical problems in a variety of situations. The case example in Figure 1-3 provides a simplified outline of one potential disability and the levels of the disablement process for an individual who has had a stroke.

Disablement models can be counterproductive if they lead to an overly reductionist approach to rehabilitation, that is, if improvements in impairments are assumed to lead to improvements in activities. This is a subtle example of the so-called medical model, in which it is assumed that curing a disease will automatically improve the patient's quality of life. PTs fall victim to the same fallacy when they focus intervention exclusively on impairments.

This pitfall can be avoided if rehabilitation is conceptualized as the reverse and mirror image of disablement (Figure 1-4). Whereas disablement begins with a disease/disorder (bottom-up), rehabilitation begins with participation—specifying the desired result in terms of personal and social roles the patient is attempting to achieve, resume, or retain (top-down). These roles require the performance of functional skills or activities—from self-care to household to community to occupation. The therapist must determine how these skills are limited in such ways as to prevent the fulfillment of the individual's roles. Then the therapist must ascertain why the specified activities are limited by determining the critical neuromotor and musculoskeletal mechanisms that are impaired. These mechanisms can be considered resources that can be used in the performance of the functional skills.

Finally, the opposite of a disease/disorder is *health*. Health is not simply the absence of disease but an active process of healing. In many instances, especially in the

acute stages, the primary goal of therapy is to promote recovery by creating an optimal environment for tissue healing and system reorganization.

For example, in a patient with an acute injury to the rotator cuff musculature, the overall goal of therapy might be to prevent disability, such as the loss of a valued recreational activity. If the patient were a recreational tennis player, the ability to perform strong and accurate overhead service swings would be an activity-level goal. The immediate impairments would likely include pain, loss of passive range of motion, and weakness. Therapy initially would be planned to promote tissue healing by avoiding strong overhead swings and encouraging pain-free motion at the shoulder. In the postacute stage of the rehabilitation process, therapy would be designed to increase strength and range of motion. As soon as practical and safe, the specific functional activities that are limited would be practiced. Isolated flexibility and strengthening exercises might be taught to the patient, but they would be validated by frequent retesting of the functional task. Finally, the patient would be taught proper techniques to avoid reinjury. In both acute and chronic stages, the clinical decision-making process is initiated by determining, in consultation with the patient, the personal and social roles that the patient wishes to fulfill.

Figure 1-4 emphasizes that a primary goal of physical therapy is to minimize participation restrictions and activity limitations. Nevertheless, the emphasis on functional outcomes should not be assumed to imply that it is enough to simply ignore impairments and focus exclusively on functional training and functional measures of performance. PTs are trained to determine the causes of movement dysfunction, usually in terms of impairments. Ignoring or neglecting this aspect of physical therapy is as much a fallacy as neglecting function.

Functional Outcomes: More Than Simply a Documentation Strategy

The organizing principles chosen by a therapist for documentation illustrate the organizing principles chosen for diagnosis and treatment. A haphazard approach to documentation is likely to reflect a haphazard approach to physical therapy evaluation and intervention. Therefore the organizational framework for documentation presented in this book represents more than simply a way to organize notes. The method of documentation is based on two assumptions: (1) a primary purpose of physical therapy evaluation is to define the specific functional outcomes that need to be achieved, and (2) the criterion for judging the effectiveness of treatment should be whether those outcomes are achieved.

ICF Clinical Example

	Body Structures and Functions	Activities and Participation	Environmental Factors
ICF Chapter and Subchapter Title	*Chapter 7* *First level: Neuromusculoskeletal and movement-related functions* *Second level: Movement functions* *Third level: Gait pattern functions*	*Chapter 4* *First level: Mobility, walking, and moving* *Second level: Walking* *Third level: Walking short distances*	*Chapter 1* *First level: Products and technology, design, construction, and building products and technology of buildings for public use* *Second level: Design, construction, and building products and technology for entering and exiting buildings for public use*
Description	**Gait pattern functions** **ICF code: b770** Functions of movement patterns associated with walking, running, or other whole-body movements. *Inclusions: walking patterns and running patterns; impairments such as spastic gait, hemiplegic gait, paraplegic gait, asymmetric gait, limping, and stiff gait pattern. Exclusions: muscle power functions (**b730**); muscle tone functions (**b735**); control of voluntary movement functions (**b760**); involuntary movement functions (**b765**).*	**Walking short distances** **ICF code: d4500** Walking for less than a kilometer, such as walking around rooms or hallways, within a building or for short distances outside.	**Design, construction, and building products and technology for entering and exiting buildings for public use** **ICF code: e1500** Products and technology of entry and exit from the human-made environment that is planned, designed, and constructed for public use, such as design, building, and construction of entries and exits to buildings for public use (e.g., workplaces, shops, and theaters), public buildings, portable and stationary ramps, power-assisted doors, lever door handles, and level door thresholds.

FIGURE 1-3   Sample descriptions from the ICF framework that could be used for a patient who has had a stroke and has gait impairments, mobility limitations, and faces environmental barriers in the workplace. (From World Health Organization: *Towards a common language for functioning, disability and health,* Geneva, 2002, World Health Organization. Retrieved January 12, 2009, from *http://www.who.int/classifications/icf/ training/icfbeginnersguide.pdf.*)

In other words, if it is accepted that physical therapy documentation should be focused on functional outcomes, then logically, physical therapy evaluation and intervention should be focused on functional outcomes. Neither the format presented here nor any functional outcomes rehabilitation format should be viewed as simply a post hoc method for justifying payment for physical therapy services in the managed care environment. Continuing to view the role of PTs as treating impairments while recasting what they do as functionally based in order to satisfy third-party payers makes no sense. The purpose of functional outcomes rehabilitation documentation is to provide an explicit and prospective framework by

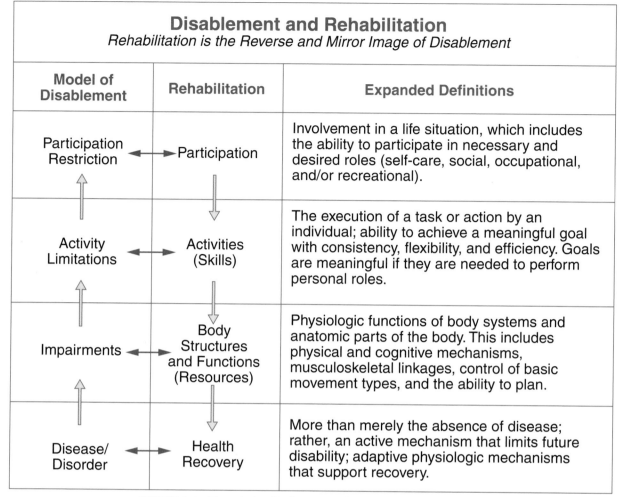

Disablement and Rehabilitation
Rehabilitation is the Reverse and Mirror Image of Disablement

Model of Disablement	Rehabilitation	Expanded Definitions
Participation Restriction	Participation	Involvement in a life situation, which includes the ability to participate in necessary and desired roles (self-care, social, occupational, and/or recreational).
Activity Limitations	Activities (Skills)	The execution of a task or action by an individual; ability to achieve a meaningful goal with consistency, flexibility, and efficiency. Goals are meaningful if they are needed to perform personal roles.
Impairments	Body Structures and Functions (Resources)	Physiologic functions of body systems and anatomic parts of the body. This includes physical and cognitive mechanisms, musculoskeletal linkages, control of basic movement types, and the ability to plan.
Disease/Disorder	Health Recovery	More than merely the absence of disease; rather, an active mechanism that limits future disability; adaptive physiologic mechanisms that support recovery.

FIGURE 1-4   The relationship between rehabilitation and disablement.

which PTs can (1) analyze the reasons for disablement in their patients, (2) formulate strategies for preventing or reversing that disablement, and (3) explain and justify the resulting clinical decisions they make.

Classification According to the ICF Framework

Writing documentation requires the PT to develop skill in classifying the various aspects of the patient's condition using the ICF as a framework. The classi-fication has two bases: the organizational level at which function is observed and the level of measurement (Table 1-1).

For example, the observation that a patient has an infection of the femur (osteomyelitis) is an example of pathologic information (at the tissue level, a health condition). The **health condition** usually includes the nature of the pathology (e.g., infection, tumor), its location, and the timing relative to onset (i.e., acute vs. chronic). Weakness of the quadriceps muscle represents a reduction in a body function (muscular); thus it is an **impairment**. It is measured in the frame of

TABLE 1-1	CLASSIFICATION OF MEASUREMENT USING THE ICF FRAMEWORK	
ICF Framework	**Organizational Level**	**Level of Measurement**
Participation restriction	Whole person in relation to society	Participation/level of assistance/quality of life
Activity limitations	Whole person	Performance/skill (goal attainment)
Impairments	Body functions or structures	Functions of specific body systems
Health condition	Tissue or cellular	Medical diagnosis

reference defined by the body system's function. The muscular system is defined by its ability to produce force over time. Weakness is measured in terms of the force output possible in a defined set of conditions.

An inability to walk is defined as an **activity limitation** because it is a deficit in the ability of the whole person to successfully perform an activity. Activity limitations are measured in terms of performance or skill. Considering whether—and to what degree—the goal of the action has been attained is most useful. A patient's inability to care for his or her child would be a **participation restriction**. It is measured at the level of the individual's social interaction, which can be quantified along three dimensions: (1) participation in desired or expected social roles, (2) the level of assistance required to achieve that participation, and (3) quality of life.

The ability to identify and classify patients' problems into each of the four main levels of the ICF model (health condition, body structures and function, activity, and participation) is a critical first step for therapists to "speak the same language" in both oral and written communication. Figure 1-5 provides clinical examples of observations or measurements and classifies them according to the ICF framework. Exercise 1-1 provides an opportunity to practice classifying various statements within the ICF framework. Chapters 5 through 8 provide more extended explanation and practice in classification and measurement according to the framework.

Summary

- This chapter has presented a conceptual framework for a specific documentation strategy organized around functional outcomes.

- Functional outcomes should be the focus of physical therapy documentation; this involves documenting limitations in activities, setting functional goals, justifying interventions, and measuring their success based on the effects on functional outcomes.

- Disablement describes the consequences of disease in terms of its effects on body structures and functions (i.e., impairments), the ability of the individual to perform meaningful tasks (i.e., activity limitations), and the ability to fulfill one's roles in life (i.e., participation restrictions).

- Rehabilitation is the reverse of disablement. Whereas disablement begins with disease/disorder, rehabilitation begins with participation—specifying the desired end result in terms of the personal and social roles that the patient is attempting to achieve, resume, or retain.

- The next chapters offer a set of guidelines for writing documentation in a functional outcomes format that should be adaptable to many different practice settings.

Health Condition ⇒	Impairments ⇒	Activity Limitations ⇒	Participation Restriction
Examples			
• Infarction of neurons in precentral gyrus of cerebral cortex • Fracture of distal tibia • Transtibial amputation of left leg • Tear of anterior cruciate ligament of knee • Viral infection of lung tissue (right lower lobe)	• Paralysis • Weakness • Sensory loss • Restriction in ROM • Hypermobility in ROM • Inadequate balance control • Gait abnormalities • Poor coordination of reaching and grasping movements • Inability to cough	• Inability to walk on level surfaces • Inability to dress oneself • Inability to prepare a meal • Inability to lift a carton weighing more than 30 pounds • Inability to walk up and down a flight of stairs	• Inability to care for oneself without assistance • Inability to work at normal occupation • Inability to fulfill role as spouse or parent • Inability to play golf (part of person's regular recreational activity)

FIGURE 1-5 Examples of classification of clinical observations or measurements using the ICF framework. *ROM,* Range of motion.

EXERCISE 1-1

Classify each statement according to the ICF model it reflects: health condition/disease (HC), impairment in body structure/function (I), activity limitation (A), or participation restriction (P). Statements may reflect positive attributes.

Statement	Classification
1. Patient has 0° to 120° of active abduction left shoulder.	_____
2. Patient can walk up to 50 feet on level surfaces indoors.	_____
3. Partial tear of right anterior cruciate ligament.	_____
4. Patient is unable to work at previous occupation of a salesperson.	_____
5. Strength right knee flexion 3/5 on manual muscle test.	_____
6. Patient needs minimal assistance to dress lower body.	_____
7. Transfemoral amputation of right lower extremity.	_____
8. Heart rate increases from 80 beats per minute to 140 after climbing one flight of stairs.	_____
9. Patient was diagnosed with multiple sclerosis October 1998.	_____
10. Patient is able to eat soup from a bowl independently.	_____
11. Left lateral pinch strength 15 lbs.	_____
12. Patient transfers from bed to wheelchair independently with use of a sliding board.	_____
13. Patient has full passive range of motion in left knee.	_____
14. Child is able to crawl distance of 6 feet on living room floor to obtain a desired toy.	_____
15. Patient is able to reach for and grasp a cup located at shoulder height.	_____
16. Patient can stand at kitchen sink for 2 minutes.	_____
17. Patient is unable to perform a straight leg raise.	_____
18. Patient has pain in right shoulder, rated 5/10, whenever he raises his arm above shoulder height.	_____
19. Patient has a personal aide for 4 hours per day to assist with daily care and household chores.	_____

Statement	Classification
20. Patient is unable to cook using the stove and needs moderate assistance to prepare all meals.	_____
21. Patient is able to transfer from floor to wheelchair within 1 minute.	_____
22. Patient was diagnosed with T8 spinal cord injury after motor vehicle accident in 2009.	_____
23. Patient is able to enter most buildings in wheelchair, provided an appropriate ramp is present.	_____
24. Partial rotator cuff tear of right shoulder.	_____
25. Patient works as a bus driver with modified work duty with limitations of 4-hour shifts.	_____

CHAPTER 2

Essentials of Documentation

LEARNING OBJECTIVES

After reading this chapter and completing the exercises,
the reader will be able to:

1. Discuss the history of the medical record and documentation.

2. Identify the four basic types of physical therapy notes.

3. List the different purposes that documentation serves.

4. Discuss the pros and cons of different documentation formats.

5. Discuss the importance of using standardized assessments as part of documentation, and describe the four types of standardized measures commonly used.

6. Describe strategies for concise documentation.

7. Appropriately use and interpret common rehabilitation and medical abbreviations.

8. Use people-first language in written and oral communication.

Documentation: An Overview

Physical therapists (PTs) and physical therapist assistants (PTAs) often view documentation as an onerous chore. At best, it is considered a necessary evil, to be accomplished as quickly and painlessly as possible. At worst, it is a conspiracy by bureaucrats to waste therapists' time and limit patient access to essential services. Despite this view, the modern medical record is one of the most important achievements in the development of twentieth-century medicine. At the beginning of the twentieth century, the notion of a patient-centered chart that stayed with the patient was almost unheard of. Instead, records were kept by individual practitioners, and often the records were haphazard. The development of a comprehensive patient-centered chart, professionally written and clearly organized, enabled direct improvements in patient care by promoting accurate and timely communication among professionals. It also allowed improvements in patient care indirectly by facilitat-

ing better review of the process. The medical chart is the collector and organizer of the primary data for clinical research. It is also an essential teaching device. Students and novice clinicians learn about how to provide patient care by reading the documentation written by expert clinicians. It is doubtful that health care would have reached the present level of accomplishment without the changes in documentation over the past century. Moreover, future improvements in patient care will be associated with, and enabled by, changes in the way the process is documented. Documentation is therefore a dynamic phenomenon, ever-changing. The dominant formats can be expected to adapt to the changes in health care.

Of course, changes in health care have occurred not just in the clinical domain, but also in the economic and social domains. The United States is in the midst of a period in which fundamental changes are occurring in the way in which health care is financed and compensated. The entire third-party payer system is likely to be overhauled in the near future, and payers may move away from reimbursing procedures (fee-for-service) and toward reimbursing outcomes. In other words, practitioners must clearly justify the treatment they are implementing in terms of the outcomes that will be achieved.

Despite its importance, documentation is often viewed negatively by therapists for at least two reasons. First, and most obvious, too little time is dedicated to documentation in the clinic. Second, therapists are given relatively little training in documentation. When proper guidelines and adequate training are provided, appropriate outcomes-based documentation does not have to be extremely labor-intensive. However, documentation is a skill that should be valued by therapists, educators, and supervisors, similar to any other physical therapy skill. Thus students and therapists must spend dedicated, focused time to learn the "skill" of documentation. Skill develops with practice, practice, and more practice.

Skill in documentation is the hallmark of a professional approach to therapy and is one of the characteristics that distinguishes a professional from a technician. Therapists should take pride in their professional writing; it is the window through which they are judged by other professionals. In fact, it could be argued that documentation of services rendered is just as important as the actual rendering of the services. Supervisors must recognize that good documentation takes time, and therapists must be provided with that time.

In this chapter, some of the essential aspects of documentation are addressed. Different classifications and formats for physical therapy documentation are presented, as well as critical aspects of information that should be included and the manner in which they should be reported.

Types of Notes

Four basic types of medical record documentation exist: the initial evaluation, treatment notes, reexamination or progress notes, and the discharge summary. The following list is adapted from *Guidelines: Physical Therapy Documentation of Patient/Client Management* (APTA, 2008).

The main aspects of this book focus on documentation of the initial evaluation components (see Chapters 5 through 11). Special considerations for writing treatment notes and progress notes are specifically covered in Chapter 12. Documentation of discharge summary and other types of documentation are discussed in Chapter 13.

INITIAL EXAMINATION/EVALUATION (WRITTEN BY PHYSICAL THERAPIST)

- Required at onset of episode of PT care
- Includes the following components:
  - Reason for referral
    - Health condition
    - Participation and social history
  - Activities
  - Systems review
  - Impairments
  - Assessment (including evaluation, diagnosis, and prognosis)
  - Goals
  - Plan of care

TREATMENT NOTES (WRITTEN BY PHYSICAL THERAPIST OR PHYSICAL THERAPIST ASSISTANT) FOR EACH THERAPY SESSION

- Identify specific interventions provided, including frequency, intensity, and duration as appropriate
- Report changes in patient/client impairment, activity, and participation as they relate to the plan of care
- Response to interventions, including adverse reactions, if any
- Factors that modify frequency or intensity of intervention and progression goals, including adherence to patient-related instructions
- Communication/consultation with providers/patient/client/family/significant other
- Documentation to plan for ongoing provision of services for the next visit(s), which should include the interventions with objectives, progression parameters, and precautions, if indicated

PROGRESS NOTES (WRITTEN BY PHYSICAL THERAPIST)

- Provide an update of patient status over a number of visits or certain period
- Should include selected components of examination to update patient's impairment, activities, and/or participation status
- Provide an interpretation of findings and, when indicated, revision of goals
- When indicated, revision of plan of care, as directly correlated with goals as documented

DISCHARGE SUMMARY (WRITTEN BY PHYSICAL THERAPIST)

- Documents current physical/functional status
- Includes the degree to which goals were achieved and reasons for any goals not being achieved or partially achieved
- Provides a discharge/discontinuation plan related to the patient's continuing care

Purposes of Note Writing

PT documentation serves many purposes. These include communication with other professionals, clinical decision making, and creation of a legal record of PT management of a patient.

COMMUNICATION WITH OTHER PROFESSIONALS

- Ensures coordination and continuity of patient care
- Organizes the planning of treatment strategies

CLINICAL DECISION MAKING

- Documents patient's problems so that an appropriate plan of care can be established

LEGAL RECORD OF PHYSICAL THERAPIST MANAGEMENT OF PATIENT

- Specifies that patient has been seen and that intervention has occurred
- Serves as a business record
- Is often used to determine how much should be billed for a visit

EXAMPLES OF USES BY OTHERS

- Make decisions about payment for services
- Decide discharge and future placement
- Used as a quality assurance tool
- Used as data for research on outcomes

Documentation Formats

Many possible formats can be used for writing notes. Sometimes a facility or institution mandates a particular format. More often, use of a particular format is not officially required but is instead established by tradition and the desire for consistency. In these cases, PTs, PTAs, and students should use the format in general use within the institution. A particular format does not guarantee well-written documentation; it just makes the process easier. The principles of well-written documentation can be applied in any format.

NARRATIVE FORMAT

The simplest form of documentation recounts what happened in a therapist-patient encounter. In this format, therapists can, and should, develop their own outline of information to cover. These outlines can be more or less detailed. The specific information listed in each heading is left to the writer's discretion, although some facilities provide guidelines for what should be covered under each heading. Because of the unstructured nature of narrative formats, the writer is prone to omissions, and there can be a high degree of variability (both within and among different writers). Furthermore, if information is not included it is assumed it was not tested, whereas the writer may have inadvertently omitted the testing information. Thus therapists must take particular care to be comprehensive in their documentation to minimize inconsistencies and maximize accuracy.

SOAP FORMAT

The SOAP note is a highly structured documentation format. It was developed in the 1960s at the University of Vermont by Dr. Lawrence Weed as part of the problem-oriented medical record (POMR). In this type of medical record, each patient chart is headed by a numbered list of patient problems (usually developed by the primary physician). When entering documentation, each professional would refer to the number of the problem he or she was writing about and then write a note using SOAP format. The SOAP format requires the practitioner to enter information in the order of the acronym's initials: subjective objective assessment plan (see Chapter 12 for more detailed information on writing SOAP notes).

The POMR was not widely adopted, perhaps because it was ahead of its time. Interestingly, however, the SOAP format did catch on and is now widely used by different professionals, despite the fact that it is no longer connected to its parent concept, the POMR. A major advantage of the SOAP format is its widespread acceptance and the resulting familiarity with the format. On the plus side, it emphasizes clear, complete, and well-organized reporting of findings with a natural progression from data collection to assessment to plan. On the other hand, it has generally been associated with an overly brief and concise style, including extensive use of abbreviations and acronyms, a style that is often difficult for nonprofessionals to interpret. On a more substantive note, Delitto and Snyder-Mackler (1995) have commented that the SOAP format encourages a sequential rather than integrative approach to clinical decision making by promoting a tendency to simply collect all possible data before assessing it. Thus, while the SOAP note does not provide the ideal format for an initial evaluation, it can be adapted to reflect functional outcomes and thus provides a useful framework for documenting treatment notes and progress notes (See Chapter 13).

FUNCTIONAL OUTCOME REPORT FORMAT

The functional outcome report (FOR) format is a relatively new documentation format. It was developed in the 1990s as changes in the economics of health care led to increased emphasis on functional outcomes. The FOR format focuses on documenting the ability to perform meaningful functional activities rather than isolated musculoskeletal, neuromuscular, cardiopulmonary, or integumentary impairments. When the format is implemented properly, FOR documentation establishes the rationale for therapy by indicating the links between such impairments and the participation restrictions they cause in the patient. FOR documentation also emphasizes readability by health care personnel not familiar with PT jargon (at the expense of increased time to write the documentation). More important, it promotes a style of clinical decision making (PT diagnosis) that begins with the functional problems and assesses the specific impairments that cause the activity limitations or participation restrictions.

Several authors have presented frameworks for FOR documentation. The most well-developed and structured format is that of Stewart and Abeln (1993). Their book has played a major role in promoting the idea that documentation should be focused on functional outcomes, and many of their ideas have been adapted in developing the format presented in this book. Their format was not adopted for this text for two reasons. First, the format is too highly structured and difficult to adapt to different clinical contexts. Second, their book and format are entirely focused on orthopedic physical therapy and thus translation into other contexts is difficult. Nevertheless, this book is highly recommended especially because of its strong emphasis on the need for FOR documentation.

What Constitutes "Documentation"?

Documentation is any form of written communication related to a patient encounter, such as an initial evaluation, progress note, flow sheet/checklist, reevaluation, or discharge summary. It encompasses the preparation and assembly of records to authenticate and communicate the care given by a health care provider and the reasons for giving that care.

Documentation takes many forms, including written reports, standardized assessments, graphs and tables, and photographs and drawings.

WRITTEN REPORTS

Most commonly, PTs use a written report to document their findings from an evaluation or convey what has occurred in a patient visit. The format of this report can take many forms; the two most common are a narrative format and a SOAP format. In this text, we use a narrative format for documenting an initial evaluation (Chapter 4). For progress notes and treatment notes, we recommend using a SOAP format (Chapter 12). Chapter 4 provides four full-length examples of initial evaluation reports, and Chapter 12 provides six examples of treatment notes and progress notes.

STANDARDIZED ASSESSMENTS

The use of standardized assessment tools is an integral part of PT documentation; however, such tools have not been universally adopted by PTs (Jette, 2009). Standardized outcome measures are measures that have been determined to be reliable and ideally validated in specific patient populations. Although outcome measures are most commonly used in PT research, their use in everyday documentation is essential. Standardized measures are very useful to be able to quantify improvements in patient performance and demonstrate the value of therapy services (to patients and third-party payers). Hundreds of outcome measures are available to therapists measuring at all levels of disablement. (Part III of the *Guide to Physical Therapist Practice* was developed as a resource on standardized tests and measures. Part III of the *Guide* is available on CD-ROM through the APTA.)

When choosing a standardized test, therapists must consider the purpose and design of the tool before using it for evaluative purposes. Following is a list of the most common types of standardized measures:

- Descriptive: a descriptive assessment provides information that describes the person's current functional status, problems, needs, and/or circumstances.
- Discriminative: a measure that has been developed to "distinguish between individuals or

groups on an underlying dimension (test score) when no external criterion or gold standard is available for validating these measures" (Law, 2001, p. 287).

- Predictive: predicts the ability or state of a person or a specific outcome in the future (Adams, 2002).
- Evaluative: used to detect change over time; undertaken to monitor a client's progress during rehabilitation and used to determine the effectiveness of the intervention.

In Chapter 6, 7, and 8, tables are provided that list many of the most commonly used measures of participation, activities, and impairments (although by no means are these lists complete). The measures listed in these chapters focus on those that may be used to assess change over time (evaluative) and those that are useful in objectively or quantitatively describing impairments, activity limitations, or participation restrictions (descriptive). Standardized tools are important for other reasons, such as to discriminate the need for services or predict risk for certain problems (e.g., in pediatric populations).

The therapist must have knowledge of the reliability and validity of an evaluation tool and understand the purpose for which the tool was designed to use it properly. In addition, therapists must consider the sensitivity of a measure: Was it designed to adequately capture changes in a patient's status that may occur as a result of intervention? It is therefore important for therapists to perform due diligence in properly researching assessment tools and ensure they are properly trained in their use. Readers are referred to Fawcett (2007) for a more detailed discussion of using outcome measures in physical therapy practice.

GRAPHS AND TABLES

Graphs can be used as a form of documentation to provide a visualization of a patient's progress in therapy. They can improve readability and readily focus a reader on the critical issues. Figure 2-1 provides an example of a graph used to chart a patient's progress. In this figure, a patient's gait speed is charted over a period of about 3 weeks. This provides an easy visualization of progress for third-party payers, other health care professionals, and most importantly the patient.

Tables are another format of documentation that can be used in the initial evaluation, both to document multiple findings of a similar impairment or functional skill and in progress reports to demonstrate changes over multiple sessions. Figure 2-2 shows two examples of tables used in an initial evaluation report. Figure 2-3 shows an example of a table used for a progress report, showing performance on the 6-minute walk test over multiple sessions.

PHOTOGRAPHS AND DRAWINGS

Some aspects of patient care are difficult to describe narratively but may be best explained visually. Photographs (obtained with the patient's written consent), can be used very effectively for documenting impairments such as posture or wound size or for documenting functional abilities. Figure 2-4 shows a child with a prosthetic arm playing the violin. Alternatively, drawings are typically used to document impairments such as extent of burn or pain (see Appendix D).

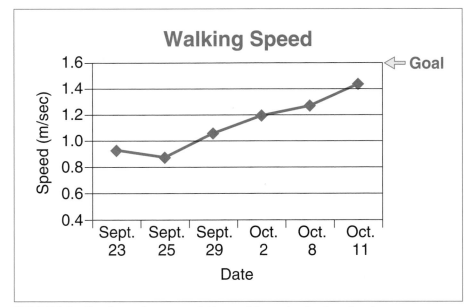

FIGURE 2-1   Graphs can be very useful in providing a visualization of patient progress.

Functional skills	Level of A	Comments
Rolling in bed	Ind.	
Positioning in bed	Min A	Needs verbal cues to use L UE and L LE to assist in movement
Supine → sitting in bed	Mod A to R Sup. to L	Can bring legs over side of bed to R, unable to use L arm and trunk to push up to sit
Sitting → supine in bed	Ind.	
Transfer bed to wheelchair	Min A c̄ sliding board	Needs A for proper setup and to initiate movement

A

Muscle Group	Strength (MMT)	
	Right	Left
Knee extension	3+/5	5/5
Knee flexion	3+/5	4/5
Ankle dorsiflexion	4/5	4/5
Ankle plantarflexion	4/5	5/5

B

FIGURE 2-2   Tables typically found in an initial evaluation report. Such tables can provide detailed information in an easy-to-read format. A, Assistance; L, left; R, right; UE, upper extremity; LE, lower extremity; Min, minimal; Mod, moderate; Sup, supine; Ind., independent; MMT, manual muscle testing.

Results of 6-Minute Walk Test				
	Feb. 5	Feb. 19	Mar. 5	Mar. 19
Distance walked (m)	205 m	262 m	301 m	355 m
Dyspnea (modified Borg)	4	4	2	2
O$_2$ sat pre/post	98/94	99/97	100/95	100/98

FIGURE 2-3   A table that could be used in a progress report demonstrating the results of the 6-minute walk test over a period of 6 weeks sat, Saturation.

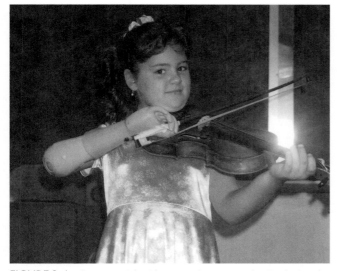

FIGURE 2-4   **A young girl with a myoeletric prosthesis playing the violin. Photographs such as this can be included as part of clinical documentation.** (Courtesy MH Mandelbaum Orthotic & Prosthetic Services.)

Evidence-Based Practice

APTA's position on evidence-based practice (HOD P06-99-17-21) states: "To promote improved quality of care and patient/client outcomes, the American Physical Therapy Association supports and promotes the development and utilization of evidence-based practice that includes the integration of best available research, clinical expertise, and patient/client values and circumstances related to patient/client management, practice management, and health policy decision making." It is therefore critical that evidence-based practice be fully integrated into clinical documentation. This is most important in documentation of the initial evaluation and plan of care as well as during documentation of treatment notes, when specific intervention strategies are reported. APTA recommends the following strategies for therapists to integrate evidence-based practice in clinical documentation:

1. By documenting tests and measures that are valid and reliable for diagnostic and/or prognostic information.
2. Through the use of standardized outcome measures, which are an effective means of evaluating and communicating changes in a patient's impairments and/or function.
3. By selecting and implementing an appropriate plan of care and interventions based on available research or clinical guidelines and that reflect patient perspectives and preferences and their influence on the plan of care (APTA, 2009).

In certain situations, it may be useful for therapists to document specific evidence or provide references. This is particularly useful when a specific treatment is not standard or when providing justification for a certain plan of care to a third-party payer (see Chapter 13 for examples of letters to third-party payers).

Strategies for Conciseness in Documentation

CONCISE WORDING

A written medical record has some specific characteristics that differentiate it from traditional narrative writing. For example, medical documentation should be appropriately concise. Time is often limited in health care settings; thus wordiness and undue lengthiness should be minimized (Figure 2-5). One way to save time in medical documentation is by not using full sentence structures and using abbreviations. Also, eliminating the words "his," "her," "a," "the," "for," and "an" can improve readibility of a medical note.

ABBREVIATIONS AND MEDICAL TERMINOLOGY

The first question that must be addressed regarding use of abbreviations is "Who will be the reader of this

Too wordy	Better
The patient can walk in the hospital corridor for 50 feet with minimal assistance	Pt. walks in hospital corridor 50 c̄ min A
Manual muscle testing was performed for right knee extension, and the strength was 5 out of 5	MMT R Knee / 5/5

FIGURE 2-5   Minimize wordiness and undue lengthiness in documentation.

note?" If the answer is "another physical therapist or physical therapist assistant (and no other person)," therapists can freely use abbreviations and appropriate PT terminology. However, if only a slight possibility exists that the note might be read by another professional (e.g., physician or nurse) or by a non-professional (e.g., administrative staff, claims auditor, member of a jury), uncommon abbreviations and jargon almost certainly will impede understanding. Furthermore, if the writer is in doubt about the use of an abbreviation, it is best to spell out the word. The time saved writing an abbreviation may not be worth it if it cannot be interpreted by anyone else.

Clearly, common medical abbreviations can be useful time-saving devices (see Figure 2-5). Appendix B provides a list of commonly accepted medical abbreviations that can be used for PT documentation in a medical chart. Although this list is not all encompassing, it represents abbreviations that are most likely to be understood by a range of medical professionals. Several books provide a more comprehensive listing of all types of medical abbreviations (Davis, 2009; Skalko, 1998). Furthermore, hospitals and health care facilities often develop their own list of abbreviations that are considered acceptable in that institution, and those lists are likely to be more encompassing than those listed here. PTs and PTAs should follow guidelines set by individual institutions when considering the appropriateness of specific abbreviations.

Certain types of documentation are intended for the primary readership of the patient. For example, a home exercise program should be written in lay terminology, avoiding abbreviations and medical jargon. Similarly, any documentation that is sent to third-party payers, and particularly to patients or their families, should make more limited use of abbreviations. If uncommon medical terminology is used, it should be defined in layperson's terms. Another example is note writing in pediatric practice, in which developmental evaluations are read primarily by parents, educators, service providers, and coordinators (Figure 2-6). Professional notes should not be written in purely lay terminology, but they can be written in such a way as to be readable by those outside the profession.

The overuse of abbreviations and jargon is a symptom of a more serious problem: the use of a private language in which much of the rationale for treatment is left implicit. If it is assumed that the reader of a note is among the *cognoscenti*, in which he or she must be able to decipher the abbreviations and strange terms, then why bother explaining what was done and why? Too often it seems as if such a philosophy guides the writing of notes. The critical elements of the clinical reasoning process cannot be omitted with the assumption that the reader will "fill in the blanks." The therapist has a professional responsibility to explain what has been done and what will be done, and why, in clear, unambiguous terms that will be understandable to all those authorized to read a therapist's notes.

OMIT UNNECESSARY AND IRRELEVANT FACTS

The *best* way to write clear, concise notes quickly is to avoid unnecessary and irrelevant facts and conclusions. Merely because the therapist has observed something does not make it appropriate to include in the note. The note should include only those observations and interpretations that are essential for documenting the patient's current medical condition. Omitting nonessential items makes the note more readable and more efficient to write.

Therapists should generally avoid, or be very careful, when including the following information in a medical note:

- Detailed social history
- Detailed living situation

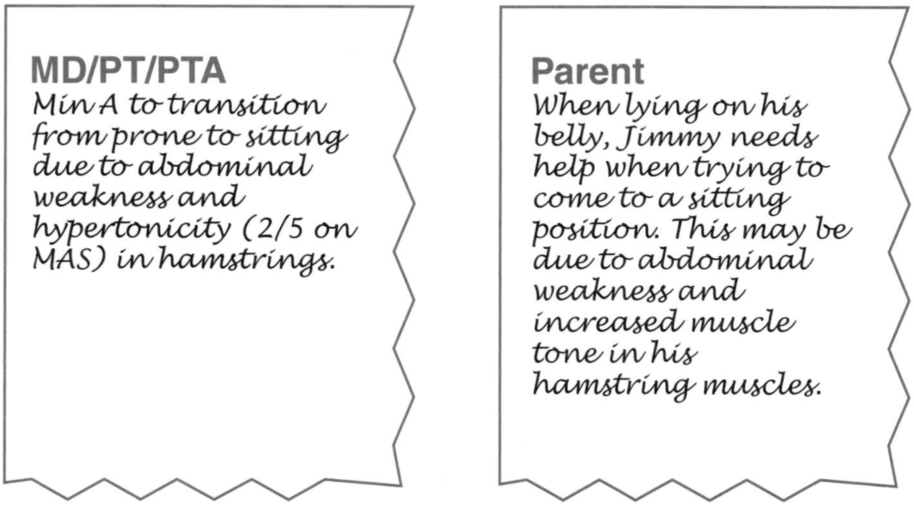

MD/PT/PTA
Min A to transition from prone to sitting due to abdominal weakness and hypertonicity (2/5 on MAS) in hamstrings.

Parent
When lying on his belly, Jimmy needs help when trying to come to a sitting position. This may be due to abdominal weakness and increased muscle tone in his hamstring muscles.

FIGURE 2-6 Notewriting is audience specific. This figure shows two different wordings for documenting mobility skills in a young child with cerebral palsy. When a note will be read primarily by a parent or professional who is not familiar with common medical terminology, terms should be defined in an understandable and meaningful way.

- Family history
- Detailed history of other medical conditions that have been resolved and do not affect the current condition

Therapists should use their knowledge of individual diseases to help guide what is considered pertinent for a medical note. In general, documentation should be kept focused to the information that directly affects that patient's current health condition.

USE OF TEMPLATES

PTs often spend a good part of their working time doing documentation. Although "paperwork" can be extremely daunting—to the experienced and inexperienced clinician alike—the work can be streamlined without sacrificing quality. While writing a long initial evaluation is not appealing to most PTs, it is equally unappealing for other medical professionals to read one. Therefore the more concise a PT's writing can be while covering all necessary and pertinent information, the better for everyone.

Templates are standard forms that therapists can use to essentially fill in the blanks. Templates ensure that pertinent items are covered and provide a consistent format for assessing different patients. Once the template is familiar to various professionals, pertinent information can be located readily within the report. Computerized documentation has facilitated the use of such templates in which therapists typically use a combination of narrative writing, check boxes, and pull-down menus from a prefabricated template to develop an individualized evaluation report. Chapter 16 provides an overview and sample templates used in computerized documentation. Other sample evaluation forms, including a template for conducting a home care evaluation, can be found in Appendix D.

If such forms are used, no line should be left blank. This way the evaluation cannot be altered by another party without the therapist's knowledge. Also, if a line is left blank, the reason it was left blank is unknown to the reader. The therapist must write one of the following on the line:

1. The results of the test, examination findings, or clinical opinion.
2. N/T (not tested), to indicate that this item was not tested. This entry in the note should be followed by a reason the item was not tested or a plan for testing in the future (e.g., "N/T 2° to time constraints—to be evaluated 11/1").
3. N/A (not applicable), to indicate that this test was not applicable for this particular patient given his or her diagnosis or condition. The

therapist should state why the test or measure is not applicable (e.g., "N/A—Pt. is currently on ventilator and unable to get out of bed").

Avoiding Labels and Derogatory Statements

People-first language is language that is used in oral or written communication that describes the disease or medical condition a person *has* without it defining who the person *is*. Terms such as *autistic, mentally retarded*, and *paraplegic* all focus on defining a person by his or her disability.

The APTA supports the use of people-first language, as described in *Terminology for Communication About People With Disabilities* (HOD P06-91-25-34, Program 50).

Physical therapy practitioners have an obligation to provide nonjudgmental care to all people who need it. They should be guided in their written and spoken communication by the *Guidelines for Reporting and Writing About People With Disabilities* (Research and Training Center on Independent Living, 2008). APTA members are encouraged to use appropriate terminology for specific disabilities as outlined in the *Guidelines*, which are available online at *http://www.rtcil.org/products/RTCILpublications/Media/GuidelinesforReportingandWritingaboutPeoplewithDisabilities.pdf*.

Patients should be thought of as people first, not their disability. Labeling patients according to their disability (e.g., stroke victim, amputee) suggests that their disability defines them. In contrast, therapists should strive to use person-first terminology in verbal and written communication (Table 2-1). Furthermore, when referring to individuals who do not have a disability, use of the term *able-bodied* (as well as *healthy* or *whole*) to contrast people without disabilities with people who have disabilities is considered inappropriate. Rather, use the term *nondisabled*.

TABLE 2-1	PERSON-FIRST TERMINOLOGY
Inappropriate Terminology	**Preferred Terminology**
Amputee	Man with amputation
Stroke victims	People who have had a stroke
Autistic	Boy with autism
Able-bodied	Nondisabled
T12 para	Woman with T12 paraplegia

Expressions such as *afflicted with, suffers from,* or *victim* focus unnecessarily on the negative aspects of a person's health condition. Rather, use a *man with post-polio syndrome,* or a *stroke survivor.* Similarly, labeling patients with terms such as *confused, agitated,* or *noncompliant,* for example, focuses the reader on the label rather than the person, and the two become invariably linked. Rather, specific behaviors of a patient should be described. Simply because a patient may not be performing a home exercise program, he or she should not be identified as a "noncompliant patient." Instead, the patient might be described as *a patient, man, or woman* and at some later point in the documentation, it could be noted that he or she *has not consistently complied with the home program.*

Therapists also should be careful to avoid derogatory statements about patients. Such terms as *Patient complains...* or *Client suffers from...* have negative connotations and should be avoided. Rather, *Patient reports...* or *Client has a diagnosis of...* reflect more objective statements.

Summary

- Documentation in physical therapy takes many forms, mainly initial evaluations, progress notes, treatment notes, and discharge summaries.
- Documentation formats include narrative, SOAP notes, and functional outcome reports.
- Within these formats, therapists can use standardized forms, tables, graphs, photographs, and drawings to improve the readability of the documentation and highlight key aspects.
- Therapists can use several strategies to write medical notes in a concise manner: concise wording, use of abbreviations, avoidance of irrelevant facts, and use of documentation templates.
- All written and oral communication should avoid labeling patients and incorporate person-first language. Patients and clients are defined *as people,* not by their disability or disease.

EXERCISE 2-1   INTERPRETING ABBREVIATIONS

For the each of the following statements, write out the entire statement, interpreting the abbreviations. Use Appendix B for assistance as necessary.

EXAMPLE: Pt. is I in all ADLs

ANSWER: Patient is independent in all activities of daily living.

1. MMT 3/5 R quads

_____

2. Pt. can stand $\bar{s}$ A for 30 sec $\bar{s}$ LOB

_____

3. Pt. can transfer bed → w/c $\bar{c}$ mod A using SB

_____

4. Pt. instructed in performing R SAQ, 3 sets × 10 reps

_____

5. PROM R ankle DF 5°

_____

6. Received Rx from MD for WBAT on L LE

_____

7. Pt. instructed to perform HEP b.i.d., 10 reps each ex

_____

8. Pt. admitted to ER 10/12/09 with GCS of 4

_____

9. Medical dx: R hip fracture $\bar{c}$ ORIF

_____

10. AROM B LEs WNL

_____

11. Pt. instructed in use of TENS unit, on prn basis

_____

12. CPT × 20 min; P&V RLL

13. Pt. was d/c'd from NICU on 3/3/09

14. PMH: IDDM ×5 yr, HBP ×10 yr

15. MRI revealed mod L MCA CVA

EXERCISE 2-2 CONCISE DOCUMENTATION AND USE OF ABBREVIATIONS

Rewrite these notes as if you were writing them in a medical record. Consider condensing sentence structure, such as eliminating unnecessary words. Use abbreviations whenever possible (see Appendix B for assistance).

EXAMPLE: Patient can walk a distance of 50 feet in the hospital corridors.

Pt. walks 50 ft in hospital corridors.

1. Patient underwent a procedure called a coronary artery bypass graft on 3/17/08.

2. Therapist will coordinate practice of activities of daily living training with occupational therapist and with nursing staff.

3. The patient's heart rate changed from 90 to 120 beats per minute after 3 minutes of walking at a comfortable speed.

4. The patient's obstetric/gynecologic doctor reported that this patient has been experiencing low back pain throughout her pregnancy.

5. Patient's daughter reports that patient has had a recent decrease in her functional abilities and has a history of falls.

6. The patient's breath sounds were decreased bilaterally. The patient was instructed in performing deep breathing exercises twice per day.

7. Patient's wife reports that the patient has had a history of chronic low back pain for the past 15 years.

_____

8. The patient's long-term goal is to be able to walk using only a straight cane.

_____

9. Deep tendon reflex of right biceps was recorded as a 2+.

_____

10. Patient can ascend and descend one flight of stairs independently, using one hand on railing.

_____

11. Prescription received for physical therapy to include therapeutic exercise and gait training.

_____

12. Resident is 82 years old and has a primary medical diagnosis of congestive heart failure.

_____

13. Electrocardiogram revealed ventricular tachycardia.

_____

14. Patient suffered a cerebrovascular accident, with resultant hemiplegia of the right upper and lower extremity.

_____

15. The home health aide was instructed in assisting patient to perform active-assistive range of motion exercises, which were straight leg raises and hip abduction in supine.

_____

EXERCISE 2-3   PEOPLE-FIRST LANGUAGE

Therapists should avoid "labeling" patients and should always use people-first language in both oral and written communication. For each of the phrases below, decide first whether the phrase is appropriate. If it is, write "OK" in the space provided. If it is not, rewrite the phrase so that it reflects person-first language or restructure the sentence to provide a more objective or positive description of the patient (much of this exercise and the answers are adapted or reprinted with permission from Martin, 1999).

1. A quadriplegic will require help with transfers.

_____

2. The patient was afflicted with multiple sclerosis when she was in her 20s.

_____

3. Many PTs are involved in foot clinics for diabetics.

_____

4. Have you finished the documentation for that shoulder in room 316?

_____

5. The patient complained of pain in the right upper extremity.

_____

6. A care plan for patients with total knee replacements involves a strong element of patient education.

_____

7. Although this computer program was designed for the disabled, able-bodied users will also find it helpful.

_____

8. Because of a spinal cord injury, the patient was confined to a wheelchair.

_____

9. Nine of 10 patients receiving physical therapy expressed interest in a group exercise session.

_____

10. The patient is behaving like a child.

_____

11. Which therapist is treating the brain-injured patient in room 216?

_____

12. The stroke victim can often return to work.

_____

13. The patient refused to modify her footwear choice even after the therapist told her not to wear 2-inch heels.

_____

14. I'll put my 10:00 on the machine while my 10:15 gets a hot pack.

_____

15. The patient suffers from Parkinson's disease.

_____

CHAPTER 3

Legal Aspects of Documentation

LEARNING OBJECTIVES

After reading this chapter, the reader will be able to:

1. List and describe the key aspects of physical therapy documentation as a legal record.

2. Use the correct method for signing notes and correcting errors in documentation.

3. Describe the Health Insurance Portability and Accountability Act (HIPAA) and the Privacy Rule and discuss the implication for physical therapy documentation.

4. Discuss the importance of appropriately documenting informed consent as part of a physical therapy evaluation.

5. Discuss the three legal reasons why a physical therapist's documentation may be scrutinized.

Documentation as a Legal Record

Documentation in a medical record is a legal document. A therapist should treat notewriting very seriously and understand that his or her notes may be scrutinized not only for payment of services, but also for legal reasons.

State practice acts define the scope of practice for PTs in each state (see *Resources* list at the end of this chapter). Therapists should be familiar with their individual state practice acts to be sure they are in compliance and that their documentation reflects practice that is within the legal description provided by their state. For example, if a state practice act requires a referral from a physician for a PT to practice, that information must be included in the medical record (regardless of whether it is required by a third-party payer).

KEY LEGAL ASPECTS OF PHYSICAL THERAPY DOCUMENTATION

Several key legal aspects pertinent to physical therapy documentation are outlined below:

- *Legibility.* Handwritten entries should be legible and written in ink.

- *Dated.* All notes must be dated with the date that the note was written. Backdating is illegal and should never be done. It is recommended that all notes be written or dictated on the date that an evaluation or intervention is performed. If a note is not written on the date, then both the date of the evaluation/intervention and the date the report was written should be indicated. For notes in an interdisciplinary medical record, the time of treatment should also be recorded.

- *Authentication.* All physical therapy documentation must be authenticated by a PT, or when appropriate,

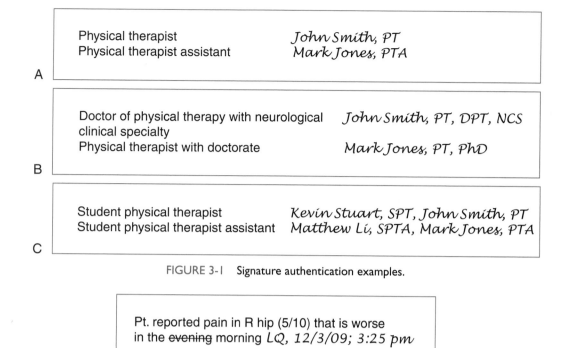

Physical therapist	*John Smith, PT*
Physical therapist assistant	*Mark Jones, PTA*

A

Doctor of physical therapy with neurological clinical specialty	*John Smith, PT, DPT, NCS*
Physical therapist with doctorate	*Mark Jones, PT, PhD*

B

Student physical therapist	*Kevin Stuart, SPT, John Smith, PT*
Student physical therapist assistant	*Matthew Li, SPTA, Mark Jones, PTA*

C

FIGURE 3-1 Signature authentication examples.

Pt. reported pain in R hip (5/10) that is worse in the ~~evening~~ morning *LQ, 12/3/09; 3:25 pm*

FIGURE 3-2 Error correction on a progress note.

a physical therapy assistant (PTA). All notes must be signed, followed by the writer's professional abbreviation, and dated. The American Physical Therapy Association House of Delegates (APTA HOD, 1999) has recommended use of standard professional designations: PT for physical therapists and PTA for physical therapist assistants (Figure 3-1, *A*).

- *Degrees and certifications.* The APTA supports the following preferred order when a therapist or assistant has additional degrees or certifications (Figure 3-1, *B*). These are not relevant legally but are important to promote consistent communication throughout the profession:
  1. PT/PTA
  2. Highest earned physical therapy-related degree
  3. Other earned academic degree(s)
  4. Specialist certification credentials in alphabetical order (specific to the American Board of Physical Therapy Specialties)
  5. Other credentials external to APTA
  6. Other certification or professional honors (e.g., FAPTA) (APTA HOD, 1999)

- *PTA authentication.* PTAs can typically sign only treatment notes; all evaluations must be written and signed by a PT. Depending on individual state practice acts, PTs may be required to co-sign each note written by a PTA.

- *Student PT and PTA authentication.* SPTs or SPTAs (individuals who are enrolled in a PT or PTA educational program) are allowed to write

notes in the medical record. These notes must be signed and dated by the student and also must be authenticated by a supervising licensed PT or PTA (see also APTA Guidelines, Appendix A) (Figure 3-1, *C*).

- *Errors.* If an error is made in a handwritten note or a printed copy of an electronic note, the therapist should place a single line through the erroneous word and write his or her initials near the crossed-out word. The date and time of correction should also be included (Figure 3-2).

- *Blank lines or spaces.* Blank lines or large empty spaces should be avoided in the record. A single straight line should be drawn through any open spaces in a report.

- *Abbreviations.* The writer should use only those abbreviations authorized by his or her facility (Appendix B provides a list of commonly used abbreviations in rehabilitation settings). Abbreviations should be kept to a minimum; if in doubt, write it out (see Chapter 2 for information on using abbreviations).

INFORMATION TO INCLUDE IN A NOTE

From a legal persepective, the medical note should provide a record of everything that was done during the therapy session. This includes what the patient did (e.g., exercises, activities) as well as specific interventions performed by the therapist (e.g., gait training, electrical stimulation). This information is not always necessary for purposes of payment, but therapists should be careful to document comprehensively for legal purposes. A therapist must ask whether his or her note, if referred to at a later date, would clearly establish what was done and why. If a therapist is being sued for malpractice, for example, the medical record will be scrutinized to determine what interventions were performed, what the patient was able to do, and how the patient reacted to the interventions.

Only information that is directly relevant to the patient's medical condition, prognosis, or intervention plan should be documented in a medical record. Sometimes conflicts or personal issues arise between therapists and patients, and between patients and their physicians or other medical professionals. Generally, information of this nature should not be included in clinical documentation. Box 3-1 contains definitions of key documentation terms.

Privacy of the Medical Record: HIPAA and the Privacy Rule

HIPAA stands for the Health Insurance Portability and Accountability Act, which was passed by Congress in 1996. There are two parts to the law. The first part is involved with the portability of an individual's health care insurance in the event of a job loss. The second part, which is pertinent to medical documentation, was designed to protect the privacy of health care data and to promote more standardization and efficiency in the health care industry.

The U.S. Department of Health and Human Services (HHS) implemented the Privacy Rule to comply with HIPAA. The Privacy Rule "address[es] the use and disclosure of individuals' health information—called *protected health information* (PHI) by organizations subject to the Privacy Rule—called *covered entities* as well as standards for individuals' privacy rights to understand and control how their health information is used" (HHS, 2003).

HIPAA rules govern only "covered entities." This includes any provider of medical or other health services, or supplies, who transmits any health information in electronic form (CMS, 2003). Therefore HIPAA applies to only those practices that submit or receive electronic documentation. In the near future, this hopefully will apply to almost all physical therapy practices.

The Privacy Rule protects all individually identifiable PHI. This is information that is held or transmitted by a covered entity in any form (electronic, paper, or oral). Such information includes a patient's demographic data (e.g., name, address, birth date, Social Security number) and information related to the following:

- The individual's past, present, or future physical or mental health or condition
- The provision of health care to the individual
- The past, present, or future payment for the provision of health care to the individual

BOX 3-1
Important Definitions

Audit: a detailed review and evaluation of selected clinical records by qualified professional personnel for evaluating quality of medical care.

Authentication: identification of the author of a medical record entry by that author, and confirmation that the contents are what the author intended.

HIPAA Privacy Rule: a component of a law passed in 1996 that is designed to protect the privacy of health care data and to promote more standardization and efficiency in the health care industry.

Informed consent: a voluntary, legally documented agreement by a health care consumer to allow performance of a specific diagnostic, therapeutic, or research procedure.

Malpractice: negligence or misconduct by a professional person, such as a doctor or physical therapist. The failure to meet a standard of care or standard of conduct that is recognized by a profession reaches the level of malpractice when a client or patient is injured or damaged because of error.

Medical necessity: services or items reasonable and necessary for the diagnosis or treatment of illness or injury or to improve the functioning of a malformed body member.

Notice of privacy practices (NPP): a notice or written document given to a health care consumer that explains the privacy policies related to his or her medical records. All patients must sign a statement acknowledging receipt of the NPP.

Third-party payer: an organization other than the patient (first party) or health care provider (second party) involved in the financing of personal health services.

Data from Reference.md (http://www.reference.md/files/D008/mD008485.html): Joint Committee on Administrative Rule (http://www.ilga.gov/commission/jcar/admincode/077/077002500L15100R.html); Centers for Medicare and Medicaid Services (www.cms.gov): Segan JC: *Concise Dictionary of Modern Medicine*, New York, 2006, McGraw-Hill; The Free Dictionary (http://legal-dictionary.thefreedictionary.com/Malpractice); Physician's News Digest (http://www.physiciansnews.com/law/802.miller.html); and *Mosby's Dental Dictionary*, ed 2, St Louis, 2008, Mosby Elsevier.

An important intention of the Privacy Rule is to limit the disclosure of any patient's PHI. A covered entity can use PHI only as the Privacy Rule permits or as the patient (or his or her representative) authorizes in writing.

The following are some basic guidelines for covered entities for maintaining patient privacy of medical records:

- Patients must be given a notice of privacy practice (NPP) document, which explains the privacy policies related to their medical records. All patients must sign a statement acknowledging receipt of the NPP.
- Therapists must obtain a patient's consent to access, use, or disclose any personally identifiable health information for purposes of treatment,

payment, and health care operations (TPO). A patient's medical record should never be disclosed to a third party (including employers and family members) without specific permission from the patient.

- Parents or guardians must grant approval for access to a minor's medical record.

For more information on HIPAA rules and compliance, refer to *www.cms.org*, which provides detailed information on HIPAA and the Privacy Rule and is updated regularly.

In addition to the HIPAA ruling, therapists should take general precautions to be sure that any documentation remains private and is not shared with unauthorized persons. The APTA Defensible Documentation (*www.apta.org*) recommends several general strategies for maintaining patient confidentiality, including the following:

- Keep patient documentation in a secure area.
- Keep charts facing down so the patient's name is not displayed.
- Patient charts should never be left unattended.
- Do not discuss patient cases in open or public areas.

Documentation of Informed Consent

Informed consent is the process by which a health care consumer is given clear information about the risks and benefits of a proposed procedure or intervention and any alternatives and the individual agrees to the proposed plan of care. In order to give informed consent, a person must have appropriate reasoning abilities and must have been provided with all relevant facts.

APTA GUIDELINES

The APTA's *Guide for Professional Conduct* does not specify the need for informed consent; however, it recommends that a PT should communicate the results of the evaluation with the patient and provide him or her with accurate and relevant information about his or her condition. Furthermore, the PT must use professional judgment to inform the patient of any risk of the proposed intervention or examination (APTA, 2004).

WORLD CONFEDERATION OF PHYSICAL THERAPY GUIDELINES

The World Confederation of Physical Therapy (WCPT) has written a more specific guideline for informed

consent by PTs. WCPT's Declaration of Principle on Informed Consent states that "A competent adult should be provided with adequate, intelligible information about the proposed therapy:

- A description of the treatment to be provided,
- A clear explanation of the risks which may be associated with the therapy,
- Expected benefits from the therapy,
- Anticipated timeframes,
- Anticipated costs, and
- Reasonable alternatives to the recommended therapy" (WCPT, 2007).

This Declaration further suggests that PTs should record in their documentation that informed consent has been obtained.

COMPONENTS OF DOCUMENTING INFORMED CONSENT

Documentation of informed consent should include the following information:

1. The PT gave the patient the necessary information to provide informed consent.
2. The patient understood the information and consented to the plan of care.

The patient/client should therefore be asked to acknowledge understanding and consent before intervention is initiated. Many facilities have a separate form for this purpose. If a separate form is not used, a statement should be included in all physical therapy evaluations (Figure 3-3), typically at the end of the plan of care.

Potential Legal Issues

In today's litigious society, PTs and other health care professionals are under continued scrutiny and potential risk for liability and malpractice. Furthermore, billing of third-party payers, such as insurance companies and Medicare, opens up therapists to claims of billing improprieties or fradulent charging.

The following sections summarize the potential legal reasons why a PT's documentation could be scrutinized.

> *The findings of this evaluation were discussed c̄ the patient, and she consented to the above intervention plan.*

FIGURE 3-3 Sample statement of informed consent.

MALPRACTICE

Malpractice suits against therapists, while rare, typically occur when an accident happens in the course of a therapy session. A patient who is recovering from an ankle injury could overexercise in therapy and reinjure the affected area, for example. Alternatively, a patient who has had a stroke could fall and sustain a fracture during gait training or transfer training.

Keeping comprehensive and up-to-date medical records is critical to minimizing liability risk. For example, if a patient has reported an increase in pain during the course of a treatment, the therapist should document the current and previous level of pain, whether the plan of care was altered, and if contact with a physician or other health care professional was made. If this information is not documented, then from a legal perspective it *did not happen*.

LAWSUITS

A patient may be involved in a lawsuit related to an accident that he or she had, such as a workplace accident or a motor vehicle accident. In such cases, the PT's records will serve as a legal record and will be scrutinized to determine the necessity of the intervention and the degree of impairments and activity limitations for a patient.

FRAUDULENT CHARGES

When billing third-party payers such as Medicare, the PT's medical records will be examined to determine whether the interventions provided match the billing for those interventions. If the PT charges for something that was not done or not supported by documentation, legal action can be taken on the part of the third-party payer or Medicare. It is critical that the PT's documentation matches exactly any *Current Procedural Terminology* (CPT) codes used (see Chapter 14). Furthermore, for payment by third parties (particularly Medicare), the physical therapy notes must justify *medical necessity*. If the treatments proposed or performed are not deemed to be medically necessary and the therapist attempts to bill an insurance company or Medicare for these services, the therapist may be vulnerable to audit or legal action by that payer.

Preventative Actions

Several actions can be taken by a therapy clinic or department to minimize the risk of an audit (by a third-party payer or government agency) or legal action. Most importantly, a clinic should stay up-to-date and in compliance with current rules related to coding, billing, documentation, and requirements for medical necessity and skilled therapy services (Fearon et al., 2009).

The following is a list of strategies that facilities or small practices can use to minimize their risk for an audit or investigation. This list was adapted with permission from presentations by Steve Levine, PT, DPT, and Helene Fearon of Fearon & Levine Consulting:

- Minimize errors and prevent potential penalties for improper billing and documentation before they occur
- Set up controls to counter risks
- Perform pre-audit self-examination to identify vulnerabilities
- Hire experts through legal counsel
- Develop compliance plans; such plans can limit your liability by providing standards of conduct for your practice or facility
- Develop corrective action plans; such plans can be used to fix any areas of weakness or vulnerability that may have been determined after a risk assessment

Summary

- Documentation in a medical note by PTs is considered a legal document.
- Documentation must comply with individual state practice acts, to which therapists should refer for information related to authentication and other specific requirements.
- Documentation of informed consent is recommended to ensure that the patient was given all necessary information pertaining to his or her condition and the results of an evaluation, and that the patient consented to the proposed plan of care.
- Although PTs and other health care professionals are vulnerable to legal actions, complete and accurate documentation practices can help to minimize legal risks.

Recommended Resources

Important resources pertaining to legal aspects of documentation:

- APTA *Guidelines for Documentation*, Appendix A
- APTA Directory of Physical Therapy State Practice Acts: *https://www.apta.org/AM/Template.cfm?Section=State_Gov_t_Affairs&Template=/TaggedPage/TaggedPageDisplay.cfm&TPLID=163&ContentID=24096*

- Centers for Medicare and Medicaid Services: *www.cms.gov*
- Health Insurance Portability and Accountability Act: *http://www.hhs.gov/ocr/privacy/index.html*
- Fearon & Levine Consulting: *www.fearonlevine.com*

- Scott RW: *Legal aspects of documenting patient care for rehabilitation professionals*, ed 3, Sudbury, MA, 2006, Jones and Bartlett.

CHAPTER 4

Clinical Decision Making and the Initial Evaluation Format

LEARNING OBJECTIVES

After reading this chapter and completing the exercises, the reader will be able to:

1. Outline a model for organizing an initial evaluation based on a functional outcomes approach.

2. Identify the basic elements for each section of the initial evaluation format.

3. Describe the relationship between the American Physical Therapy Association's *Guide to Physical Therapist Practice* patient/client management model and the sections of the initial evaluation format.

4. Categorize components of an initial evaluation into the initial evaluation format.

This chapter presents a format for organizing physical therapy documentation that is based on two important models for physical therapy: the International Classification of Functioning, Disability and Health (ICF) framework and the patient/client management model from the American Physical Therapy Association's (APTA) *Guide to Physical Therapist Practice* (the *Guide*). The format is based on three fundamental assumptions presented in previous chapters:

1. Documentation both shapes and reflects clinical problem-solving strategies.

2. A top-down model of disablement provides a useful framework for clinical problem solving, and thus documentation.

3. Documentation should be organized around functional outcomes.

The format presented herein is intended to provide a set of general guidelines for organizing documentation that can be adapted to different practice settings. It is not intended to be a rigidly applied procedure for writing documentation. PTs practice in a variety of settings, encounter many different types of patients and clients, and write documentation for many different reasons. No single format could be applicable to all these situations. Nevertheless, the general principles of functional outcomes documentation can be captured in a generic format and adapted to different purposes and contexts.

Two main formats for documentation are presented in this book: (1) a format for writing the initial evaluation of a patient and (2) a format for writing progress and treatment notes. Other types of documentation, such as discharge summaries, letters to referral sources, and others, can easily be constructed from these two main types. **The major focus of this book is on the initial evaluation format because it is the most critical to establishing a framework for clinical decision making.** Each section of the initial evaluation format is further detailed in separate chapters (Chapters 5 to 11). The format for progress and treatment notes is a modified form of the SOAP note (see Chapter 2) and is presented in Chapter 12. Practice exercises in categorizing statements into the different sections of the initial evaluation format are provided at the end of this chapter.

The format for an initial evaluation is based on the top-down disablement model presented in Chapter 1. There are six main sections (Table 4-1). The first three sections include information related to the ICF framework: health condition and participation (Reason for Referral section), activities (Activities section), and body structures and functions (Impairments section). The next three sections present the diagnosis (Assessment), the Goals, and the Plan of Care.

One of the important contributions of the *Guide* is the "patient/client management model." This model describes the process by which a PT determines the critical problems that require intervention and develops an intervention plan to address those problems. The model defines five integrated elements of the

TABLE 4-1	**SIX SECTIONS OF THE INITIAL EVALUATION FORMAT**
Section	**Information Included**
Reason for referral	**Health condition** • Current condition • Past medical history • Medications **Social history and participation** • Living environment, work status (job/school/play), community, and leisure integration or reintegration • Prior level of functioning • Environmental factors
Activities	*Can include any of the following subheadings, as appropriate:* Self-care and home management (including activities of daily living and instrumental activities of daily living) Assistive and adaptive devices Environmental, home, and work (job/school/play) barriers Listing of specific skills assessed (e.g., ambulation, stair climbing, feeding, bed mobility)
Impairments	Systems review *Can also include any the following subheadings, as appropriate:* Aerobic capacity/endurance Anthropometric characteristics Arousal, attention, and cognition Circulation (arterial, venous, lymphatic) Cranial and peripheral nerve integrity Ergonomics and body mechanics Gait, locomotion, and balance Integumentary integrity Wound Joint integrity and mobility Motor function Muscle performance Neuromotor development and sensory integration Orthotic, protective, and supportive devices Pain Posture Prosthetic requirements Range of motion (including muscle length) Reflex integrity Sensory integrity Ventilation and respiration
Assessment	Includes evaluation, diagnosis, and prognosis
Goals	Participation goals Activity goals Impairment goals (optional)
Plan of care	Coordination/communication Patient-related instruction Direct interventions

process: examination, evaluation, diagnosis, prognosis, and intervention. The model is illustrated and each of the elements is defined in Figure 4-1.

The initial evaluation format fits very closely with the patient/client management model (Table 4-2). In this format, examination and evaluation are combined. As is emphasized in the patient/client management model, evaluation is a dynamic process—not something that is initiated only after all data have been collected. Therefore there is an interplay between examination and evaluation.

Data are collected and evaluated, and then decisions are made about what additional data to collect. This process often may involve hypothesis testing. In the functional outcomes approach the starting point for data collection is the Reason for Referral, which establishes both the primary reasons for referral and the patient's participation restrictions. This then leads to specific examination procedures to determine which activities are related to the participation restriction and which impairments are leading to activity limitations.

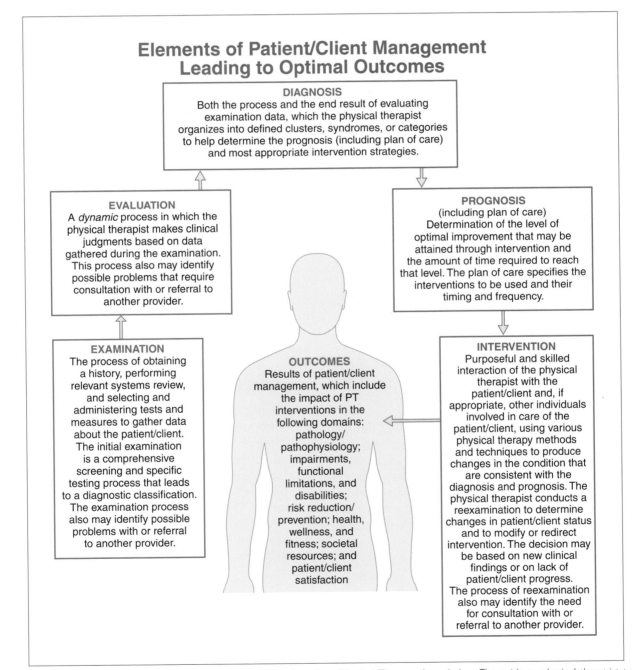

Elements of Patient/Client Management Leading to Optimal Outcomes

DIAGNOSIS
Both the process and the end result of evaluating examination data, which the physical therapist organizes into defined clusters, syndromes, or categories to help determine the prognosis (including plan of care) and most appropriate intervention strategies.

EVALUATION
A *dynamic* process in which the physical therapist makes clinical judgments based on data gathered during the examination. This process also may identify possible problems that require consultation with or referral to another provider.

PROGNOSIS
(including plan of care)
Determination of the level of optimal improvement that may be attained through intervention and the amount of time required to reach that level. The plan of care specifies the interventions to be used and their timing and frequency.

EXAMINATION
The process of obtaining a history, performing relevant systems review, and selecting and administering tests and measures to gather data about the patient/client. The initial examination is a comprehensive screening and specific testing process that leads to a diagnostic classification. The examination process also may identify possible problems with or referral to another provider.

OUTCOMES
Results of patient/client management, which include the impact of PT interventions in the following domains: pathology/pathophysiology; impairments, functional limitations, and disabilities; risk reduction/prevention; health, wellness, and fitness; societal resources; and patient/client satisfaction

INTERVENTION
Purposeful and skilled interaction of the physical therapist with the patient/client and, if appropriate, other individuals involved in care of the patient/client, using various physical therapy methods and techniques to produce changes in the condition that are consistent with the diagnosis and prognosis. The physical therapist conducts a reexamination to determine changes in patient/client status and to modify or redirect intervention. The decision may be based on new clinical findings or on lack of patient/client progress. The process of reexamination also may identify the need for consultation with or referral to another provider.

FIGURE 4-1   **The patient/client management model.** (From American Physical Therapy Association: *The guide to physical therapist practice,* ed 2, Alexandria, VA, 2001, American Physical Therapy Association.)

TABLE 4-2	RELATIONSHIP OF THE *GUIDE*'S PATIENT/CLIENT MANAGEMENT MODEL TO THE DOCUMENTATION FORMAT	
Patient/Client Management Model	Components of the Initial Evaluation	Process
Examination/evaluation	Reason for referral	Explain medical and health conditions that are pertinent to patient's current problems
	Participation	Determine restrictions in participation in work or personal roles
	Activities	Measure patient performance on the activities that the individual needs to perform to overcome or prevent participation restrictions
	Impairments	Identify and measure the impairments that contribute to the observed functional activities
Diagnosis	Assessment	Establish a diagnosis and justify necessity of physical therapy intervention
Prognosis	Goals/plan of care	Develop a set of goals in consultation with the patient
Intervention	Plan of care	Plan an intervention strategy that will help the patient achieve the goals

Thus the functional outcomes format applies a logical sequence to the reporting of the data that were collected.

The critical step in clinical reasoning is establishing a diagnosis. The diagnosis establishes the causes of specific problems that the PT or PTA will address in the intervention strategy. Sometimes the diagnosis may be a statement of the nature and location of the health condition that is causing the problem. More commonly it is a statement of the causal links between impairments and activity limitations. Diagnosis is considered in more detail in Chapter 9.

After a diagnosis has been established, the PT determines the expected outcomes, based on the history, examination, and other factors. In the functional outcomes format these outcomes are organized into three sets of goals: participation goals, activity goals, and impairment goals. This organization clarifies the distinct nature of these goals and encourages the formulation of goals at each level.

In the last section of the initial evaluation the PT plans a strategy for intervention. As noted in the *Guide*, intervention involves three processes: coordination and communication, patient-/client-related instruction, and direct interventions. Again, each is given a separate subsection in the initial evaluation format to encourage explicit documentation of these categories.

A Description of the Initial Evaluation Format

The following sections discuss each of the main components of the initial evaluation format in some detail. Each component is further detailed in Chapters 5 to 11, and case examples of complete intial evaluations can be found at the end of this chapter.

Ideally, the format of your intial evaluation should *guide* your clinical decision making. Table 4-3 summarizes the evaluation process, emphasizing clinical decision making. This process uses a *top-down model*. After obtaining patient history and pertinent medical information, therapists ask patients about their *participation restrictions*, and then ascertain which *activities* are limited, and whether *impairments* exist in body structures and functions that contribute to these activity limitations and participation restrictions. This leads to a process of developing an *assessment*, which includes a diagnosis and prognosis, setting of *goals*, and developing a *plan of care*.

REASON FOR REFERRAL

The Reason for Referral typically entails a short narrative summary of the reason for evaluating a particular patient in physical therapy (see Chapters 5 and 6). This includes defining any previously established diagnosis and pertinent medical history, as well as the patient's social history and current level of participation. This information is linked together in this one section as it provides the rationale for why the patient was referred for evaluation. The following two sections are therefore included in the reason for referral.

Current Condition

The current condition section includes the following information (as pertinent):

- Patient information, such as name, age, and gender

TABLE 4-3	PROCESS USED TO EVALUATE A PATIENT AND DEVELOP A PLAN FOR INTERVENTION
Main Sections of Initial Evaluation	**Questions the Physical Therapist Asks**
Reason for referral	What is the primary health condition? What other medical conditions may affect the primary health condition? What was the individual's prior level of functioning? What is the individual's current life situation—home environment, work, social support? How is the current condition affecting the individual's life and life roles?
Activities	What specific activities (or functional skills) does the individual need to learn (or relearn) to be able to accomplish his or her life roles? How does inadequate performance in specific activities prevent the individual from fulfilling life roles?
Impairments	How are/why are the individual's movements dysfunctional? What neuromuscular, sensorimotor, or cardiovascular mechanisms are inadequate (e.g., range of motion, strength, sensation, pulmonary function)?
Assessment	What is the patient's diagnosis, or can the current diagnosis be modified? What is the justification for physiotherapy intervention? What are the causal links between activity limitations and participation restrictions? Between impairments and activity limitations? Between health condition and impairments?
Goals	What goals have the therapist and patient agreed on? What level of participation does the patient need/want to achieve? What activities will be used to benchmark the patient's progress toward accomplishing the overall goals? Are there any impairment goals that are critical to be achieved?
Plan of care	What musculoskeletal, neuromotor, and physiologic resources must be enhanced to enable the individual to relearn the specified functional skills? What sequence of tasks will optimally challenge the patient? What should be done to promote tissue healing or prevent damage?

- Current condition (history of present illness): medical diagnosis/pathology information
- Past medical history, identifying source: patient report, chart review, or both, or other
- Medications

Social History and Participation

The principal purpose of this section is to establish the patient's current level of participation in life roles and document pertinent social history. *Participation* refers to the ability of an individual to fulfill desired or required personal, social, or occupational roles or to achieve personal goals. *Social history* includes information about a person's living environment and situation (such as where he or she lives and with whom) and current work or employment situation. This section should also encompass information pertaining to a patient's general health status, including participation—or restriction in participation—in recreational and social activities. It would be pertinent to include information about how the patient's current level of functioning in his or her life roles has changed because of the current medical condition. Standardized outcome measures that describe a person's quality of life or level of participation in work, home, and social/recreational activities are also reported in this section.

ACTIVITIES

Information in the Activities section is intended to identify the critical activity limitations that contribute to participation restrictions (see Chapter 7). What are the functional skills that (1) the individual needs to perform to fulfill his or her goals and required roles and (2) are they now in some way less than adequate? Activities should be reported concretely and completely and should be quantified to the degree possible. This can be done by use of quantifiable measurements (such as walking speed or distance walked), or by use of standardized tests that measure the activity level.

IMPAIRMENTS

This section identifies those impairments, such as range of motion limitations or strength deficits, that have a causal relationship to the observed activity limitations or might cause activity limitations in the future if not treated (see Chapter 8). This information should be documented using objective measures, such as degrees of range of motion or manual muscle testing grade, whenever possible.

ASSESSMENT

The Assessment section typically begins with an overall impression: a brief statement summarizing the patient's reason for being referred for physical therapy. The PT then outlines a diagnosis that includes three components: differential diagnosis, classification based on etiology or movement system (if pertinent), and the relationship of the problem with activity limitations and participation restrictions (see Chapter 9). Normally this diagnosis will link either a health condition or impairment to activity limitations. APTA *Guidelines for Physical Therapy Documentation* state that a physical therapy diagnosis is required for all initial evaluations. The assessment concludes with a statement summarizing the PT's recommendations and the necessity of physical therapy intervention (if applicable).

GOALS

This section identifies the expected outcomes of physical therapy intervention, the ends toward which physical therapy intervention is directed (see Chapter 10). Specific *goals* are written that are related to these outcomes. All goals must be measurable and must include a time frame. The goals can have several levels:

- **Participation goals:** Typically one or two participation goals are useful to highlight the overall level of participation in work, social, recreational, and home activities that a patient is expected to achieve.

- **Activity goals:** Activity goals state the predicted functional performance at the end of therapy. These goals must be related to a specific activity, skill, or task that can serve as a **benchmark** for an individual's progress.

- **Impairment goals:** Impairment goals document expected improvements or changes in impairments that will result at the end of therapy. These goals should have a clear relationship to the stated activity goals. For example, achieving a certain shoulder range of motion may be critical to the functional task of lifting or reaching.

All three levels of goals are not required for each documentation. The type and number of goals written depends on the setting and context. However, at a minimum, activity goals should be included in an initial evaluation documentation.

INTERVENTION PLAN

This section outlines the plan for achieving the goals listed in the previous section and presents a concise rationale for the intervention strategy chosen (see Chapter 11). It is useful to begin with the proposed frequency of treatments, as well as a tentative date for reevaluation. Many institutions mandate this approach. The intervention plan should then be documented in the following three categories:

- **Coordination and communication:** Services that require coordination or communication with other providers, agencies, departments, and so on should be included here.

- **Patient-related instruction:** The PT should document specific instruction or teaching of the patient or of the patient's caregivers.

- **Direct interventions:** These interventions are performed by the PT or PTA (e.g., therapeutic exercise, functional training, manual therapy techniques). (See Figure 11-1 for appropriate categorization and terminology from the *Guide*.)

Case Examples

Four examples are included here to illustrate how the initial evaluation format might be used in actual practice.* Readers, especially beginning students, should not see this format as a rigid blueprint to be copied exactly in other situations. Rather, this format should be perceived as a starting point, a set of guidelines to be used for designing effective physical therapy documentation.

Case Examples 4-1 through 4-4 show the variability in how the same format can be applied in different settings and for different patient populations. Some evaluations are shorter, some longer, and include different evaluative information (particularly in the Activities and Impairments sections) as is pertinent for each specific case.

Conclusion

This chapter has outlined the initial evaluation format for functional outcomes documentation. This format is designed so that physical therapy documentation reflects the evaluative, diagnostic, and planning processes that PTs and PTAs use in modern practice. Indeed, as evident in the *Guide to Physical Therapist*

---

*All cases presented in this book may be loosely based on actual patients. However, all names are fictitious and identifying information has been deleted or changed.

Practice, practice is moving from a format based on medical models to a more patient-centered, top-down approach. The format outlined in this chapter attempts to capture both of these aspects of physical therapy practice (see Table 4-3).

Summary

- The format for writing functional outcomes reports is based on (1) clinical problem-solving strategies, (2) a top-down model of disablement, and (3) organization around functional outcomes.

- The format provides a set of general guidelines that can be adapted to different practice settings.

- The format has six main sections: Reason for Referral, Activities, Impairments, Assessment, Goals, and Plan of Care (see Table 4-1).

- The critical step in the evaluation process and clinical reasoning is establishing an assessment and diagnosis. The diagnosis states the causal links among impairments, activities, and participation and justifies the need for intervention. The diagnosis therefore establishes the specific problems that the PT or PTA will address in the Plan of Care.

CASE EXAMPLE 4-1

Physical Therapy Initial Evaluation
Setting: Outpatient

Name: Smith, Herbert   **D.O.B.:** 6/4/50   **Date of Eval.:** 07/29/09

REASON FOR REFERRAL

Health Condition: CURRENT CONDITION: Mr. Smith is a 59 y.o. male s/p L TKR on 7/21/09. Pt. reports gradually increasing pain in B knees for the last 2-3 yr, c̄ L knee becoming severe within the last 2 mo. **PMH:** OA B knees diagnosed 3 yr ago; controlled HTN. **MEDICATIONS:** Lopressor (for high blood pressure), Coumadin (blood thinner post surgery), Percocet (for pain, 2.5 mg/325 mg 1-2 tablets q6h)

Social History/Participation: Pt. lives c̄ wife in 2-story home; 5 steps to enter, 12 steps (8-in height) in between floors. Before surgery pt. was unable to stand s̄ UE support for >30 min. Pt. reports walking "very slowly" before surgery and had "sharp" L knee pain when putting weight on L leg. Pt. required A from wife when walking long distances. At present, pt. is unable to perform household tasks such as cleaning and assisting with house maintenance. Pt.'s wife assists c̄ household tasks and ADLs as needed. Pt. is employed as a surgeon. Prior to this surgery, pt. worked FT, up to 12 hr/day, and was required to stand for up to 1½ hr at a time. Pt. has not returned to work 2° to standing and walking limitations postsurgery. Pt. reports that for many years he enjoyed playing golf 2×/wk but has been unable to do so for the last 4 mo before surgery 2° to pain and walking limitations.

ACTIVITIES

STANDARDIZED TESTS: *Optimal Score:* Difficulty 57/105; self-confidence 62/105. *Lower Extremity Functional Scale:* Preop 39, current 28. **AMBULATION:** Walks c̄ 2 str canes using 4-point gait pattern c̄ S for indoor distances; can amb. 50 ft in 60 sec before needing to sit 2° to pain. Pt. demonstrates ↓ L stance time and antalgic gait pattern. Has not attempted outdoor ambulation. **STAIR CLIMBING:** ↓↑ 12 steps of 8-in height using arm railing and 1 str cane c̄ step-to-step pattern c̄ S within 2 min; unable to negotiate stairs using a step-over-step pattern. **SELF-CARE:** Pt. reports he is I in dressing x̄ requires min A to don/doff L sock and shoe. Pt. reports he showers in a stall shower holding onto grab bar; needs min A of wife (to reach LEs and occasionally to maintain balance). **STANDING TASKS:** Able to stand for 10 min at countertop (kitchen or bathroom) while reaching c̄ either hand, using other hand for support, limited 2° to pain (6/10). Reaching for objects above shoulder height c̄ UE support with cane or using countertop. Unable to reach for objects below knee height to either side.

IMPAIRMENTS

SYSTEMS REVIEW: Resting vitals: HR 76 bpm; BP 128/84 mm Hg; RR 16. Vitals postambulation (50 ft): HR 84 bpm; BP 132/84 mm Hg; RR 22. (+) blood supply and venous return in distal L LE. No evidence of cognitive or neurologic impairments; able to communicate effectively.

AROM	Left	Right
Knee ext	–18°	–10°
Knee flex	18°-68°	10°-100°
Ankle DF	–5°	0°-5°

MUSCLE PERFORMANCE (MMT): Knee ext: L 3+/5; R 4/5; Knee flex: L 3+/5, R 4/5.

ANTHROPOMETRIC CHARACTERISTICS: Height 5′ 8″; weight 220 lb; circumferential measurements: mid-patella L > R by 1.5″, mid-malleoli L > R by 0.75″.

PAIN: Pt. has experienced pain around entire L knee joint since surgery 8 days ago; gradually improving. Pain at rest is described as "aching" (3/10 on pain scale), c̄ occasional "sharp" pain c̄ WB (6/10), and at end ROM (8/10). Pain in R knee 2/10 described as "constant, dull pain."

INTEGUMENTARY: Observation reveals L knee is edematous c̄ significant rubor; surgical site is clean, dry, and intact c̄ Steri-Strips in place. No observable exudates present.

ASSESSMENT

Pt. is a 59 y.o. male, who is moderately obese, s/p L TKR who presents c̄ limitations in L knee ROM and strength and postsurgical edema. This has resulted in an inability to ambulate and climb stairs independently, c̄ reduced speed and limited distance, and limited independence in dressing and bathing. Edema, pain, and ↓ L knee strength have also resulted in reduced ability to bear weight on L side, which is evident by pt.'s impaired gait pattern and standing tolerance. Pain and ↓ R knee strength 2° to OA may additionally limit pt.'s functional recovery. Based on pt.'s preop Lower

CASE EXAMPLE 4-1

Physical Therapy Initial Evaluation—*cont'd*
Setting: Outpatient

Name: Smith, Herbert   **D.O.B.:** 6/4/50   **Date of Eval.:** 07/29/09

Extremity Functional Score (LEFS) and his relatively young age, pt. is expected to achieve >60 points on LEFS and at least 600 m on 6-min walk text within 6 mo postop.* Pt. requires outpatient PT to address the above impairments and activity limitations to facilitate functional independence and return to work and previous recreational activities.

GOALS

PARTICIPATION GOALS:
1. Pt. will return to work at the same capacity as 6 mo ago, within 4 mo.
2. Pt. will be able to participate in household chores and moderate-intensity home maintenance.

ACTIVITY GOALS:
1. Pt. will be able to don/doff shoes and socks independently 3/3 days within 1 wk.
2. Pt. will ambul 500 ft inside clinic corridors, gait speed at least 1.0 m/sec $\bar{s}$ an assistive device independently within 2 wk.
3. Pt. will stand $\bar{s}$ UE support for up to 30 min, pain <2/10 within 4 wk.
4. Pt. will ↑ 4 flights of stairs (48 stairs; 8″ height) using a railing and step-over-step pattern in <5 min, within 4 wk.
5. Pt. will ambul outside on varied terrain using str cane within 4 wk.

IMPAIRMENT GOALS:
1. Pain <3/10 in L knee during WB activities within 2 wk.
2. AROM L knee ext −5°, L knee flex 5-85° within 3 wk.
3. PROM L knee ext 0°, L knee flex to 0-95° within 4 wk.
4. Strength L knee flex/ext 4/5 within 3 wk.
5. Strength R knee flex/ext 5/5 within 3 wk.

PLAN OF CARE

Pt. will be seen 3×/wk for 45 min each session. Pt. will be reevaluated in 4 wk.

COORDINATION/COMMUNICATION: Order will be placed through medical supplier for shower chair for stall shower.

PATIENT-RELATED INSTRUCTION: Pt. instructed in pain/edema management activities $\bar{c}$ elevation and ice, ther ex emphasizing quadriceps and hamstring flexibility, strength and function in both open and closed kinetic chains (supine, seated, and standing). Patient also instructed in safety precautions on stairs and uneven surfaces. Patient verbalized understanding of all instructions. Will continue to progress pt. $\bar{c}$ HEP, and instruct pt. in importance of proper diet and long-term exercise.

DIRECT INTERVENTIONS:
- Cryotherapy to L knee followed by quadriceps/hamstring/calf stretching and A/PROM activities in supine, sitting, and standing to B knees.
- Gait trng indoors and outdoors on a variety of surfaces and inclines to improve safety, endurance, speed, and ↓ need for A device.
- Stair climbing trng to improve endurance and independence.
- Functional trng in variety of activities incorporating UEs in standing (including kitchen tasks, self-care activities, and golf swings) to improve standing tolerance, knee strength, and stability.

The findings of this evaluation were discussed $\bar{c}$ the patient, and he consented to the above intervention plan.

_____   _____

Jen L. Therapist   Date

_____

*Kennedy DM et al: Assessing recovery and establishing prognosis following total knee arthroplasty, *Phys Ther* 88:22, 2008.

CASE EXAMPLE 4-2

Physical Therapy Initial Evaluation
Setting: Inpatient Rehabilitation

Name: Rizzo, Rachel   **D.O.B.:** 2/7/63   **Date of Eval.:** 07/10/09

REASON FOR REFERRAL

Health Condition

CURRENT CONDITION: Pt. is a 46 y.o. female admitted to County Rehabilitation Center on 7/9/09 c̄ dx of exacerbation of relapsing/remitting MS (initial diagnosis 1996). Pt. admitted to County Hospital 7/4/09 for IV steroid treatment. Referral by primary MD requests gait trng 2° to recent exacerbation leading to difficulty walking.

PMH: R ACL repair 15 yr ago.

MEDICATIONS: Avonex (30 mcg IM; interferon beta 1a for MS), Baclofen (10-mg tablets i.d. for spasticity)

Social History/Participation

Before this hospitalization, pt. performed ADLs I'ly and ambulated with a str cane. Pt. lived c̄ 21 y.o. son in ground floor apartment c̄ no steps; responsible for light housekeeping & some cooking. Her son assisted c̄ some housekeeping & daily chores; he states he is available to assist c̄ other tasks as needed when she returns home. Pt. has not been employed for past yr 2° to disability. Pt. reports fatigue is 1° limiting factor. Volunteers 1 day/wk for 4 hr at local library sorting books and assisting c̄ computer searches.

KURTZKE EDSS: 6.5

ACTIVITIES*

ADLs: BED MOBILITY: Pt. positions self comfortably in bed & rolls B I'ly. Supine ↔ sitting on bed c̄ min A for B LE.
TRANSFERS: Pt. transfers from sit ↔ stand @ bed c̄ min A. Uses B arms to assist c̄ push off but needs min A to stand. W/C ↔ bed c̄ min A c̄ RW; able to transfer using SB c̄ CG. **SELF-CARE:** Bathing requires mod A from nurse's aide for tub transfers and to bathe completely; remains seated 2° to fatigue. Dressing c̄ mod A.

SITTING ABILITY: Sitting balance on edge of bed upright for 5 min s̄ UE support (time limitation due to fatigue). Can sit I'ly in W/C for >30 min.

STANDING ABILITY: Pt. can stand for up to 3 min. at bathroom sink and perform simple one-handed self-care activities using R UE for support with c̄Ⓢ. Can stand 3 min c̄ Ⓢ using RW.

MOBILITY: Pt. walks 50 ft c̄ rolling walker and min A on a smooth floor hospital corridor in 2.25 min (average 2 trials). HR increased to 130 bpm. Pt. can propel W/C for distances in hospital corridor up to 100 ft, limited by fatigue.

IMPAIRMENTS

SYSTEMS REVIEW: HR 72 bpm; BP 130/84 mm Hg, RR 20 at rest. Pt. reports STM loss, mild deficit noted during interview and evaluation. Pt. able to communicate effectively.

REFLEX INTEGRITY: Modified Ashworth Scale (muscle tone) 2/4 B hip adductors and ankle plantarflexors.

SENSORY INTEGRITY: Impaired sensation to light touch (5/8 correct responses) and pin prick (4/8 correct responses) below knees B.

MUSCLE PERFORMANCE

MMT	Left	Right
Hip flexion	2/5	3/5
Hip extension	2/5	3/5
Hip abduction	2+/5	3/5
Hip adduction	3/5	3/5
Knee extension	3–/5	3+/5
Knee flexion	3/5	3/5
Ankle dorsiflexion	2/5	3/5
Ankle plantar flexion	2/5	3/5

PROM
- Hip abd: L 0°-25°; R 0°-30°
- Ankle DF L 0°; R 0°-5°

---

*This patient would also be scored on the Functional Independence Measure (FIM), which would be reported separately and would be used for outcomes measurement.

CASE EXAMPLE 4-2

Physical Therapy Initial Evaluation—*cont'd*
Setting: Inpatient Rehabilitation

Name: Rizzo, Rachel **D.O.B.:** 2/7/63 **Date of Eval.:** 07/10/09

Gait, Locomotion, and Balance

GAIT: Has difficulty advancing L leg during swing c̄ ↓ hip & knee √ & foot drop noted; pt. requires min A to advance L LE 25% of the time. Trendelenburg gait to compensate for L abd. weakness during L stance.

BALANCE: Berg Balance Score: 7/56 *Sitting*: Can reach 5 in outside arm's length to front and both sides. Able to maintain balance to mod. external perturbations c̄ recovery in all directions (5/5 trials). *Standing*: Reach 3 in. outside arm's length to front and both sides. Pt. able to maintain bal. c̄ mod ant. & post. perturbations 3/5 trials; stepping strategy used 2/3 trials to post. perturbation. Able to stand 10 sec s̄ walker; reports fear of falling.

AEROBIC CAPACITY/ENDURANCE: Fatigue avg. 6.5/7 on Fatigue Severity Scale (scale 1-7, 7 = highest severity); fatigue has worsened since recent exacerbation.

INTEGUMENTARY INTEGRITY: Edema B ankles, L < R (28 cm circumference L malleoli, 26 cm R).

PAIN: Pt. reports no pain at time of eval.

ASSESSMENT

Pt. is a 46 y.o. female who presents c̄ symptoms of an acute exacerbation of MS. Pt. presents c̄ LE weakness (L>R), impaired balance, fatigue, and limited PROM B hip abd and ankle DF, which have led to limitations in performing bed mobility, self-care, and ambulation. Limited endurance and LE weakness have led to limitations in pt. using ambulation as her primary means of mobility. Pt. is at ↑ risk for falls 2° to ↓ symmetry and rhythmicity of gait. Pt. requires inpatient rehabilitation to address this recent decline in functional abilities and to assist patient in returning to prior functional level.

GOALS

PARTICIPATION GOAL:
1. Pt. will carry out self-care activities & mobility within the home c̄ supervision of an HHA aide in 1 mo.

ACTIVITY GOALS:
1. Pt. will rise from supine → sitting on edge of bed I'ly 5/5 trials within 20 sec (1 wk).
2. Pt. will maintain sitting on edge of bed for 10 min I'ly (1 wk).
3. Pt. will transfer sitting on bed → standing (c̄ walker) I'ly, 5/5 trials (1 wk).
4. Pt. will stand for 10 min at bathroom sink while performing self-care tasks (2 wk).
5. Pt. will walk 200 ft within 2 min, in hospital hallway c̄ supervision using a rollator, c̄ HR <110 bpm (2 wk).

PLAN OF CARE

Pt. will be seen b.i.d. 7 days/wk during inpt rehab stay. Full reeval. in 2 wk. PT should continue on daily basis s/p DC.

COORDINATION/COMMUNICATION: Trng in bathing and other self-care activities will be coordinated c̄ OT. Will request compression stockings from MD and training in proper use via Nursing. Consider referral to orthotic clinic within 1-2 wk for possible L AFO.

PATIENT-RELATED INSTRUCTION: Pt. and nursing aides will be instructed in optimal strategies for performing functional activities, esp. transfers. Pt. and family will be instructed in p.m. and weekend exercises to increase PROM hip abd. and ankle DF, and for guarding during transfers and ambul. Fatigue management and energy conservation discussed c̄ pt. and will continue to be incorporated t/o PT sessions.

DIRECT INTERVENTIONS: Stretching exercises to ↑ PROM hip abd & ankle DF. AROM & strengthening exercises in supine & standing for B LE musculature, focusing on hip √ & abd, knee √/, and ankle PF/DF. Trng in bed mobility, transfers, and sitting (to increase endurance). Standing bal training to address standing balance limitations and improve endurance. Gait training in different environments to improve speed, safety stability, and endurance, and ↓ need for assist. Progress pt. with AD to use of a 4-wheeled rollator, to consider for home use.

The findings of this evaluation were discussed c̄ the patient, and she consented to the above intervention plan.

_____   _____
Jen L. Therapist   Date

CASE EXAMPLE 4-3

Physical Therapy Initial Evaluation
Setting: Outpatient

Name: Jones, Susan   **D.O.B.:** 6/17/65   **Date of Eval.:** 7/18/08

REASON FOR REFERRAL
Health Condition

CURRENT CONDITION: Ms. Jones is a 43 y.o. female c̄ dx of cervical sprain/strain s/p MVA on 6/15/08. Pt. reports cervical pain radiating into L shoulder since the accident, with increasing intensity during the last week.

PMH: C-section 2004 otherwise uneventful.

MEDICATIONS: Flexoril (10-mg tablets t.i.d.).

Social History/Participation

Pt. lives with husband & 10 y.o. daughter in 2-story home. Pt. limited in performing household tasks such as cleaning and cooking due to L hand dominance and limited endurance with any task >20 min. Pt. is employed as an administrative assistant with marketing firm for 30 hr/wk with current schedule reduced to 15 hr/wk 2° to limited tolerance c̄ computer tasks, phone calls, and other administrative duties. Pt. with computer postioned to R and not equipped with headset.
Neck disability scale: 56%

ACTIVITIES

AMBULATION AND STAIR CLIMBING: Unaffected

SELF-CARE: Pt. reports ↑ time necessary to complete dressing, from 5 to 10 min 2° to pain. Pt. with limitations in reaching above shoulder height on L side.

DRIVING: Pt. reports difficulty driving and limits most car rides to <30 min 2° to pain.

IMPAIRMENTS

SYSTEMS REVIEW: HR 60 bpm; BP 120/72. Pt. reports being a visual learner.

AROM: Cervical flexion 50%, cervical extension 25%, L cervical sidebend 25%, R cervical sidebend 50%, B cervical rotation 50%

MUSCLE PERFORMANCE: Bilateral C1-4 myotomes: 5/5; R C5-T1 myotomes: 5/5; L C5-T1 myotomes: 4/5; B scapular musculature grossly 3+/5 with lower traps 3/5 B

CIRCULATION: Negative vertebral artery, Roos test B and Adson test B.

PAIN: Central posterior c-spine, C5-6 spinous processes tender upon palpation (4/10 on pain scale) with occasional radiation into L upper trap. Pain at rest rated as 3/10 on pain scale with ↑ to 6/10 c̄ attempted L sidebend and L rotation.

JOINT INTEGRITY AND MOBILITY: Hypomobility noted at C2-3 segment B and hypermobility noted with C5-6 and C6-7 segments B.

POSTURE: ↑ forward head and ↑ thoracic kyphosis noted with static and dynamic sitting and standing postures.

REFLEX INTEGRITY: Biceps, bracioradialis and triceps 2+ B.

SENSORY INTEGRITY: Dermatomes C1-T1 intact B to light touch.

CASE EXAMPLE 4-3

Physical Therapy Initial Evaluation—*cont'd*
Setting: Outpatient

Name: Jones, Susan   **D.O.B.:** 6/17/65   **Date of Eval.:** 7/18/08

ASSESSMENT

Pt. is a 43 y.o. female who presents with pain and limitations in cervical ROM, cervical and scapular musculature strength, static and dynamic postures, and hyper and hypo joint mobility resulting from MVA. This has resulted in reduced capacity to perform computer and phone activities related to work as well as self-care limitations and decreased ability in performing household tasks. Pt. requires outpatient PT to address these impairments and activity limitations to facilitate functional independence and return to work full capacity.

GOALS

PARTICIPATION GOALS:
1. Pt. will return to working 30 hr/wk schedule in 4 wk.

ACTIVITY GOALS:
1. Pt. will perform household tasks including cleaning and cooking s̄ pain in 4 wk.
2. Pt. will be I in self-posture correction s̄ cues in 4 wk.

IMPAIRMENT GOALS:
1. Pain will be 0/10 at rest and upon palpation of c-spine with ↑ to <3/10 with attempted L sidebend and rotation in 3 wk.
2. Full and pain-free AROM of c-spine in 4 wk.
3. Normal joint mobility at C2-3 B directions 4 wk.
4. Increase scapular musculature strength by 1 grade B in 6 wk.

PLAN OF CARE

Pt. will be seen 3×/wk for 45-min sessions. Pt. to be reevaluated in 4 wk.

COORDINATION/COMMUNICATION: Ergonomic assessment will be performed at pt.'s work site.

PATIENT-RELATED INSTRUCTION: Pt. instructed in postural exercises, pain management with cryotherapy and heat as needed, ther ex for cervical myotomes and scapular musculature and AROM exercises. Pt. also instructed in general ergonomic concepts and given pt. educ pamphlet with pictures of proper postures and techniques. Pt. verbalized understanding of all instructions. Will continue to progess pt. with exercises and HEP as tolerated.

DIRECT INTERVENTIONS: Postural instruction to increase overall endurance with static and dynamic postures. Prone and sitting exercises to target scapular and cervical musculature. AROM exercises to increase mobility and increase flexibility. Cryotherapy to c-spine.

The findings of this evaluation were discussed with the pt. and she consented to the above intervention plan.

_____   _____
Mark O. Therapist   Date

CASE EXAMPLE 4-4

Physical Therapy Initial Evaluation

Name: Robert LaGrange   **D.O.B.:** 5/16/37   **Date of Eval.:** 6/9/09   **Time:** 11:45 AM

REASON FOR REFERRAL

Health Condition

CURRENT CONDITION: Pt. was admitted to ICU following CABG ×4 6/4/09. Pt. had renal failure and contracted pneumonia following surgery and on day 4 was still intubated. PT eval and Rx ordered 6/8/09.

PMH: Angioplasty (March 2005) and IDDM (×12 yr).

MEDS: Cephalosporin infusion with 0.9% sodium chloride 20 mg/mL.

Social History/Participation

Pt. works part-time in retail home-building store; lives with wife in a retirement community; elevator in building and no stairs.

ACTIVITIES

Required assist ×2 to roll to side and come to sit on edge of bed. Required assist ×1 to maintain sitting position on edge of bed (BP: 136/94). Posture in sitting noted excessive kyphosis, moderate sidebending to L $\bar{c}$ R shoulder elevated. Pt. was able to sit for 2 min $\bar{c}$ mod A before reporting fatigue.

IMPAIRMENTS

SYSTEMS REVIEW: Pt. is alert but pale; appeared to be resting comfortably. Communication was established using eye blinks (yes/no responses).

STATS: Pt. on ventilator (CPAP). RR 18 bpm, TV 8 mL/kg, PEEP 7.0 cm H2O, PSV 10 cm.

VITALS: HR 98 (supine), BP 126/90 (supine).

AUSCULTATION: Crackles noted right middle and lower lobes. Heart sounds normal.

PALPATION: Pt. had normal chest motion but excessive use of accessory musculature was noted. No pain reported on palpation.

SKIN INTEGRITY: Sternal incision site and bilateral femoral graft site with staples and healing well; no signs of infection.

RANGE OF MOTION: Pt. demonstrated full AROM ×4 extremities against gravity. Limitation PROM noted in R ankle DF −5°, L ankle DF 0°.

GOALS

ACTIVITY GOALS (15 DAYS):
1. Pt. will sit on edge of bed for 5 min $\bar{s}$ assistance.
2. Pt. will transfer from supine → sitting $\bar{c}$ min A ×1.

IMPAIRMENT GOALS (10 DAYS):
1. Maintain clear airways daily.
2. Successful extubation.

CASE EXAMPLE 4-4

Physical Therapy Initial Evaluation—*cont'd*

Name: Robert LaGrange   **D.O.B.:** 5/16/37   **Date of Eval.:** 6/9/09   **Time:** 11:45 AM

PLAN OF CARE

COORDINATION/COMMUNICATION: Coordinate with nursing staff for positioning schedule, out-of-bed schedule, and suctioning.

PATIENT-RELATED INSTRUCTION: Pt. to be instructed in AROM exercises within 1 wk.

DIRECT INTERVENTIONS: Focus on maintaining clear airways and moving toward extubation. Respiratory Rx b.i.d. to include positioning, percussion, and vibration. Suctioning prn following Rx to assist with airway clearance. Inspiratory resistance training and use of pressure support ventilation to begin weaning from ventilator. AAROM strengthening to minimize atrophy and deconditioning, including quad sets, gluts sets, ankle pumps, and AAROM for hip flexion (heel slides) and shoulder flexion (to 90°). Mobility training to include positioning in side lying and semisupine, bed mobility training, and transfers to sitting.

The findings of this evaluation were discussed with the pt. and he consented to the above intervention plan.

_____   _____

Michael Schultz, Therapist   Date

EXERCISE 4-1

In the space provided, identify in which of the six sections of the initial evaluation model the following statements belong (R = Reason for Referral; Ac = Activities; I = Impairments; As = Assessment; G = Goals; PC = Plan of Care). The statements are taken from a variety of initial evaluation reports. See Tables 4-1 to 4-3 and Case Examples 4-1 to 4-4 for help completing this exercise.

1. Child will ride an adaptive tricycle independently for 25 ft in the gym in 8 wk.   _____

2. ROM R knee flexion 95°.   _____

3. BP 150/90, HR 96.   _____

4. Pt. has a 2-yr history of seizures occurring approximately 2×/mo.   _____

5. Pt. education will include instructions in home program for walking with self-monitoring of HR and perceived exertion.   _____

6. Pt. works as a secretary full-time but is currently restricted to part-time (½ days) due to wrist pain.   _____

7. Pt. is able to climb 10 stairs with left hand holding railing in 25 sec.   _____

8. Pt. presents with poor expiratory ability 2° to pneumonia, resulting in an ineffective cough and lowered endurance for daily care activities.   _____

9. Pt. is a 23 y.o. professional dancer who works 7 days/wk.   _____

10. Pt. will be able to stand at bathroom sink for 5 min to brush teeth and wash face and comb hair in 2 wk.   _____

11. Intervention will include therapeutic exercise: progressive resistive exercises to quadriceps and strengthening in standing position via squatting and lunging exercises.   _____

12. Strength R shoulder flexion 3+/5.   _____

13. The pt.'s ineffective right toe clearance and weak hip musculature are resulting in slow and unsafe ambulation indoors.   _____

14. Pt. can lift a 10-lb box (maximum weight) from floor to waist height.   _____

15. Therapist will coordinate training for dressing and bathing with pt.'s OT and nursing staff.   _____

Components of Physical Therapy Documentation

CHAPTER 5

Documenting Reason for Referral: Background Information and Health Condition

LEARNING OBJECTIVES

After reading this chapter and completing the exercises, the reader will be able to:

1. Identify and classify various aspects of documenting a patient's background information and health condition.

2. Explain the three key elements of describing a patient's current health condition.

3. Discuss the implications of direct access for documenting medical diagnoses.

Within the scope of their practice, PTs encounter patients with a variety of health conditions. *Health condition,* as defined by the ICF framework, is an umbrella term for disease (acute or chronic), disorder, injury, or trauma (Figure 5-1). It may also include other circumstances, such as pregnancy, aging, stress, fitness level, congenital anomaly, or genetic predisposition. Health conditions can result from infections, acute injuries, metabolic imbalances, or degenerative disease processes.

Any physical therapy initial evaluation note must provide specific information about the medical diagnosis or known or suspected pathologic conditions. Because it may be pertinent to the patient's referral to physical therapy, the health condition must be presented in a clear and concise fashion in the PT's documentation.

In the *Guide to Physical Therapist Practice* (American Physical Therapy Association [APTA], 2001; the *Guide*), information pertaining to a patient's health condition is categorized under "History" in the Examination Section. The *Guide* defines history as follows:

The history is a systematic gathering of data—from both the past and the present—related to why the patient/client is seeking the services of the physical therapist.... While taking the history, the physical therapist also identifies health restoration and prevention needs and coexisting health problems that may have implications for intervention (p. S34).

Thus the relevance of history taking, as it relates to the health condition, is that it provides the foundation for why the patient or client is referred for physical therapy, thus setting up the reason for referral. What are the specific medical diagnoses, health problems, or health risk factors that bring the patient to seek the services of a physical therapist?

This chapter discusses documentation of Reason for Referral as it relates to the health condition. Readers will have an opportunity to practice writing statements related to health condition and appropriately identify information that belongs in this section of a report.

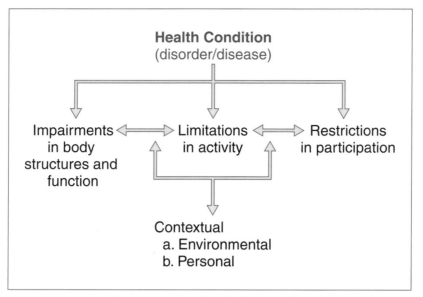

FIGURE 5-1   This chapter discusses documentation pertaining to Health Condition (disorder/disease) based on the ICF framework.

Documenting Elements of Health Conditions

In general, health condition information is included early in an evaluation because these data are critical to determining how the PT should proceed with the examination. Therapists perform a process known as differential diagnosis, in which they gather information to confirm or modify any previously determined diagnoses (from other health care professionals) or develop their own diagnosis (see Chapter 9 for more information on diagnosis by PTs). In addition, therapists will ask pathology-related questions, which help identify possible problems that require consultation with or referral to another provider. Certain conditions raise concerns about whether an underlying condition exists in which physical therapy may be contraindicated or in which referral to another health professional would be warranted.

Detailed information about the health condition is therefore an important part of determining the appropriateness of physical therapy as an intervention. Certain health conditions are appropriate for physical therapy; others are not. However, diagnosis alone does not determine the appropriateness of intervention; instead, the associated or secondary limitations or impairments related to a diagnosis warrant physical therapy intervention.

In some ways, the health condition information documented by the PT in this section is somewhat limited. At this point, the therapist simply classifies any facts he or she has available before the examination is performed. As the examination proceeds, the PT may uncover information that may help to refine any previously given diagnosis. Any new information obtained during the course of the physical therapy examination

that confirms, clarifies, elaborates on, or possibly contradicts the established diagnosis and health condition should be documented in the appropriate section (e.g., Impairments, see Chapter 8) and summarized in the Assessment section (see Chapter 9). Thus information about health conditions and diagnosis does not begin and end in this section.

Information about a patient's health condition can be organized in the initial evaluation note in many ways. Different institutions frequently mandate a certain organizational structure, and this is often preprinted on customized initial evaluation forms. The degree to which each of these headings is used differs depending on the institution and patient population. For the general initial evaluation, the following categorization of information is recommended to document health condition and the reason for referral:

- Patient information and demographics
- Current condition
- Past medical history
- Medications
- Other (family or developmental history, as pertinent)

Table 5-1 provides a detailed listing of the types of information that can be included in each of these categories. Case Examples 5-1 through 5-3 at the end of this chapter provide sample documentation in different clinical settings.

PATIENT INFORMATION AND DEMOGRAPHICS

General patient information and demographics are the first items included in any medical documentation and typically include the patient's name, date of

TABLE 5-1	COMPONENTS OF DOCUMENTING REASON FOR REFERRAL
Component	**Information Included**
Patient information and demographics	Patient's name Date of birth Sex Demographic information, such as race or ethnicity (if relevant)

Current condition	Reason patient is referred, if not evident
	Concerns that led the patient to seek services of a physical therapist
	Current and prior therapeutic interventions (if any)
	Mechanisms of injury or disease, including (see Table 5-2):
	    Underlying disease process
	    Location
	    Time course
	Previous occurrence of current condition

Past medical history	Any prior surgeries, other diagnoses, or pre-existing conditions The date or the time course of the medical condition
Medications	Name of the medication Dosage (if known) What the medication is prescribed for

Other	Growth and development
	    Developmental history
	    Hand dominance
	Family history
	    Familial health risks

This table incorporates terminology found in the APTA *Guide to Physical Therapist Practice*, 2001, p S36.

birth, date evaluation was done, and any pertinent demographic information. If the patient's race or ethnic background is relevant to the patient's diagnosis, it can be included here.

CURRENT CONDITION

This section includes information pertaining to why the patient or client was referred for physical therapy and by whom if it is not evident. This sets the framework for the reason this evaluation is being performed. Next, information about the current health condition (e.g., diagnosis) for which the patient is being referred for physical therapy is included. In fact, this section of a note is sometimes simply titled "medical diagnosis." In most cases, the PT should go beyond simply restating any previously determined diagnosis and describe a specific precipitating incident, if any, or mechanism of injury. The therapist should also report what other treatments have been performed (e.g., consultation with other medical professionals). If a diagnosis is not provided by a referring health care professional, the therapist should document any information provided by the patient identifying the primary problem or chief complaint—what is the reason the patient is seeking the PT's services?

Information about the patient's health condition sets the foundation for the physical therapy examination. The PT must gather all relevant information to develop an accurate picture of the patient's medical condition that warrants referral to physical therapy. Whenever possible, three key elements of the patient's current health condition should be specified: the underlying disease process, its location, and the time course (Table 5-2).

If a physician or other health care professional referred the patient to physical therapy, this information should be documented in this section. If applicable, the name of the referring professional should also be listed here in addition to any specific information, orders, or contraindications that he or she communicated.

PAST MEDICAL HISTORY

Information documented in this category should include any medical history that may be relevant (even indirectly) to the current condition. Past medical history (PMH) can include the following:

- Any prior surgeries, other diagnoses, or pre-existing conditions
- The date or the time course of the medical condition or surgery (e.g., ACL repair 12/2/09, IDDM ×10 yr, h/o coronary artery disease ×8 yr)

When the PT writes as part of a medical chart in a hospital setting or uses computerized documentation, PMH may be found in another part of the chart to which all medical professionals can refer. In this case, the therapist should document that the PMH was noted and confirmed by the patient, and a reference to where this information can be found should be documented.

MEDICATIONS

Therapists should document medications the patient is taking for the current condition, as well as any medications taken for other medical conditions. It is important to document (1) the name of the medication, (2) the dosage (if known), and (3) the reason the medication is being prescribed (e.g., Zoloft 50 mg q.i.d. for depression). Vitamins and over-the-counter medications may also be included, especially if they have known side effects that would be important to consider.

OTHER INFORMATION

Several other types of information can be included in this section of a report. These include developmental history and family history. A developmental history can be used in certain pediatric settings and involves information related to a child's growth and overall development (e.g., the age at which a child first sat up or walked alone). This information would not be pertinent, however, for most adolescent or adult evaluations. A family history may be helpful for understanding the patient's medical diagnosis (e.g., a strong family history of heart disease or a history of certain musculoskeletal abnormalities).

Obtaining Health Condition Information

Information about the patient's health condition can be obtained in different ways. First, the information can be obtained directly from the physician, either by referring to the medical record or by personal communication. Second, it can be provided directly by the patient, but this method can be less reliable than obtaining it directly from medical personnel or a medical record. Third, information can be obtained through a third party such as a family member. This method is useful when the patient is unable to provide an accurate account of his or her own medical condition.

Because of the differences in how health condition information and medical history can be obtained, documentation of the source(s) of information is important and should be made in this section. For example, if information about a patient's medical history is obtained directly from the patient, the PT could write "Pt. reports having had a L ACL reconstruction in 1996." Otherwise, those who read the record typically assume that the information is obtained from medical personnel or a medical record. Ideally an evaluation report should include information obtained from both the patient (or caregiver/family member) and medical record or personnel to provide the most comprehensive and complete accounting of the patient's current medical status.

Diagnoses and Direct Access

Therapists who practice in direct-access states face additional issues regarding diagnoses. In many situations under direct access, no medical diagnosis is available. Therapists must then determine the diagnosis and health condition through their own evaluation. In some cases, this is not possible within the scope of tests and measures available to PTs and referral to a physician or other health care personnel is warranted. Reports from diagnostic tests such as magnetic resonance imaging scans (MRIs) and x-ray films may be necessary to clarify the patient's health condition.

All PTs, but particularly those who practice in direct-access states, must clearly document all known aspects of a patient's health status and must be able to make a reasonable differential diagnosis. An important question that each therapist must ask is "Is the health condition one that is within the scope of practice for a physical therapist, and is it amenable to physical therapy intervention?" Therefore clear, concise, and accurate documentation of the health condition (including disease process, location, and time course) is of utmost importance. In direct-access cases in which the patient has not been referred by a physician, aspects of the medical condition obtained from a patient/family interview and chart review should be documented in this first section of the note. However, the PT's final diagnosis should not be documented until the Assessment section because it may depend on physical findings not yet presented.

Prevention and Health Promotion

Many therapists are currently involved with prevention: primary, secondary, and tertiary. This raises specific issues regarding documentation. For *primary prevention*, there is no presenting diagnosis or illness. For example, if a therapist performs an evaluation or intervention for a client who is at risk for developing osteoporosis, documentation of pathologic information should include why the client is at risk for developing this problem and a discussion of the potential consequences.

TABLE 5-2	ELEMENTS OF HEALTH CONDITION
Element	**Description**
Underlying disease process	Type of pathology, such as infection, tumor, or trauma Results of any diagnostic tests (e.g., laboratory tests, MRI scans, or x-ray films) Any information provided directly from the referring physician that identifies the specific pathology
Location	Specific origin of pathology Includes specific area of the brain, spinal cord, muscles, nerves, joints, or tissues that are affected
Time course	How long the problem has existed Include date of injury or surgery, or date a diagnosis was made

Secondary and tertiary prevention are related to current disease processes. *Secondary prevention* consists of decreasing the duration of illness, severity of disease, and sequelae through early diagnosis. This would apply, for example, to individuals with certain types of cardiac disease. *Tertiary prevention* consists of limiting the degree of disability and promoting rehabilitation and restoration of function in patients with chronic and irreversible diseases, such as multiple sclerosis. Documentation in such cases needs to focus not only on the specific referring health condition (e.g., multiple sclerosis), but also the subsequent health conditions and/or impairments that can be prevented (e.g., muscle contractures). This can be a tricky situation because documentation of prevention is not always well accepted by third-party payers. However, the more that therapists can document the need for and purpose of preventative intervention, the more likely it will become standard practice.

Summary

- Health condition, including current condition and past medical history, provides the foundation for the reason for referral.

- Medical information and any previously determined diagnosis are included early in an evaluation report because of their importance in shaping the therapist's examination.

- Information in this section can typically be organized into the following categories: patient information and demographics, current condition, past medical history, medications, and other (e.g., family or developmental history).

- Documentation of specific health condition information is important (Current Condition); this includes providing information about the underlying disease process, the location of the pathologic condition, and its time course.

CASE EXAMPLE 5-1

Setting: Outpatient

Name: Ally McCarthy   **D.O.B.:** 9/25/44   **Date:** 12/11/09   **Sex:** F

CURRENT CONDITION: Pt. was referred by Dr. Hull for eval and Rx related to low back dysfunction. Pt. reports sudden onset of LBP after lifting heavy boxes 12/1/09. Pt. sought medical advice from Dr. Hull 3 days later on 12/4/09. Dr. Hull prescribed x-rays, which revealed L2-5 DDD as per phone conversation with Dr. Hull. Pt. was then prescribed Flexoril and referred to PT. Pt. reports h/o generalized LBP over past 10-15 yr; Rx $\bar{c}$ various anti-inflammatories and several episodes of PT intervention $\bar{c}$ symptoms resolving $\bar{p}$ 1 mo. on average.

PMH: NIDDM ×5 yr; R ACL reconstruction Nov. 2000; no complications and no limitations on activities related to this surgery.

MEDS: Flexoril (muscle relaxant for LBP; 10 mg table, 3 t.i.d.).

CASE EXAMPLE 5-2

Setting: Outpatient

Name: Lucy Quick   **D.O.B.:** 9/24/67   **Date:** 9/29/09   **Sex:** F

CURRENT CONDITION: Pt. is self-referred. RA diagnosed 7/03, primarily affecting hands, wrists, and knees B. Pt. reports recent flare-up approx. 4 wks. ago which required course of prednisone (20 mg ×1 wk and then tapered to 5 mg) and has resulted in pain, stiffness, and residual ↓ in wrist ROM B.

PMH: Pt. reports L knee arthroscopic surgery ×10 yr, 2° to meniscal tear.

MEDS: Embrel IM anti-TNF for Rx of RA; 50 mg 1×/wk

FAMILY HISTORY: Pt. has family history of autoimmune diseases, including thyroid disease and pernicious anemia.

CASE EXAMPLE 5-3

Setting: Acute Rehabilitation

Name: Tara Smith   **D.O.B.:** 6/19/78   **Date:** 10/4/08   **Sex:** F

CURRENT CONDITION: Pt. is a 30 y.o. female who was admitted to North Haven Rehabilitation Center on 10/3/08 for multidisciplinary rehab. Pt. sustained an incomplete ASIA D C6 SCI s/p MVA 9/24/08. She was sent to North Haven Hospital for 9 days. X-rays and MRI revealed nondisplaced fx of C6 vertebral body requiring no surgical intervention. Referral received for Philadelphia cervical collar when OOB with no active or passive ROM to c-spine and no heavy lifting (>5 lb).

PMH: Pt. denies any significant PMH; confirmed by chart review.

MEDS: Colace (stool softener; 100 mg); Tylenol prn.

EXERCISE 5-1

The following statements are from various sections of an initial evaluation report at a pediatric rehabilitation center. Extract the information that would be appropriate to include in the History section of the report. Indicate to which section each statement belongs according to the following codes: PI = patient information, CC = current condition, PMH = past medical history, MED = medications, OTHER = other (e.g., family history, developmental history) or N/A = not appropriate to include in this section.

1. Chelsea had a fall 4 years ago resulting in R humerus fracture, requiring casting; healed with residual problems. _____

2. Chelsea has 3/5 strength (MMT) in B quadriceps. _____

3. Chelsea has a diagnosis of myotonic dystrophy, a form of muscular dystrophy resulting in muscle weakness and accompanied by myotonia (delayed relaxation of muscles after contraction). _____

4. She is not currently taking any medications. _____

5. Chelsea enjoys math and art classes at school. _____

6. There is a history of myotonic dystrophy in Chelsea's family, so Mrs. Green (mother) and Chelsea were very familiar with related symptoms and problems. _____

7. Chelsea first began showing symptoms of myotonic dystrophy when she was in third grade. _____

8. Chelsea was referred by the Smithtown School District for this independent PT evaluation to assist in educational planning. _____

9. Chelsea has not had any surgeries or hospitalizations. _____

10. Chelsea is able to ascend and descend a full flight of stairs. _____

11. Chelsea is a 12 y.o. girl who attends Jonesbridge Middle School. _____

12. Chelsea's primary concern is that she gets fatigued when walking between classes. _____

EXERCISE 5-2

Each of the following statements could be found in the Current Condition section of an initial evaluation. First, identify what is wrong with each statement, using the following key to indicate which components are not specified in enough detail: DP = disease process, L = location, or TC = time course. Any one or all three components may be problematic. Rewrite a more appropriate and plausible statement in the space provided.

NOTE: A certain amount of clinical knowledge is necessary to provide a clinically plausible statement. It may be necessary to consult textbooks or other resources based on your current knowledge base in a particular area; however, the purpose of these exercises is not to test your clinical knowledge but to obtain practice in appropriate documentation.

Statement	What Is Wrong?	Rewrite Statement
EXAMPLE: Patient has a strained muscle.	L, TC; also more detail regarding nature of strain could be provided, if known.	Pt. has grade II strain of R quadriceps, sustained 10/1/00.
1. Pt. had heart surgery yesterday.		
2. Pt. reports pain starting 5/10/09.		
3. Pt. had a right-sided stroke.		
4. Pt. is an amputee.		
5. Pt. has typical problems related to aging.		
6. Pt. complains of fatigue.		
7. Pt. has a broken leg.		
8. Pt. diagnosed with cancer 11/07.		

■ EXERCISE 5-3

Each of the following statements could be found in either the Past Medical History or Medication sections of an initial evaluation. None the statements provides enough detail. Rewrite a more appropriate and plausible statement in the space provided.

Past Medical History

1. Pt. has h/o cardiac problems.

_____

2. Pt. has h/o several surgeries.

_____

3. Pt. is a diabetic.

_____

Medications

4. Pt. is taking multiple medications for various medical conditions.

_____

5. Pt. is taking antispasticity meds.

_____

CHAPTER 6

Documenting Reason for Referral: Participation and Social History

LEARNING OBJECTIVES

After reading this chapter and completing the exercises, the reader will be able to:

1. Describe the components of documenting participation, social history, and general health status.

2. Describe the usefulness of standardized outcome measures for documenting participation.

3. Describe the process of conducting an interview to obtain information pertaining to level of participation, social history, and general health status.

4. Document these components with accuracy and specificity.

Chapter 5 discussed documentation of reason for referral as it pertains to medical information and health condition. A second important part of documenting reason for referral relates to social history and participation (Figure 6-1). This addresses both environmental and contextual factors and describes the ability of a patient or client to perform the specific functions pertinent to his or her everyday life. How is the current condition affecting the individual's life? What are the patient's current life roles, and is the patient able to perform his or her roles as a husband/wife or father/mother? What is the person's home and/or work environment, and how does it affect his or her ability to function independently? Can he or she work in either a paid or volunteer position? Is he or she able to engage in social and recreational activities?

How is this information best obtained? The first step is to obtain as much information as possible from the patient's medical record. This minimizes repetitive interviewing of the patient and helps prepare the therapist to better organize the examination.

The second step is to spend time talking with, and listening to, patients. Although time is often limited in rehabilitation settings, physical therapists (PTs) can prevent many missed diagnoses and develop an appropriate plan of care from the onset if they spend an adequate amount of time gathering pertinent information about their patients. Simply asking some basic questions can provide the therapist with valuable information about the problems affecting a patient's life. Indeed, asking these questions early often saves time because it enables the therapist to be more selective in his or her examination.

Assessment of participation clearly sets the rehabilitation professional apart from many other medical professionals. Medical doctors, for example, spend much of their time determining an accurate health condition and relating the patient's impairments to that condition. Conversely, PTs should (and often do) spend a significant amount of their time at the other end of the disability spectrum—focusing on the interrelationship between participation and activities and between activities and impairments. Obtaining this information that encompasses a patient's specific life roles provides the foundation for shaping the rehabilitation process. As noted in Chapter 1, it is the starting point for the process of rehabilitation.

Components of Documenting Participation and Social History

The *Guide to Physical Therapist Practice* (APTA, 2001) outlines various aspects of patient history taking that are part of the examination process. Table 6-1 details aspects of the patient history that can be categorized in this section of a note. Depending on the patient's problems and length of the evaluation, each component can be documented independently (Case Examples 6-1 and 6-2) or generally combined (Case Example 6-3). The degree to which the headings Participation and Social History are used may differ depending on the institution and patient population. In addition, other information can be included here. General Health Status is often included in this section and includes information pertaining to the patient's overall health and wellness. This information could include physical and psychological functioning, level of fitness, and behavioral health risks (e.g., history of smoking) or growth and development (in pediatric cases, e.g., date

at which child began sitting or walking). Case Examples 6-1 through 6-3 provide sample documentation of participation and social history in different clinical settings (also see Case Examples 4-1 to 4-4).

The *focus* of documentation of participation and social history varies for different patients and in different settings. Certainly, the primary concern for patients who are very sick in the hospital is working toward attainment of an independent functional status, such as their ability to dress themselves and shower. In fact, in a *hospital* setting, documentation of a patient's work status, home situation and environment, and general health status often refers to what the patient was doing before being admitted to the hospital (What was his or her job? What sports and recreational activities did he or she enjoy participating in?). When the patient is receiving *outpatient* or *home-based services,* the focus of documentation should reflect current issues (Is the patient currently working and, if so, at what functional level? Can he or she return to recreational sports?).

PARTICIPATION

Measurement of participation encompasses a person's involvement in community, leisure, and social activities, which are essential to an individual's quality of life. Providing accurate and reasonable documentation

TABLE 6-1	COMPONENTS OF DOCUMENTING REASON FOR REFERRAL: PARTICIPATION AND SOCIAL HISTORY
Component	**Information From Guide Included in Each Component**
Social history	Living environment and community characteristics Family and living situation Family and caregiver resources, devices, and equipment (e.g., assistive, adaptive, orthotic, protective, supportive, prosthetic) Projected discharge destination Cultural preferences

Participation	Work status
	Community, leisure, and social activity
	Physical function (mobility, sleep patterns, restricted bed days)
	Psychological function (depression, anxiety)
	General health perception/quality of life
	Level of physical fitness
	Prior functional status
	General health status
	    Physical and psychological functioning
	    Level of fitness
	    Behavioral health risks

Additional components (if pertinent):	
Growth and development	Developmental history as pertinent

This table incorporates terminology found in American Physical Therapy Association: *The guide to physical therapist practice,* ed 2, Alexandria, VA, 2001, American Physical Therapy Association, p S36.

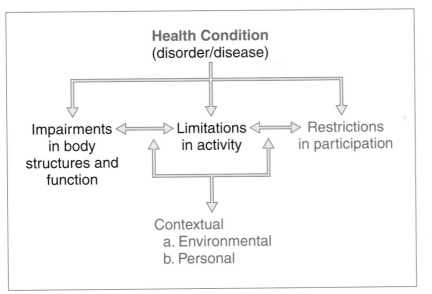

Health Condition
(disorder/disease)

Impairments
in body
structures and
function

Limitations
in activity

Restrictions
in participation

Contextual
a. Environmental
b. Personal

FIGURE 6-1   This chapter discusses documentation pertaining to Restrictions in Participation, as well as Contextual Factors (environmental and personal), based on the International Classification of Functioning, Disability and Health framework.

about a person's ability to participate in these activities is critical, particularly to justify services for many patients who may appear "high functioning."

If a patient or client is working or has recently stopped working because of an injury or illness, the nature of the work should be documented in sufficient detail. Such notations typically include a listing or description of the tasks or activities the patient performs in a typical day (e.g., typing, writing, lifting) and any unique requirements to the patient's job (e.g., "lifting >50 lb," "standing for >1 hr at a time"). The therapist should also document here any volunteer work in which the patient is or was participating (e.g., "volunteers at hospital transporting patients 1 ×/wk") and any of the patient's social activities, if this information is pertinent to rehabilitation.

It is important to contrast *current* level of functioning and participation with *prior* level of functioning and participation. *Prior functional status* refers to the degree of functional skill of a patient in self-care, leisure, and social activities before the onset of the current medical diagnosis or health condition. Determination of prior functional status is particularly relevant for older patients or those with previous medical conditions. Such patients may not have been independent in all activities before the onset of their current condition; they may have had some limitations as a result of other medical conditions or problems related to their current medical condition. For example, a patient who has had a stroke may have had a preexisting condition of emphysema. This may have limited the patient's walking distance as a result of pulmonary limitations even before the stroke.

The goal of therapy is often to restore the patient to at least the level of prior functioning. Sometimes the goal is to restore the patient to a higher level of functioning, as in the case of a patient with arthritis who elects to have a total knee replacement. Because that patient's functional abilities may have been significantly limited by the arthritis, the knee replacement may enable the patient to improve to a significantly higher functional level.

SOCIAL HISTORY

The PT documents a wide range of information pertaining to the patient's home and living situation under this heading, often including details about the type of home, the number of floors, and the number and type of stairs. If a patient uses certain medical equipment, such as a wheelchair or a raised toilet seat, this is reported here. The PT should describe the equipment and how it is used in sufficient detail. (Example: "Pt. uses a lightweight wheelchair, with gel cushion and swing-away leg rests, for mobility within the home.")

Descriptions of the patient's family and caregiver resources are also components of the home environment. Cultural beliefs and behaviors, as they are relevant to the rehabilitation process, should also be included here. However, specific details about a patient's personal life that are not pertinent to his or her current medical condition or reason for referral should not be included in patient documentation. For example, it would rarely be necessary to refer to a patient as "divorced" or to identify a person's specific religious affiliation unless it affected his or her evaluation and treatment in some way.

Specificity of Documentation

Information in this section of the report should be sufficiently detailed that it is useful to the therapist or other personnel reading the report. The information presented in this section helps to shape both the patient's prognosis and the intervention plan. Furthermore, it provides the foundation for developing appropriate and realistic goals that will be based on the patient's current level of participation and his or her lifestyle.

An example could be a patient who has had a recent heart attack (myocardial infarction [MI]) and is undergoing cardiac rehabilitation. Consider the specificity of these examples:

- POOR EXAMPLE: *Pt. worked full time prior to MI.*
- BETTER EXAMPLE: *Pt. worked 50+ hr/wk as a bank VP; pt. reports job was "stressful" and required frequent traveling (3-4×/mo).*
- POOR EXAMPLE: *pt. led an active lifestyle prior to MI.*
- BETTER EXAMPLE: *Before heart attack, pt. ran 4 miles 4×/wk and enjoyed sailing his sailboat 1-2×/wk in summer.*

If a goal of this patient is to return to his active lifestyle and level of occupation, documentation of the details of these activities is important. Case Examples 6-1 through 6-3 at the end of this chapter further illustrate this point.

Interviewing Strategies

The therapist can begin the inquiry by asking the patient some simple questions. Table 6-2 lists various questions that could be asked to ascertain this information. The type of questions asked during an interview should vary depending on the age and medical diagnosis of the patient. Specifically, the therapist needs to determine the patient's premorbid lifestyle and the patient's current goals for regaining that lifestyle. The interview can be conducted with either the patient, a caregiver, or both. For young children, interviews are often conducted with the parent or guardian.

TABLE 6-2	SAMPLE INTERVIEW QUESTIONS TO ASCERTAIN PARTICIPATION-BASED INFORMATION	
	Young Child	**Older Man**
Patient	5 y.o. boy with cerebral palsy, lives at home with parents (interview directed at parent)	64 y.o. semiretired carpenter, with rotator cuff tear, divorced, lives alone, has 2 grandchildren
Social history	• Describe your child's home and living situation. • Do you have any stairs? How many? • Does your child have any siblings? • Who else provides care for your child? • Do you have any cultural or religious beliefs that may affect this evaluation or any future treatment?	• Describe your home and living situation. • Do you have any stairs? How many? • Do your children live close by? • Are they able to assist you in any way with household tasks?
Participation	• Is your child able to participate fully in all school activities, including sitting at his desk during lesson plans and participating in gym class? • What types of play or recreational activities does your child engage in? • Does he have any difficulties or limitations in activities he would like to engage in but is unable? • Does your child participate in age-appropriate chores in the house, such as helping to clean his room? • What types of social interactions does your child engage in? Does your child have any difficulty engaging in play with his peers? • How would you describe your child's overall health?	• To what extent have you recently been involved in your work as a carpenter? • To what degree are you limited in your ability to work? • Are you able to maintain the basic upkeep of your apartment, for example, doing the cleaning or the laundry? • Has your social activity (e.g., time spent with family and friends) changed at all because of your current condition? • What recreational activities (e.g., sports, leisure activities) did you engage in before this recent injury? Are you having any difficulty or limitations performing those activities now? • How would you describe your overall health? • Do you smoke?
Growth and development	• At what age did your child first sit up; walk; talk? • How would you describe his development?	Not applicable.

Outcome Measures

Although conducting a basic interview often is the quickest way to obtain participation information, the use of standardized assessment tools can provide a more reliable and systematic measure. Because the International Classification of Functional Disability and Health (ICF) has been used more frequently by health care professionals, new research efforts have been undertaken to identify outcome measures that distinctly measure the levels of participation, activities, and body structures and function. In particular, several new tools have been designed to specifically measure aspects of participation. Table 6-3 provides a list of some commonly used standardized outcome measures that are primarily designed to assess participation. Some of these measures were designed before the implementation of the ICIDH-2 and thus use the term *disability* rather than *participation.*

It is important to note that most of these measures, indeed probably all, do not measure only participation, but also some aspects of activity and body structures and function (Perenboom & Chorus, 2003). Those instruments that most closely measure only participation are the Perceived Handicap Questionnaire and the London Handicap Scale (Perenboom & Chorus, 2003). In fact, participation and activities may not be able to be truly differentiated into distinct domains (Jette, Tao & Haley, 2007). Until these constructs can be more clearly defined through research, the authors recommend the two should be documented independently to the extent possible.

Several measures listed in Table 6-3 attempt to measure a construct known as *quality of life.* Quality of life is the degree of well-being felt by an individual or group of people. Although quality of life itself cannot be directly measured, a patient's perception of his or her quality of life can. Quality of life and participation are distinct entities, but they are clearly related and for purposes of documentation, information pertaining to quality of life—and outcome measures related to quality of life—should be included in this section. (For additional information about choosing appropriate outcome measures, see Chapter 2.)

HOW IS LIFE PARTICIPATION MEASURED?

The tools listed in Table 6-3 measure life participation obtained by patient self-report. Self-report is a very important piece of an examination, particularly in assessment of outcomes. Patients sometimes have little or no improvement in impairments or even in particular functional abilities, but they may have significantly improved their quality of life or ability to engage in life roles. For example, a patient may have developed strategies of coping with pain or effective compensatory strategies to accomplish tasks. Alternatively, he or she may show improvement in impairments, such as weakness or limited range of motion, with no corresponding reduction of participation.

Self-report measures are often thought to be less valuable because they are not "objective." Self-report measures are inherently subjective, which increases the chance that the patient will provide inaccurate or exaggerated information. Nevertheless, a patient's perception of his or her limitations or problems is just as important as other components of the assessment process, albeit not the only measure. For example, the Oswestry Disability Questionnaire (Roland & Jenner, 1989) was designed for use in patients with back pain and evaluates a person's perceived limitations in various life activities. Such limitations often are difficult to ascertain by physical examination, in part because they measure activities that are not readily evaluated in a clinic setting (e.g., sleeping and traveling).

DOCUMENTING THE RESULTS OF OUTCOME MEASURES

For documentation purposes, only the scores from standardized tests should be reported in the body of an evaluation report. The therapist may choose to summarize components from the tests that are pertinent or provide a brief interpretation of the test results (see Case Example 6-3). This applies to all forms of standardized testing, including tests used for activity limitations and impairments (see Chapters 7 and 8, respectively). The completed standardized test form should be included in the patient's record, although third-party payers may not see it. Often third-party payers see only an evaluation report or summary.

Preventing Participation Restrictions

In some therapist-patient encounters there is no clear restriction in participation. The most obvious example is primary prevention, in which the patient is a healthy individual with only the risk of developing a disabling illness. In addition, therapists often see patients in the acute stages of an illness or immediately after an injury when a participation restriction is not yet fully understood. Indeed, in such instances the therapist actively intervenes to prevent these restrictions from occurring (secondary prevention) or limit their severity (tertiary prevention). For example, a patient who sees a PT for acute low back pain

TABLE 6-3	SOME COMMONLY USED STANDARDIZED MEASURES OF PARTICIPATION*
Outcome Measure	**Description**
Craig Handicap Assessment and Reporting Technique (CHART) (Whiteneck et al., 1992)	Consists of 32 items across the six WHO domains of handicap, including physical independence, cognitive independence, mobility, occupation, social integration, and economic self-sufficiency.
London Handicap Scale (LHS) (Harwood et al., 1994)[†]	Measures handicap in six subscales: mobility, physical independence, occupation, social integration, orientation, and economic self-sufficiency. Also provides an overall handicap severity score.
Nottingham Health Profile (NHP) (Hunt et al., 1980)	Provides a brief indication of a patient's perceived emotional, social, and physical health problems. Part I consists of 38 questions in six subareas: energy level, pain, emotional reaction, sleep, social isolation, and physical abilities. Part II evaluates seven life areas: work, looking after home, social, home life, sex life, interests, and vacations.
Oswestry Disability Questionnaire (Fairbank et al., 1980)	Used extensively for evaluation of disability in people with low back pain. Assesses disability/participation in 10 functional areas with 6-item responses each.
Participation Measure for Post-Acute Care (PM-PAC) (Gandek et al., 2007)	Relatively new measure that evaluates participation with 51 items covering nine domains: mobility; role functioning; community, social, and civic life; domestic life/self-care; economic life; interpersonal relationships; communication; work; and education.
Quebec Back Pain Disability Scale (QBPDS) (Kopec et al., 1995)	20-item self-administered test designed to assess the level of functional disability in individuals with back pain. Patients rate level of difficulty in performing various functional tasks.
Rehabilitation Activities Profile (Jelles et al., 1995)	Consists of 21 items divided into a total of 71 subitems. Covers the domains of communication, mobility, personal care, occupation, and relationships. Severity of problem as perceived by the patient is rated on a 4-point Likert scale.
Re-Integration to Normal Living Index (RNL Index) (Wood-Dauphinee et al., 1988)	Consists of 11 questions covering eight dimensions. It considers both patients' perceptions and objective indicators of physical, social, and psychological dimensions.
Roland Morris Questionnaire (RDQ) (Roland & Morris, 1983)	A self-report, self-completed questionnaire designed to assess the degree of functional limitation in patients with low-back pain in primary care. 24 items selected from Sickness Impact Profile with the term "because of my back" added to each to make it specific to lower back pain.
SF-36 (Stewart et al., 1988)[†]	Includes 36 items pertaining to general well-being and frequency and degree of participation in daily living, social, and recreational activities. Role and social functioning subscale measure at level of participation.
Sickness Impact Profile (Bergner et al., 1981; van Straten et al., 1997)[†]	A 136-item questionnaire. Includes everyday activities in 12 subscales (sleep and rest; emotional behavior; body care and movement; home management; mobility; social interaction; ambulation; alertness behavior; communication; work, recreation, and pastimes; and eating).
WHO Disability Assessment Schedule 2 (WHODAS II) (www.who.int/icidh/whodas/generalinfo.html)	Assesses day-to-day functioning in six activity domains: understanding and communicating, getting around, self-care, getting along with people, life activities, and participation in society. It provides a profile of functioning across the domains and an overall disability score.
WHO Quality of Life (WHOQOL) (WHOQOL group, 1998)	Consists of 26 items in four domains: physical health, psychological health, social relationships, and environment. Designed to measure the level of satisfaction in carrying out activities or tasks, or in participating in these activities. Abbreviated version of the WHOQOL.

*Refer to references listed to determine each measure's proper use and measurement properties.
†This measure is approved by the Scientific Advisory Committee of the Medical Outcomes Trust.
WHO, World Health Organization.

is at risk for developing chronic low back syndrome, which might lead to loss of employment or inability to fulfill other roles. An athlete with a tendon injury might need carefully controlled rest and stabilization to prevent long-term loss of the ability to participate in competitive sports. A newborn with spina bifida may exhibit few current restrictions in life skills but is clearly at risk for future restrictions; early intervention is designed to minimize these future restrictions.

Identifying potential participation restrictions is therefore an important component of PT practice and affects the plan of care. As an example, consider again the patient with acute low back pain. If the potential restriction in participation is occupational in nature, intervention might be focused on teaching the patient to perform certain work-related skills safely and alternative ways to accomplish certain tasks. If, however, the potential restriction involves competitive athletics, a very different approach would be used—one with greater emphasis on strengthening muscles and fine-tuning movement strategies so that the patient could continue to perform at a high level without causing further injury.

Clinicians can use a considerable database of evidence to support this concept. Numerous studies have shown that the natural history of certain diseases (and risk factors) lead to predictable participation restrictions (Incalzi et al., 1992; Adams et al., 1999; Curtis & Black, 1999; Feuerstein et al., 1999; Stuck et al., 1999; Lamb et al., 2000; Westhoff et al., 2000). Clinicians can use this evidence to determine whether a significant risk of future participation restriction exists and justify intervention on that basis.

Summary

- Documentation of *participation* and *social history* ascertains critical information about a patient's life, including his or her home situation and work.

- Participation is specific to an individual and his or her environment. In a pediatric setting, participation is often related to a child's ability to play or attend school. For an adult patient, participation encompasses the ability to perform specific functions related to daily care, work/occupation, social life, and leisure.

- Participation information is most commonly obtained through patient and family interviews and from the medical record. Through the interview process the therapist ascertains the patient's *premorbid lifestyle* and determines the patient's *current goals* for regaining that lifestyle.

- Standardized questionnaires use self-reporting to determine a patient's health perception and participation in recreational, social, occupational, and personal activities.

CASE EXAMPLE 6-1

Setting: Outpatient

Name: Rick Quincy   **D.O.B.:** 12/29/63   **Date of Eval.:** 6/14/08

CURRENT CONDITION: L4-5 disk herniation, onset of current symptoms 5/20/08.

PARTICIPATION: Oswestry Disability Questionnaire 28/50 (indicating severe disability). He is currently unable to perform daily household duties (e.g., gardening, taking out trash) 2° to pain. Prior to onset of LBP, pt. enjoyed watching sports (currently able to sit for only 30 min) and attending daughter's softball games (has not attended a game for 2 wk due to inability to sit on bleacher-style seats). Pt. works as an independent building contractor. He is currently doing paperwork at his desk and making phone calls but has not yet returned to any physical labor. Job entails 60% moderate-heavy lifting (up to 100 lb) and 40% desk work, requiring sitting at desk and phone for 1-2 hr at a time.

GENERAL HEALTH STATUS: Before onset of LBP, pt. led relatively sedentary lifestyle. Hx of smoking 1 pack/day for past 20 yr.

SOCIAL HISTORY: Lives with wife and 2 children in 2-story home. His wife has taken responsibility for all household duties and has hired some outside help to assist with gardening and other chores.

CASE EXAMPLE 6-2

Setting: Inpatient Acute Care

Name: Lisa Jeter   **D.O.B.:** 5/20/59   **Date of Eval.:** 12/10/09

CURRENT CONDITION: s/p aortic aneurysm, 12/5/09.

PARTICIPATION: Pt. employed as data analyst; works out of her home 4 days/wk using computer, fax machine, and telephone. Before hospitalization, pt. and her husband split daily household duties. Pt. was responsible for the family's money management, laundry, cooking, and shopping. Pt. led active lifestyle—enjoyed jogging every morning with her daughter; actively coached daughter's soccer team, and her husband reports her health as being excellent. Previous recreational activities include camping trips, skiing, and going to the theatre.

SOCIAL HISTORY: Pt. lives c̄ husband and 2 teenage children in 2-story home; 5 steps to enter c̄ 2 railings and 12 steps to 2nd floor with 1 railing (on R to ↑). Bedrooms and bathroom are on 2nd floor. Pt.'s husband works full-time and states that he would need additional support to assist in pt.'s daily care skills if she is not independent when she returns home.

CASE EXAMPLE 6-3

Setting: Outpatient

Name: Anita Garcia   **D.O.B.:** 1/3/90   **Date of Eval.:** 1/10/09

CURRENT CONDITION: s/p Colles fracture of R distal radius 12/1/08

PARTICIPATION/SOCIAL HISTORY: Pt. attends Southern State University; lives in first-floor apartment with 2 roommates. Unable to perform daily activities with R hand (e.g., brushing teeth and blow-drying hair) 2° to pain. Pt. is R handed but primarily is using L hand to write and type, with considerable difficulty. Before injury, pt. played intramural volleyball 2×/wk.

EXERCISE 6-1

Identify the errors in the following statements documenting Reason for Referral: Participation and Social History. Rewrite a more appropriate statement in the space provided.

Statement	Rewrite Statement
EXAMPLE: Pt. cannot return home.	Pt. cannot return home at this time; there are 2 flights of stairs leading to her apt. and no modifications can be made.
1. Pt. is confined to a wheelchair.	
2. Has poor motivation to return to work.	
3. Works on a loading dock.	
4. Client enjoys sports.	
5. Pt. cannot return to work 2° to architectural barriers.	
6. Pt. was very active before her injury.	
7. Pt. is in poor shape.	
8. Pt. lives in an apartment.	
9. Pt. has a history of bad health habits.	
10. Pt. uses adaptive equipment.	

EXERCISE 6-2

Indicate which classification component should be used for each statement. Participation = P, Social History = S, NP = not pertinent. Statements that either do not belong in this section or are not relevant to be reported in an evaluation should be classified as NP.

1. Pt. lives with her daughter in an apartment building on the 2nd floor. There is an elevator that sometimes doesn't work.   _____

2. Pt. has a raised toilet seat, grab bars, and shower chair in shower.   _____

3. Pt. enjoys watching *Jeopardy* and *Wheel of Fortune* every evening.   _____

4. Pt. is not currently working 2° to walking and standing limitations.   _____

5. Before surgery, pt. enjoyed 2-3 outings per month to mall or to visit friends.   _____

6. Pt. will be independent in outdoor ambulation for distances >1000 ft.   _____

7. Before surgery, pt. was working 3 days/wk as a retail sales clerk, which required standing and walking most of the day.   _____

8. Pt. has a hx of IDDM ×10 yr; HTN ×5 yr.   _____

9. Pt. reports leading a relatively sedentary lifestyle and does not participate in regular exercise program.   _____

10. Pt. lives in 1-story home with 5 steps to enter.   _____

EXERCISE 6-3

This exercise is designed to practice patient-interiew techniques for obtaining participation and social history information, and to document the findings in the Reason for Referral section of an initial evaluation. Students should form groups of pairs. **Two case reports (A and B) can be found in Appendix C for this exercise.** One student (acting as patient) should carefully read Case Report A in Appendix C. The second student (acting as therapist) will ask the patient questions aimed at obtaining a comprehensive assessment of social history and participation. The patient should be careful to answer directly only those questions asked by the therapist, based on information provided in the Case Report, but can improvise as needed. Then students should switch roles for Case Report B. The therapist may choose to record answers on a separate sheet of paper, and write the final documentation in the space provided.

CASE REPORT A

Setting: Outpatient

Name: Terry O'Connor   **D.O.B.:** 3/23/43   **Date of Eval.:** 7/2/09

Reason for Referral

CURRENT CONDITION: R hip bursitis, onset around 5/10/09. Pt. is a 66 y.o. female who had a gradual onset of pain approximately 2 mo ago in her R thigh, which progressed to a continuous "throbbing pain." Pain radiates from the R hip to the R knee. Pt. does not attribute it to any particular incident.

Social History

Participation

Health Status

CASE REPORT B

Setting: Inpatient Rehabilitation*

Name: Tommy Jones   **D.O.B.:** 5/12/89   **Date of Eval.:** 7/2/09   **Admission Date:** 7/2/09

Reason for Referral

CURRENT CONDITION: C7 incomplete SCI 2° to MVA on 6/15/09. Pt. was transferred this morning from County Acute Care Hospital, where he has been since his accident. Medical records reveal one episode of orthostatic hypotension on coming to sitting and two episodes of autonomic dysreflexia. Pt. underwent surgery on 6/16/09 for anterior cervical fusion. Currently cleared for all rehabilitation activities per Dr. Johnston (per phone conversation this morning).

Social History

Participation

Health Status

*NOTE: Patient is in a hospital setting, so participation/social history information will be based mainly on patient's abilities and activities before admission to hospital.

CHAPTER 7

Documenting Activities

LEARNING OBJECTIVES

*After reading this chapter and completing the exercises,
the reader will be able to:*

1. Define activities and function.

2. Discuss the factors involved in deciding which activities should be included in documentation.

3. Identify and classify various aspects of documenting activities.

4. Appropriately categorize activities of daily living and instrumental activities of daily living.

5. Document activities using a skill-based framework.

Defining and Categorizing Activities

This chapter discusses documentation and categorization of Activities (Figure 7-1). *Activity* as defined by ICF is the execution of a task or action by an individual. Many therapists typically refer to this as *function, functional ability, functional status,* or *functional activities.* As discussed in Chapter 1, the ICF has an inherently positive approach toward disablement. Thus therapists should be encouraged to document those activities a person is *able* to perform. In most cases, documentation should include abilities *and* limitations as they relate to function. However, the primary purpose of the ICF is to shed a positive light on disablement. In this book, we use the term *Activities,* in accordance with ICF terminology, as a global category for documenting skills, abilities, and limitations related to function.

The term *function* is typically used by rehabilitation professionals to describe a person's performance of skills or tasks that are pertinent to his or her daily life. *Function* can be defined as "the action for which a person is fitted or employed" (Davis, 2000). If an action is to be considered functional, it must (1) be meaningful to an individual and (2) help an individual to fulfill

his or her roles (e.g., spouse, parent, volunteer, worker, student, pet owner).

In the current edition of the *Guide to Physical Therapist Practice,* the list of tests and measures is not distinguished based on Participation, Activities, and Body Structures and Functions. Rather, the tests and measures are listed alphabetically, which is not necessarily conducive to providing a logical organization for a patient evaluation (Gordon & Quinn, 1999). Five of the 24 groupings in the list of tests and measures presented in the *Guide* have components that measure functional abilities:

- Aerobic capacity and endurance
- Gait, locomotion, and balance
- Neuromotor development and sensory integration
- Self-care and home management (including activities of daily living [ADLs] and instrumental activities of daily living [IADLs])
- Work (job/school/play), community, and leisure integration or reintegration (including IADLs)

In several of these categories the differentiation between Body Structures and Functions and Activities is difficult, as in the case of "gait, locomotion, and balance." The task of walking is certainly an activity, but

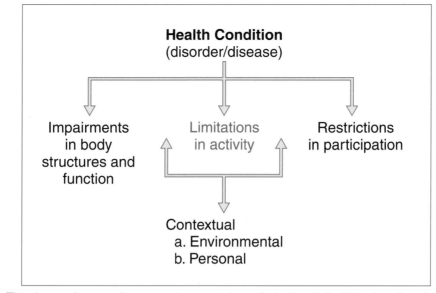

FIGURE 7-1   This chapter discusses documentation pertaining to limitations in Activities, based on the ICF framework.

describing the details of the gait pattern or the balance needed to maintain walking is more closely related to impairment of body functions. In fact, the differentiation between impairments and activities may be considered as a continuum rather than a strict separation. Figure 7-2 and Box 7-1 illustrate this concept. This continuum is discussed in more detail below.

Activities are arguably the most important component of physical therapy documentation, particularly when they pertain to function. Performance in functional activities is used to justify the need for physical therapy services as well as to show a patient's improvement over time. From a PT's perspective, health conditions and the resulting impairments are important insofar as they affect a patient's daily functioning. Functional activities are those that are meaningful to patients: Can they walk, run, get dressed, reach, and grasp for objects? Improvements in these activities should be a primary outcome of physical therapy intervention.

Documenting Task Performance

Physical therapy intervention often entails practice of specific actions, such as walking, squatting, lifting, reaching, and grasping. In effect, these actions are **tasks** that are used in a wide range of activities. Therapists often quantify and qualify performance on tasks as a measure of a patient's functional ability. Reaching, grasping, walking, and many other types of movement patterns are *elements* of functional activities; they are not functional activities per se. They are not considered activities because they do not have a clearly definable and meaningful goal or purpose.

For instance, gait evaluation describes the *movement patterns* used for walking. Gait deviations (e.g., Trendelenburg, excessive circumduction, foot drop) are therefore impairments. Walking to the bathroom and walking outside on grass to move through a yard describe *activities* because they have a meaningful goal. As stated earlier, functions are actions that are meaningful to an individual and help an individual to fulfill his or her roles in life. In certain situations, documentation of a patient's performance of tasks outside the context of specific functional activities may be useful. For example, a therapist could document a person's ability to reach forward into space or to take steps in the parallel bars. For documentation purposes, such elemental tasks are most logically reported in the Activities section of the report.

Tasks represent the interface between activities and body structures and functions (see Figure 7-2). Evaluation of the movement patterns and strategies used to perform such tasks provides important insight into the underlying impairments that affect activities. Task evaluation may bridge many functional skills. For example, the ability to squat is an important task for functional activities ranging from using the bathroom to picking up an object. Importantly, therapists may use task analysis to derive a deeper understanding of the contribution of various impairments to activity performance. Documentation of tasks therefore often includes information about how the movement was performed and the effect of any impairments on functional performance.

Although evaluation of task performance is an important aspect of the physical therapy evaluation process, therapists should give priority to

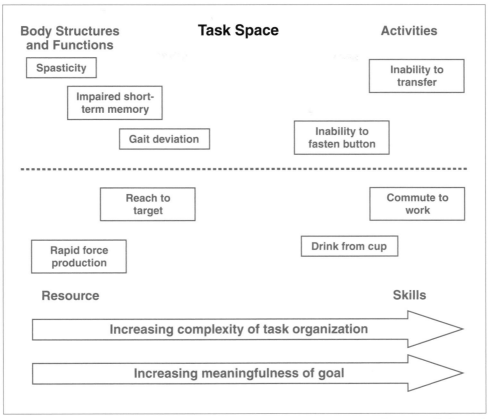

FIGURE 7-2   This task space represents the interface between body structures and functions and activities. Tasks can have stronger components of either activities or body functions depending on the nature and goal of the task.

context-based activity assessment. For example, tasks such as reaching and grasping often can be assessed within the context of a functional activity, such as eating or brushing teeth. A person's ability to perform reaching and grasping behaviors is affected by the context in which they are performed (e.g., in a sitting or standing position). Similarly, assessment of gait abnormalities may differ depending on the context in which walking occurs (e.g., walking on tile vs. carpeting).

Documenting Performance of Functional Activities

One of the important roles of a PT is to determine *which* activities are meaningful to a specific individual and help that person achieve independence and skill in these activities. Many possible activities could be important for an individual. Pertinent functional activities are those that are related to a person's specific life roles and relevant to the patient's therapeutic goals. Functional activities can be categorized in each of the three life roles: personal, occupational, and leisure. Some activities are common to almost everyone. Other activities are more specific to a person's life roles, such as those required for work or recreational sports.

Box 7-2 presents examples of common activities related to personal, occupational, and leisure roles. Personal Activities are further divided into ADLs and IADLs. ADLs are the basic tasks of everyday life—eating, dressing, bathing, and so on. IADLs are not necessarily critical for everyday functioning but are important for independent functioning within a community—answering the telephone, managing finances, and so on. This list can be used as a guide to documentation of activities. PTs can create subheadings within this section of the report to better organize the information and improve readability (Case Examples 7-1, 7-2, and 7-3). It is often useful to group activities or tasks together (e.g., ambulation or transfers) and include all related tasks under their appropriate headings.

Documentation of activities should be customized to the particular setting. The focus of activity documentation for a patient who resides in a nursing home would likely be on ADLs. In contrast, a therapist may perform a specific worksite evaluation for a patient; in this case, the activity documentation would be limited to occupational activities.

BOX 7-1

The Gray Line Between Activities and Impairments in Body Structures/Functions

As mentioned in Chapter 1, the ICF model affords different perspectives to describe physical therapy patients and their conditions. A patient's condition can be described in terms of the health condition, body structures and functions, activities, or participation. These are not separate and distinct characteristics of the patient; they are all aspects of the same disabling condition, described in different measurement systems. Furthermore, some overlap occurs between levels of the ICF model. For example, the classification of an evaluation finding as an impairment versus an activity limitation, and between and activity limitation and participation, is often a slightly gray area.

The crucial distinction between impairments and activity limitations is between means and ends. Activities are described in terms of goals or ends. The impairment level describes means to an end: by what mechanisms the goal is accomplished. This important distinction can be illustrated with reference to two movement systems: balance and walking.

Balance

Balance is a perfect example of a characteristic that is difficult to categorize. In its purest sense, balance is described at the impairment level, reflecting the ability of an individual to maintain an upright position against gravity. However, balance is often evaluated through a set of tasks that might be considered "functional." For example, the ability to stand in one place for more than 30 sec is certainly an activity, as is the ability to reach to the floor to pick up an object. Thus if balance is described in terms of the goal, it is an activity. If it is analyzed in terms of the component mechanisms (e.g., increased sway, role of vision), then it is at the impairment level.

Walking

Walking is another example of a task that combines both impairments and activity limitations. Therapists often describe walking in functional terms—how long a patient can walk, how quickly, with how much assistance. However, another important component of walking is evaluation of how a person walks—his or her gait pattern. Gait analysis can be considered a measure at the impairment level. Therapists often describe gait deviations (such as a Trendelenburg gait) that reflect the presence of an underlying impairment (gluteus medius weakness). Again, if the walking is measured in terms of goal attainment (e.g., distance, speed), then it is a function. If gait is analyzed in terms of why the goal is not being achieved (e.g., insufficient knee flexion during swing or inadequate stance phase control of knee extensors), then walking is being described in terms of impairments.

Classification

Even more problems arise in classification of standardized tests and measures. Standardized tests sometimes measure across different levels of the ICF framework (e.g., measuring some components of activities and some of impairments). This in fact may be desirable when a global standardized test is needed.

These difficulties with classification and distinction may seem academic, but documentation can be frustrating if therapists are searching for clear-cut answers (e.g., Is balance an activity or an impairment?). The following strategy is suggested.

All information about a topic (e.g., standing ability, balance control) should be included under one subheading (e.g., standing balance). Even if a particular topic mixes function and impairments, cohesive presentation of that information in the written report is of primary importance (see Case Example 7-1, where standing and sitting ability include components of a balance assessment). Reading a report with information about a single component scattered throughout the report is difficult. Whether the information is categorized under "activities" or "impairments" can depend on the focus of information being written.

For most patients who reside at home or will be returning home, the therapist is responsible for evaluating those activities that are pertinent to different environmental situations. Therapists must ask themselves "In what types of environments will the patient function?" Most activities can be performed in many different environments. For instance, the task of "walking" can occur in a controlled, closed environment, such as the physical therapy gym in a hospital. Walking also can occur in a more variable and open environment, such as walking across a busy street. Thus simply documenting the task of "walking" is not particularly meaningful if it is devoid of environmental context. Therapists must take care to assess a range of environmental contexts as they are *meaningful* to a specific patient. (See Gentile's "Taxonomy of Tasks" for more information on environmental and task classification [Gentile, 2000]).

Functional skills for children assume a slightly different meaning. Throughout the course of childhood, the activities and environments that children encounter can change greatly. In early childhood, children need to access various environments—for example, playground, play group, getting into/out of the car, or using public transportation—and they can perform a wide variety of tasks within those environments, such as climbing, getting up and down from the floor, and walking. As a child gets older the school environment becomes important, and he or she would perform activities such as retrieving books from a library shelf, carrying a lunch tray, navigating hallways, and so on.

BOX 7-2

Documenting Activities: A Suggested List of Activities Related to Personal and Occupational Roles*

Personal Activities

Activities of Daily Living

- Bed mobility
- Transfers
- Dressing
- Toileting
- Grooming
- Oral care
- Bathing
- Self-care
- Eating
- Ambulation
- Climbing stairs

Instrumental Activities of Daily Living

- Ability to use telephone
- Shopping
- Food preparation
- Housekeeping
- Laundry
- Transportation
- Management of medications
- Management of finances

Other Personal Activities (Other Possible Categories)

- Sitting ability
- Standing ability
- Mobility within the home
- Wheelchair mobility
- Household activities

Occupational and Work Activities

Work/School Activities

These activities vary depending on occupation and can include the following:

- Traveling to work/school
- Sitting at desk
- Moving around office/school
- Writing, using computer
- Lifting objects
- Other specific work-related or school-related tasks

Volunteer Work/Community Service

Play activities

For children, "play" is their "work"

- Ball playing
- Jumping
- Running
- Doing puzzles
- Stacking blocks
- Stringing beads

Leisure Activities

Leisure Activities

These activities vary depending on patient interest and can include the following:

- Going to the movies
- Socializing with friends
- Hobbies (e.g., sewing, stamp collecting)

Recreational Activities

These activities vary depending on patient interests and can include the following:

- Exercising
- Playing recreational sports

*This box provides a suggested list of activities related to personal, occupational, and leisure roles. Therapists can use this list a guideline when determining which activities to document for a patient.

In addition, although children generally perform many of the same personal roles as adults (e.g., bathing, dressing, eating, and general mobility), their work and leisure activities clearly differ. "Play skills" encompass a child's work and leisure activities, particularly for younger children. In physical therapy, such skills are often categorized as gross motor skills. Documentation of pediatric evaluations often includes a section on gross motor skills and a separate section on self-care or self-help skills (as they are sometimes termed).

CHOOSING WHICH ACTIVITIES TO DOCUMENT

Many possible activity limitations can be documented by the PT. A patient may have limitations in personal, occupational, and/or leisure activities. How does a therapist choose which activities to document? In some situations, occupational, therapists (OTs) will be involved in functional assessment, particularly for ADLs and IADLs. In such cases, PTs and OTs should collaborate and coordinate their documentation of functional abilities to avoid overlap.

When a PT is the only rehabilitation professional working with a patient, many functions may be relevant to the patient's care. Evaluation and documentation of all functions would be impractical and unnecessarily time consuming. In those cases, therapists must **prioritize** the functions that are most critical to the patient at the present time. For example, an individual who has had a severe brain injury and is just learning to sit and stand without assistance will likely be unable to perform most or all of the personal, work, and leisure activities that he or she was able to perform before the injury. Documentation at an early point in the patient's recovery would likely focus on his or her ability to perform basic daily care skills. As the patient begins to recover from the head injury, the therapist may begin to evaluate and document different types of skills, such as those related to IADLs or occupational activities. Conversely, a patient with rotator cuff tendonitis may have minimal limitations in functional abilities. The patient may be able to perform all daily living, work, and most leisure activities, and he or she may be limited only in the ability to participate in a specific recreational sport activity.

Often the purpose of documenting activities is to demonstrate, at some later point, improvement in these activities over time. In many situations in which a large number of possible functional activities can be measured, therapists can choose to measure and document performance on a few activities that can be used as **benchmarks** (Box 7-3). These activities serve as measures of progress. Therapists should carefully choose as benchmarks those activities that are most meaningful to the patient and sensitive to showing improvement as a result of intervention.

DOCUMENTATION IN THE ABSENCE OF ACTIVITY LIMITATIONS

Sometimes therapists report that patients have no specific activity limitations, only impairments that could lead to a potential limitation at some later point if intervention is not provided. For patients and clients who are seen for a current medical condition, it may be argued that there should be an activity limitation to justify skilled intervention by a PT. If no activity limitation is present, then the therapist should question why skilled services are needed. For example, an elderly client with lack of range of motion of the shoulder joint may be referred for physical therapy. The client has no limitation in performing any functional activity but lacks several degrees of joint range of motion in shoulder flexion and abduction (an impairment). The therapist would be prudent to instruct the patient in range of motion and other therapeutic exercises to prevent further loss of range of motion and maintain shoulder strength. However, if

---

BOX 7-3

Choosing Which Activities to Measure

The following guidelines should be used in deciding which activities should be measured and documented:

- Consider the practice setting—hospital, outpatient, home care. It will most significantly influence the PT's choice of functional skill documentation. Some agencies/hospitals mandate evaluation of specific functional skills. Collaboration with other health professionals, such as OTs, will eliminate unnecessary redundancy.

- Choose activities that are meaningful to the patient, family members/caregivers, or both.

- Prioritize activities that are most critical to the patient at this time in his or her rehabilitation.

- Choose **benchmark** activities—those that are amenable to showing improvement as a result of physical therapy intervention. This will differ depending on the patient and his or her stage of learning. Simple tasks like transfers may be most useful early in rehabilitation, whereas more complex tasks like shopping or preparing meals are usually more appropriate later.

---

this impairment in range of motion does not result in activity limitations or participation restrictions, justifying the need for extended skilled services to third-party payers may be difficult.

Many therapists provide intervention aimed at *preventing* participation restrictions and activity limitations. Although it is currently difficult to justify the medical necessity for such services, PT intervention may nonetheless be appropriate. Preventative intervention is an important part of PT practice; however, most current third-party payers will not pay for it. Therapists are encouraged to document *potential* participation restriction, activity limitations, or both that may occur if the underlying pathologic condition or impairments are not addressed. In fact, such documentation may be helpful in justifying the role of preventative physical therapy services as standard of care. In the current health care climate, however, if a medical necessity for intervention cannot be justified based on the evaluation, the patient may need to be informed that his or her problems do not meet the standards for third-party payment. The patient can then choose to pay for services on a cash payment basis.

Measurement of Activities

LEVEL OF ASSISTANCE

Functional activities can be measured at varying levels of complexity. The simplest measure of activity performance is *whether the goal was achieved*. This question can often involve *level of assistance*—how much assistance or what type of assistive device did the individual need to successfully complete the task? Level of assistance is typically measured by determining an estimated percentage of assistance provided by the therapist or caregiver for performing ADLs (O'Sullivan & Schmitz, 2006). The Functional Independence Measure (FIM) is a tool used in rehabilitation settings that provides a reliable measure of level of assistance on ADLs on a scale of 1 (total assistance) to 7 (complete independence). This scale is the most commonly used and accepted terminology for measuring level of assistance in rehabilitation. Figure 7-3 presents the different levels of assistance and how they are defined.

A tool by Lawton and Brody (1969) has gained acceptance for documenting level of assistance in IADLs on three more broadly defined levels: needs no help, needs some help, unable to do at all. Figure 7-4 presents this tool in a table format that can be used for documentation purposes.

SKILL-BASED ASSESSMENT

Goal achievement and level of assistance provide a relatively small component in the evaluation of a person's functional abilities. In almost all cases, documentation of activities—ADLs, IADLs, or other activities—should exceed simple qualitative assessment and level of independence and assess some components of skilled performance. *Skill* can be defined as the ability to achieve a desired outcome with *consistency*, *flexibility*, and *efficiency*. Table 7-1 outlines a skill-based model for evaluation of functional activities and provides examples of objective ways in which functional abilities can be documented.

The particular aspects of a skill that a therapist chooses to measure depend on the task and the patient's level of skill. If a patient requires a high level of assistance to accomplish a task, a skill-based

assessment may be limited (see Case Example 7-1). Furthermore, documentation of skill can involve any *one* or *all* of these three components: consistency, flexibility, and efficiency. For example, in early skill learning the level of assistance and consistency of performance may be more valuable measures than efficiency and flexibility. Such measures may not be meaningful until a higher level of skill is achieved.

Standardized Tests and Measures

Many different standardized tests and measures are useful in assessing functional skills. Table 7-2 lists some commonly used tests of functional performance. Several books and resources provide detailed information on the many functional assessment tools in current use, including their intended purpose (*Guide to Physical Therapist Practice*, part 3, 2001; Cole, 1995; Enderby, John & Petheram, 2006, Lewis & McNerney, 1994, Lewis & McNerney, 1997).

As discussed in Chapter 6, many standardized assessment tools measure across more than one level of the ICF model. For example, some tests measure both impairment and activities. An example of such a test is the Berg Balance Scale (Berg et al., 1992). This scale measures standing balance at the impairment level, as in standing with eyes closed or with a narrowed base of support, and at the functional activity level, as in picking up an object from the floor. The tests and measures presented in Table 7-2 *primarily* measure performance in functional activities but may have components of participation or impairment assessments or both.

Standardized functional measures are an important aspect of physical therapy documentation; however, they should never be used *in place of* an evaluation tailored to the specific activities pertinent to a patient. If a standardized test is conducted as part of an evaluation, the therapist should report summary scores in

---

FIM LEVELS

No Helper
   7 Complete Independence (Timely, Safety)
   6 Modified Independence (Device)
Helper—Modified Dependence
   5 Supervision (Subject = 100%)
   4 Minimal Assistance (Subject = 75% or more)
   3 Moderate Assistance (Subject = 50% or more)
Helper—Complete Dependence
   2 Maximal Assistance (Subject = 25% or more)
   1 Total Assistance or not testable (Subject less than 25%)

FIGURE 7-3 Definitions of level of assistance based on the Functional Independence Measure (FIM). The FIM measures level of assistance in various domains on a 7-point scale. (From Uniform Data System for Medical Rehabilitation: *Guide for the Uniform Data Set for Medical Rehabilitation*, Version 5.0, Buffalo, 1996, State University of New York at Buffalo.)

Instrumental Activities of Daily Living

Please check the box that most applies for each activity:

Activity	Need No Help (2 pts. each)	Need Some Help (1 pt. each)	Unable to Do at All (0 pts. each)
1. Using the telephone			
2. Getting to places beyond walking distance			
3. Grocery shopping			
4. Preparing meals			
5. Doing housework or light repair work			
6. Doing laundry			
7. Taking medications			
8. Managing money			
Total Score: ___ =	(___ × 2 =) ___ +	(___ × 1 =) ___ +	0

FIGURE 7-4 A table such as this can be useful for documenting level of assistance needed for various instrumental activities of daily living. (From Lawton MP, Brody EM: Assessment of older people: Self-maintaining and instrumental activities of daily living, *Gerontologist* 9:179–186, 1969.)

TABLE 7-1	A SKILL-BASED MODEL OF DOCUMENTING FUNCTIONAL PERFORMANCE		
Skill Component	**Definition**	**Examples**	**Documentation Example**
Consistency	Ability to successfully perform a skill repeatedly over multiple trials or days	• Rate of goal achievement (number of successes/number of attempts) • Number of days/week able to perform • Accuracy (spatial measures of errors) • Accuracy (number of errors)	*Patient is able to transfer from bed to wheelchair using sliding board 3 out of 5 mornings with assistance of husband only for setup.*
Flexibility	Ability to perform a skill under a variety of environmental conditions	• Height, surface, position of equipment/objects • Environment (e.g., open vs. closed) • Ability to do two tasks at once	*Patient walks up 6 steps in home (8" high) with railing; unable to carry anything in hands. Requires verbal reminders for foot placement to walk up 4 outside steps (10" high) with railing.*
Efficiency	Ability to perform a skill within a certain level of energy expenditure (cardiovascular and musculoskeletal)	• Time to complete task • Distance completed • Speed of movement • Heart rate, respiratory rate, or blood pressure changes	*Patient can walk from bed into bathroom (10 ft) in 14.2 seconds (average time/3 trials), with increase in HR to 100 bpm*

TABLE 7-2	A LIST OF SOME COMMONLY USED STANDARDIZED MEASURES OF ACTIVITIES*	
Measure	**Population/Setting**	**Purpose**
Acute Care Index of Function (ACIF) (Van Dillen & Roach, 1988)	Patients in acute care hospitals	20-item scale designed to measure functional status at levels appropriate to acute care setting. Items are divided into four categories: mental status, bed mobility, transfers, and mobility (wheelchair and ambulation).
Barthel Index (Mahoney & Barthel, 1965)	Rehabilitation centers	Consists of 10 items that measure a person's daily functioning, specifically ADLs and mobility.
Cincinatti Knee Rating Scale Function Assessment (CKRS) (Barber-Westin et al., 1984).	Patients with knee pain or dysfunction	Includes a functional assessment based on six abilities important for participation in sports (walking, using stairs, squatting and kneeling, straight running, jumping and landing, and hard twist cuts and pivots).
Emory Functional Ambulation Profile (EFAP) (Wolf et al., 1999)	General rehabilitation	Assesses performance of walking ability based on varying environmental contexts.
Functional Independence Measure (FIM) (Keith et al., 1987)	Rehabilitation centers	18-item, 7-level ordinal scale measuring level of assistance on various functional tasks. Developed to provide a uniform measurement and data on functional and rehabilitation outcomes.
Instrumental Activities of Daily Living (Lawton & Brody, 1969)	General	Rates ability to perform eight different instrumental ADLs on a 0 or 2 scale.
Jebsen test of hand function (Jebsen et al., 1969)	Orthopedic hand and upper extremity impairments	Timed pegboard test with norms established; primarily manipulation and reaching.
Motor Assessment Scale (MAS) (Carr & Shepherd, 1998)	Stroke	Evaluates performance of seven functionally based tasks. Rating is based on movement patterns used to accomplish the task.
Outpatient Physical Therapy Improvement in Movement Assessment Log (OPTIMAL) (Guccione et al., 2005)	Outpatient centers	Measures difficulty and self-confidence in performing 21 movements that are necessary components of various functional activities.
6-minute walk test (6MWT) (Guyatt et al., 1985)	Cardiac, adult neurologic	Measures the distance a patient can quickly walk on a flat, hard surface in 6 minutes.
Timed up and go test (Podsiadlo & Richardson, 1991)	Geriatric, rehabilitation, falls risk assessment	Measures time to stand up from a chair, walk 10 feet, turn around, walk back, and sit down.
Tuft's Assessment of Motor Performance (TAMP) (Gans et al., 1988)	Rehabilitation—stroke, brain injury	Motor assessment for use with adults, with 32 mobility, ADL, and communication test items rated on a 6-point proficiency scale and time recorded for task completion.

*Refer to references listed to determine each measure's proper use and measurement properties.

the evaluation report and attach the scoring form to the report. Reporting results of the entire test as part of the body of an evaluation report is too cumbersome, but therapists may choose to highlight specific components or provide a brief summary of the patient's performance on the test (see Case Example 7-3).

Summary

- Documenting activities, and in particular functional activities, is likely the most important component of physical therapy documentation and is used to justify the need for physical therapy services.

- For an activity to be considered functional, it must (1) be meaningful to an individual. and (2) help an individual to fulfill his or her roles.
- A specific function cannot be separated from the context in which it was performed. Thus context-specific documentation is a critical feature of reporting a patient or client's functional status.
- Rather than document all possible activities, the PT should prioritize the activities that are most meaningful to the patient and are amenable to change.

- Therapists must document specific activity limitations that are related to certain impairments or a health condition. In preventative care this may include documenting *potential* participation restriction, activity limitations, or both.
- Skill can be defined as the ability to achieve a desired outcome with *consistency, flexibility*, and *efficiency*. These components can be used to provide reliable and measurable documentation of activities beyond level of assistance.

CASE EXAMPLE 7-1

Setting: Home Care

Name: Maureen Smith **D.O.B.:** 5/12/48 **Date of Eval.:** 7/3/09

CURRENT CONDITION: A 61 y.o. woman c̄ L-sided cerebral hemorrhage 5/14/09 with resulting R-sided hemiparesis; discharged from Rehab Center on 7/1/09 where she spent 4 wk after acute care stay at Community Hospital.

ACTIVITIES

STANDARDIZED TESTS: Barthel Index: 25/100, Motor Assessment Scale: 16/54

BED MOBILITY: Pt. rolls to R I'ly; rolls to L c̄ min A to bring R leg over. Needs mod A to position self in bed c̄ use of trapeze.

SITTING ABILITY: *On bed:* Bed needs to be positioned so pt.'s feet are flat on floor. Able to sit for 10 min independently (limited due to reported fatigue). Unable to reach >1″ outside arm's length in all directions. *In wheelchair:* Can sit in W/C for up to 30 min; begins to lean to R side and cannot straighten self s̄ A.

STANDING ABILITY: Requires mod A to stand for 20 sec c̄ R AFO.

TRANSFER W/C ↔ BED: Uses SB to transfer from bed to W/C (toward the L side only) and back with min A to set up SB and begin initial movement on board. Completes task in approx. 1 min.

MOBILITY: Pt. uses W/C as primary means of mobility in home. Can propel W/C with one-arm drive in home except into bathroom (too narrow). Outside mobility limited to propulsion on level surfaces for 5 min, c̄ HR ↑ to 110 bpm. Requires A to negotiate curbs, ramps, and uneven terrain.

FEEDING: Pt. needs A to set up plate, utensils, and cup but can eat with spoon or fork with L hand. Uses modified scoop-plate to get food onto utensil. Needs A to cut foods. Can drink using a light cup or with a straw. Self-care, grooming, and bathroom transfers: Refer to OT eval.

CASE EXAMPLE 7-2

Setting: Outpatient

Name: Rich Green   **D.O.B.:** 8/2/45   **Date of Eval.:** 6/15/09

CURRENT CONDITION: Pt. is a 63 y.o. male carpenter s/p R rotator cuff repair on 4/2/09 $\bar{p}$ fall from ladder (8-wk postop).

ACTIVITIES

TRANSPORTATION: Pt. able to drive up to 45 min at a time. Pt. reports pain ↑ from 2/10 at rest to 5/10 while driving >15 min. Reports needing to frequently rest R arm.

AMBULATION: No limitations in amb. when not carrying items. Pt. is able to carry up to 3 lb item in R hand while walking for up to 1 min before reports of fatigue.

HOUSEHOLD ACTIVITIES: Pt. is able to reach 2nd shelf (26″ above waist) in cupboard with only minimal elevation of shoulder, with pain rating of 2/10. Able to ascend/descend full flight of stairs (12 stairs) carrying only up to 5 lb (e.g., tray, laundry basket) with both hands $\bar{s}$ ↑ in pain.

DRESSING: Able to don a button-down shirt or pullover shirt I within 30 sec.

CASE EXAMPLE 7-3

Setting: Inpatient Acute Rehabilitation

Name: Kareem Patel   **D.O.B.:** 3/23/35   **Date of Eval.:** 6/21/09

CURRENT CONDITION: Pt. is s/p AAA repair, 10 days postop.

ACTIVITIES

FIM AMBULATION SCORE: 5

AMBULATION: Pt. walks within room unassisted. Requires supervision for ambulation outside room for fatigue monitoring.

RESULTS OF 6-MINUTE WALK TEST:
Distance Walked: 150 ft; **Surface:** Indoor/level/tile; **Device:** Rolling walker; **Bracing:** None
Assistance: CG; **Supplemental Oxygen Used:** 2 L/m NC; **Borg Rating of Perceived Fatigue/Exertion:** 11; **Posttest:** HR 70 bpm; BP 142/70 mm Hg; RR 24 breaths/min; O_2 saturation 91%

STAIRS: Able to ascend/descend 6 steps $\bar{c}$ CG, step to step with 1 hand on railing. HR post: 96 bpm; BP: 140/82.

ADLs: Pt. is I in all ADLs. Able to stand for up to 2 min at a time for daily care routine (brushing teeth, combing hair, shaving); takes 2 breaks in a 5-min period. IADLs assessed by OT.

EXERCISE 7-1

Identify the errors in the following statements documenting Activities. Rewrite a more appropriate statement in the space provided.

Statement	Rewrite Statement
Example: Demonstrates poor sitting balance.	Pt. is able to sit for 10 seconds on side of bed, feet flat on floor, before losing balance to the right side. Needs assistance to return to an upright sitting position.
1. Able to walk 50 ft.	
2. Able to eat with a spoon with occasional assistance.	
3. Pt. is confined to using a wheelchair for long-distance mobility.	
4. Able to climb a few stairs.	
5. Can throw a ball but cannot catch one.	
6. Can walk on uneven surfaces.	
7. Pt. is not motivated to walk.	

Statement	Rewrite Statement
8. Dresses upper body with difficulty.	_____
9. Walks slowly.	_____
10. Pt. doesn't drive.	_____
11. C/o pain during standing.	_____
12. Transfers with assistance.	_____
13. Pt. can lift various sized boxes.	_____
14. Pt. can't get up from a low chair.	_____
15. Pt. is having trouble sitting for extended periods at work.	_____

EXERCISE 7-2

The following statements are from an initial evaluation report written in a hospital setting. For statements that do not belong in the Activities section, write NA (not appropriate) on the line provided. For statments that do belong in the Activities section, use Box 7-2 to determine a probable subheading (e.g., transfers, ambulation) under which this information could be listed.

Example: Pt. is able to use commode in her bedroom with min A to transfer: toileting.

1. Pt. walks 100 ft in hospital hallway c̄ supervision, c̄ ↑ in HR to 120 bpm.   _____

2. Pt. performs daily morning routine of brushing teeth and shaving within 5 min s̄ SOB while sitting 2/3 days.   _____

3. Pt. can ↑↓ 10 stairs with 1 railing, step over step, in 22 sec.   _____

4. Strength B knee extension 4/5.   _____

5. Pt. has 20 yr history of IDDM.   _____

6. Pt. transfers from bed to W/C c̄ supervision.   _____

7. Able to stand with min A in hospital room for up to 2 min; limited due to fatigue (HR increase to 102 bpm).   _____

8. PROM R knee flexion 110°.   _____

9. Pt. can ↑↓ 6″ and 8″ curbs c̄ CG.   _____

10. Pt. performed ADLs I before surgery.   _____

11. Able to dress upper body independently; requires mod A to reach down to put on pants and don shoes and socks from a seated position.   _____

12. Able to come from supine to sitting on edge of bed with contact guarding.   _____

13. Pt. is able to prepare simple meals not requiring stove-top cooking or carrying pots/pans > 2 lb.   _____

EXERCISE 7-3

For each of the occupations listed below, write a list of functional activities that would be most appropriate to document in the Activities section for a theoretical patient. They should be activities specific to the patient's particular life role.

Bus driver

_____

_____

Homemaker

_____

_____

College student

_____

_____

Administrative assistant

_____

_____

Professional basketball player

_____

_____

CHAPTER 8

Documenting Impairments in Body Structure and Function

LEARNING OBJECTIVES

After reading this chapter and completing the exercises, the reader will be able to:

1. Define impairments in body structure and function.

2. Appropriately classify impairments into categories for documentation purposes.

3. Document impairments concisely using appropriate terminology and abbreviations.

Defining and Categorizing Impairments

According to the ICF model, body structures are defined as anatomic parts of the body such as organs, limbs, and their components. Body functions are physiologic functions of the body (including psychological functions) (Figure 8-1). Thus **impairments** are problems in body function or structure such as a significant deviation or loss.

PTs evaluate the functioning of a wide range of body structures, including those related to the musculoskeletal, neurologic, cardiopulmonary, and integumentary systems. In evaluating these systems, therapists attempt to ascertain the nature and extent of any impairments that may be contributing to a patient's activity limitations or participation restrictions. The body structures and functions that a therapist chooses to evaluate for a particular patient are based on the patient's activity limitations and his or her underlying health condition. A comprehensive consideration of all possible impairments is beyond the scope of this chapter, but the key aspects of documenting commonly assessed impairments are discussed (see O'Sullivan & Schmitz, 2006).

The *Guide to Physical Therapist Practice* (the *Guide*; American Physical Therapy Association [APTA], 2001) provides a list of the tests and measures typically used by PTs. Of the 24 groupings in Chapter 2 of the *Guide*, 18 include some components of impairment-based tests and measures (Box 8-1). As emphasized in Chapter 7, the *Guide* does not organize tests and measures according to impairment and activity. This differentiation is often difficult and may be perceived as a continuum rather than a strict separation (see Figure 7-2).

When categorizing impairments, it can be useful to create headings that organize impairment documentation in an evaluation report or progress note. The *Guide* presents a categorization of the tests and measures used in physical therapy. These headings can be used for documentation purposes and provide a reasonable approach to organizing this section of an evaluation. However, impairments may be categorized in many ways depending on the patient's medical condition, the facility, and the personal preferences of the therapist (see Case Examples at the end of this chapter).

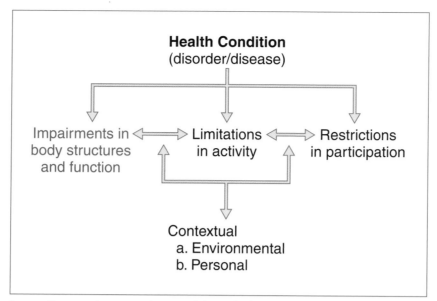

Health Condition
(disorder/disease)

Impairments in body structures and function ⟺ Limitations in activity ⟺ Restrictions in participation

Contextual
a. Environmental
b. Personal

FIGURE 8-1   This chapter discusses documentation pertaining to body structures and functions, based on the ICF framework.

BOX 8-1

Components of Documenting Impairments in Body Structures and Function

- Aerobic capacity/endurance
- Anthropometric characteristics
- Arousal, attention, and cognition
- Circulation (arterial, venous, lymphatic)
- Cranial and peripheral nerve integrity
- Ergonomics and body mechanics
- Gait, locomotion, and balance
- Integumentary integrity
- Joint integrity and mobility
- Motor function (motor control and motor learning)
- Muscle performance (including strength, power, and endurance)
- Neuromotor development and sensory integrity
- Pain
- Posture
- Range of motion
- Reflex integrity
- Sensory integrity
- Ventilation and respiration/gas exchange

From American Physical Therapy Association: *The guide to physical therapist practice*, ed 2, Alexandria, VA, 2001, American Physical Therapy Association.

Systems Reviews

A PT decides which impairments to measure based on the patient's activity limitations and his or her underlying health condition. However, all PTs must perform certain basic assessment procedures and document them accordingly. One such set of measures includes a **systems review**.

A systems review is a "brief or limited examination of the anatomical and physiological status of the cardiovascular/pulmonary, integumentary, musculoskeletal, and neuromuscular systems and the communication ability, affect, cognition, language, and learning style of the patient/client" (*Guide to Physical Therapist Practice*, 2001, p. S34). This may include communication skills, cognitive abilities, factors that might influence care, and learning preferences. A systems review typically also includes a cardiovascular screening for each patient, which can include an assessment of blood pressure and heart rate, and a general screen of range of motion and muscle strength. It is important to note that the information included in a systems review is a screening, and depending on the nature of the patient's condition and the results of this screening, a more detailed assessment of these areas may be necessary.

For example, if an elderly patient is referred with shoulder pain, the following information would be important to include in a systems review: blood pressure/heart rate (cardiovascular), communication, and cognition (communication ability). In addition, skin assessment (integumentary), range of motion (ROM) and strength in the lower extremities in addition to the upper extremities (musculoskeletal), and any neurologic signs such as sensory changes or reflexes (neuromuscular), should also be assessed as part of a general screening.

The cases at the end of this chapter and in Chapter 4 provide examples of systems review documentation for different patient populations.

Strategies for Documenting Impairments

CHOOSING WHICH IMPAIRMENTS TO DOCUMENT

The general approach of this text is to evaluate and report those results that are relevant to the patient's current condition and that are necessary to develop an adequate rationale for the diagnosis and intervention plan. If a patient is *at risk* for developing an impairment because of a particular medical condition, the absence of impairment should be documented. For example, in a patient with severe diabetes and associated peripheral vascular disease, the skin condition of the toes should be checked regularly and documented because tissue necrosis is a genuine risk in these patients.

SPECIFICITY OF DOCUMENTING IMPAIRMENTS

Quantifiable and objective data should be provided for impairment measures to be useful for diagnostic or evaluative purposes. Therapists should take care to document impairments with clarity and precision, avoiding vague and ambiguous terminology. Terms such as *minimal, moderate,* and *maximal* or *good, fair,* and *poor* are not particularly useful in descriptions of impairments and should be used sparingly in favor of more measurable, quantifiable assessments. Case Examples 8-1 to 8-3 give examples of documenting commonly assessed impairments in a concise but specific manner.

DOCUMENTING NORMAL FINDINGS

An assessment of body structures and functions must include documentation of the results of every test or measure that the therapist has performed, even if the findings were negative (i.e., normal). Documentation of normal findings can occur when the findings are directly relevant to confirming, refuting, or reshaping the medical diagnosis. For example, if a patient has pain in his or her shoulder and strength and ROM of the neck and shoulder are normal, these specific findings would be very important to document.

Therapists sometimes use two general terms, WNL (within normal limits) or WFL (within functional limits), to indicate "normal" or "typical" findings. The authors strongly discourage the use of WFL, as there is no accepted definition for this term and different professionals reading a note may interpret it in different ways. WNL should also generally be avoided, except when used to describe the results of a quick screening examination.

Standardized Tests and Measures

Many impairment-based measures used in physical therapy are quantitative. Therapists should carefully choose impairment-based measures that have established reliability and validity. Examples of some commonly used standardized tests and measures are listed in Table 8-1.

Documenting Strength and Range of Motion

DOCUMENTING STRENGTH

ROM assessment and muscle strength testing are two of the most common impairment measures for PTs. Both provide numeric data, in number of degrees and strength grade, respectively. Although ROM measurements generally have been found reliable (Mayerson & Milano, 1984), manual muscle testing has more limited reliability (Frese et al., 1987; Escolar et al., 2001), and its utility as a screening tool for muscle weakness has been questioned (Bohannon, 2005). Despite this limitation, manual muscle testing continues to be the most commonly used method by PTs to measure strength (see Case Example 8-1). Other measures, such as handheld dynamometers or isokinetic measurements (e.g., peak torque or torque curves), can provide more reliable and quantitative data to evaluate muscle strength and measure its change over time.

Functional strength tests, such as the Sit-to-Stand test (Csuka & McCarty, 1985) and functional hop test (Booher et al., 1993), can also provide useful information related to muscle strength (Davies, et al., 1996). (See Malone et al., 1996, for more information on strength measures and documentation.) In certain cases, a description of functional strength or motor control is most appropriate (see Case Example 8-2).

DOCUMENTING RANGE OF MOTION

Reporting joint range of motion, most commonly in number of degrees, can be susceptible to certain ambiguities. For example, consider the following statement:

Knee extension-flexion ROM is 10°-150°

The end of flexion range in this statement is clear (150°), but the end of extension range is ambiguous. Does this statement mean that the individual cannot fully extend the knee (10° knee flexion contracture), or does it mean that the individual has 10° of extension beyond the neutral?

The ambiguity arises in trying to report flexion-extension as a single range of values. Although there

TABLE 8-1	STANDARDIZED ASSESSMENTS OF IMPAIRMENTS	
Measure	**Population**	**Purpose**
Berg Balance Scale (Berg et al., 1992)	Any neurologic condition, the elderly, individuals with balance problems	Measures balance ability on 14 balance items, such as standing with eyes closed, turning in place, and standing on one leg.
Cincinnati Knee Rating System (symptoms) (Barber-Westin et al., 1984)	Patients with knee dysfunction	Measures symptoms related to knee pain, including pain, swelling, and giving way, on a 6-point scale.
Constant Murley Score (Constant & Murley, 1987)	Patients with shoulder dysfunction	100-point scoring system: 35 points derived from patient's reported pain and function; 65 points from assessment of ROM and strength.
Fugl-Meyer (Fugl-Meyer et al., 1975)	Stroke	Based to a large extent on Brunnstrom's (1996) description of the stages of stroke recovery; most items scored on a 3-point scale (0, 1, 2); includes motor function, sensation, ROM, and pain
Glasgow Coma Scale (Jennett & Teasdale, 1977)	Brain injury	Rates alertness and cognitive awareness in three categories (eyes, verbal, and motor).
Mini-Mental State (Folstein et al., 1975)	Any individual with cognitive deficits or dementia	Assesses several categories related to cognition, including memory, recall, and language.
NIH Stroke Scale (Goldstein et al., 1989)	Stroke	11-item clinical evaluation tool used to assess neurologic outcome and degree of recovery. Includes evaluation of level of consciousness, motor function, and language, among others.
Rate of Perceived Exertion (Borg & Linderholm, 1970)	Cardiopulmonary	Patients rate their perceived exertion level on a 15-point scale.
Short physical performance battery (Guralnik et al., 1994)	General population; elderly patients	Evaluates balance, gait, strength, and endurance by examining a patient's ability to stand with the feet together in the side-by-side, semitandem, and tandem positions, time to walk 8 feet, and time to rise from a chair and return to the seated position five times.
Tinetti Gait and Balance (Tinetti, 1986)	Any neurologic condition, the elderly, individuals with balance problems	Developed as a screening tool to identify older adults at risk for falls. Balance component measures balance on eight specific tasks; gait component measures specific gait parameters during ambulation. All are scored on a 0 to 2 scale.

are accepted ways to do this (see Reese & Bandy, 2002, for an excellent discussion of the different methods of recording ROM values), the best way to avoid ambiguity is to separate the range into two separate components, one for each direction of movement. For example:

Knee flex: 0°-150°
Knee ext: 0°-10°

This unambiguously states that the individual has 150° of flexion range and 10° of extension beyond neutral. If, instead, the individual has a 10° knee flexion contracture, it would be reported in this way:

Knee flex: 10°-150°
Knee ext: –10°

Note that ROM is always stated as a range of values (e.g., 0°-150°), except when the individual cannot reach the neutral value, in which case the range is stated as a single negative value (see Case Examples 8-1 and 8-2).

A second problem that sometimes arises with reporting of ROM is confusion between active and passive. When the term "range of motion" or abbreviation "ROM" is used without a modifier, it implies *passive* ROM. If the writer of the note means active ROM, then the word "active" must be stated. However, in all cases use of PROM and AROM is preferable so that is it clear whether passive or active ROM was measured.

USING TABLES AND CHECKLISTS

Tables or checklists can be useful to manage a large amount of data. Such forms can be appended to an initial evaluation to simplify it and not clutter the text. This strategy is useful for measures such as ROM or manual muscle tests, which can be cumbersome to document (see Appendix D). In such cases, pertinent findings could be highlighted in the initial evaluation note while referring the reader to additional documentation.

If such forms are used, no line should be left blank so that the evaluation cannot be altered by another party without the therapist's knowledge. Also, if a line is left blank, the reason it was left blank is unknown to the reader. The therapist must write one of the following on the line:

1. The results of the test, examination findings, or clinical opinion.

2. *N/T* (not tested) indicates that this item was not tested. This entry in the note should be followed by a reason the item was not tested or a plan for testing in the future (e.g., *N/T 2 ° to time constraints—to be evaluated 11/1/09*).

3. *N/A* (not applicable) indicates that this test was not applicable for this particular patient, given his or her diagnosis or condition. The therapist should state why the test/measure is not applicable (e.g., *N/A—Pt. is currently on ventilator and unconcious; unable to get out of bed*).

Documenting Pain

Pain is probably the single most common reported problem that a PT encounters in clinical practice. It is not enough to write merely that "Pt. c/o pain in L shoulder" or some similar statement. Instead, the pain symptoms should be documented precisely and completely. Bickley and Hoekelman (1999) have nicely outlined the seven characteristics of a symptom that need to be clarified. Based on their formulation, the essential characteristics of pain that should be documented are as follows:

1. *Location:* Where is the pain? Does it radiate? Is there a discrete locus or an indefinite area? Use precise anatomic terminology or include a drawing of the precise locus and extent. Many clinics have forms with outlines of the body (anterior and posterior) that can be used to mark the location of the pain. It is best if the patient marks this directly on a form (see Appendix D).

2. *Quality:* What does it feel like? The nature of the pain sensation can vary widely. For example, it may be sharp, burning, stabbing, aching, or throbbing, to name just a few descriptors. It is best to ask the patient to describe the pain and to use the patient's own words in the documentation.

3. *Severity:* How bad is it? The intensity of the pain sensation is often assessed verbally by using a numeric scale (usually 0 to 10, where 10 is the "worst possible pain") or a visual analog scale (VAS) (see Appendix D). The severity is then documented as n/10 in the case of the numeric scale or as a percentage of maximal pain in the case of the VAS.

4. *Timing:* When did the pain start? When and how often does it occur? Is it getting better or worse with time?

5. *Factors that make it better or worse:* How is the pain affected by different movements or activities or rest?

6. *Setting in which pain occurs:* Are there environments, personal activities, emotional situations, or other circumstances that bring about the pain?

7. *Associated manifestations:* Are there other symptoms that occur in conjunction with the pain?

EXAMPLE: Pt. reports sharp, stabbing pain in right knee (localized to discrete point in center of patella) during stance phase of walking (3/10 at comfortable walking speed). Pain increases as walking speed increases, is most intense (8/10) during running, and is absent at rest. Onset of pain "about 3 months ago." Pain is gradually worsening and is now preventing her from exercising or engaging in recreational sports (e.g., tennis).

For documentation of an initial evaluation, the first five characteristics listed above are almost always included. However, sometimes not all of these characteristics require documentation. For example, settings and associated manifestations may be unremarkable in a specific case and therefore do not need to be included in the documentation. When documenting a progress report or treatment note, it would be redundant for the therapist to document each of these characteristics, particularly if they had not changed. In a treatment note, a therapist may choose to document only the patient's pain rating on a 0 to 10 scale or VAS if all other aspects remain the same.

For children and individuals for whom English is not a first language, ascertaining the type and degree of pain can be difficult. In such situations, facial expressions are frequently used and should be included in an evaluation report. The Wong-Baker FACES Pain Rating Scale is a useful tool that has demonstrated validity and reliability (Wong & Baker, 1988) (see Appendix D).

Summary

- Impairment-based documentation should be categorized into test and measure headings to provide a concise and organized written report.
- Therapists should document a systems review, which is a screening of key body systems that may or may not be related to the patient's current condition.
- Impairment documentation should include all tests and measures that were performed but should highlight impairments that contribute to the observed activity limitations or participation restrictions.
- Whenever possible, impairment documentation should be quantitative. Standardized tests and measures can provide a reliable means for reporting impairments quantitatively.

CASE EXAMPLE 8-1

Setting: Outpatient

Name: Jose Rodriguez   **D.O.B.:** 12/29/86   **Date of Eval.:** 2/25/09

CURRENT CONDITION: 22 y.o. male college student c̄ medical diagnosis of R partial ACL tear 2/22/09.

IMPAIRMENTS

SYSTEMS REVIEW: Skin intact. No evidence of cardiovascular problems; HR 60; BP 120/78. Cognition and communication intact.

Measure	Left	Right
PROM		
Knee ext	0–10°	–5°
Knee flex	0–145°	5–120°
Strength (manual muscle tests)		
Knee ext	5/5	4/5
Knee flex	5/5	4/5
Reflex integrity		
Patellar tendon	2+	2+
Achilles tendon	2+	2+
Special tests		
	–Lachman	+Lachman (grade 2 with firm end point)
	–Pivot shift	+Pivot shift (grade I)
Anthropometric characteristics		
Inferior pole of patella	34.0 cm	35.0 cm
Superior pole of patella	35.0 cm	36.0 cm
3 cm proximal to superior pole of patella	36.5 cm	37.5 cm
15 cm proximal to superior pole of patella	43.0 cm	42.5 cm

INTEGUMENTARY: Moderate color and tenderness along the anteromedial joint line as well as MCL and medial meniscus.

PAIN: Pain 3/10 at rest; throbbing, aching pain midpatellar region. 7/10 while ↑↓ stairs and doing any twisting motion; described as jabbing pain midpatellar region.

CINCINNATI KNEE RATING SYSTEM (SYMPTOMS): 24/40

CASE EXAMPLE 8-2

Setting: Nursing Home

Name: Marjorie Jones   **D.O.B.:** 5/12/27   **Date of Eval.:** 7/3/09

CURRENT CONDITION: Pt. is an 82 y.o. female c̄ dx PD c̄ history of multiple falls.

IMPAIRMENTS

SYSTEMS REVIEW: HR 68 bpm; RR 15 breaths/min; BP 120/78 mm Hg. **INTEGUMENTARY:** +2 Pitting edema noted in both lower legs and feet. **POSTURE:** Forward head, thoracic kyphosis, posterior pelvic tilt, and flexion at B hips and knees in standing. **ROM:** Limited PROM as follows: B hip extension −10°; B hip flexion 10-100°; −10°; B knee extension −10°; R shoulder flexion 0-160°, ER 0-45°, abduction 0-140°; L shoulder flexion 0-140°, ER 0-40°, abduction 0-120°. **MUSCLE TONE:** Moderate rigidity (cogwheel) evident in PROM ×4 extremities, all directions. **MOTOR CONTROL:** Able to move all 4 extremities against minimal resistance. Rapid alternating movements of UEs are slowed. Resting tremor B hands; does not interfere c̄ hand fx. **SENSATION:** Intact to light touch B UEs and LEs. **GAIT/LOCOMOTION*:** 25 sec. *10 m walk gait speed:* 1.2 ft/sec. *Tinetti Gait*[†]: 5/12. Walks without an assistive device for short distances on floor (approximately 100 ft to go to nurses' station or recreation room). Pt. exhibits a shuffling gait with foot flat initial contact; takes small steps, and has a fast cadence (140 steps/min). She also has a narrow step width c̄ R foot occasionally crossing midline. Pt. demonstrates occasional freezing episodes while ambulating in room. Hips and knees are flexed, and there is no visible trunk rotation and only slight arm swing. **BALANCE:** *Tinetti Balance:* 9/16; pt. had particular difficulty with turning and attempting to rise.

---

*Includes assessment of gait impairments and activity level measurements (e.g., walking speed distance).
[†]The complete scoring sheet for the Tinetti Gait and Balance tests would be included as part of the documentation, typically attached to the evaluation report.

CASE EXAMPLE 8-3

*Setting: Hospital Inpatient**

Name: Gareth Jones   **D.O.B.:** 6/12/38   **Date of Eval.:** 8/2/09

CURRENT CONDITION: Pt. is a 71 y.o. male c̄ dx of COPD c̄ h/o frequent acute exacerbations.

IMPAIRMENTS

SYSTEMS REVIEW: ROM no limitations noted. B UE and LE; pt. is communicative and alert and oriented ×3. HR 130 bpm; RR 20 breaths/min; BP 148/88 mm Hg.

VENTILATION/RESPIRATION: Dyspnea, wheeze, productive cough (mucopurulent sputum); chest pain left side. Use of accessory muscles of inspiration, hyperinflated chest, Hoover's sign, peripheral cyanosis, raised jugular venous pressure, pursed-lip breathing.

PALPATION: Limited thoracic expansion, decreased movement noted at the left lower zone, vocal fremitus on left. **PERCUSSION:** Hyperresonant ++ all zones although ↓ resonance (dull) left base. **AUSCULTATION:** Fine crackles and wheeze all zones, c/o plural rub left base.

TEST RESULTS: Spirometry: FEV_1 <40%. Arterial blood gases: pH 7.28, Pao_2 8 kPa, Pco_2 7.5 kPa, HCO_3^- 32 mmol/L, base excess +4 (F_io_2 0.28). Chest radiograph: hyperinflated thorax, flattended diaphragm, consolidation/pleural effusion left base.

INTEGUMENTARY: Peripheral pitting edema noted in B LEs BK.

AEROBIC CAPACITY: Unable to stand due to breathlessness.

---

*Note that in this example some different headings than those recommended by the *Guide to Physical Therapist Practice* are used. Therapists should choose headings that best fit the clinical setting in which they are working.

■ EXERCISE 8-1

The following statements could be written in an Impairment section of an evaluation report. In the space provided, classify each of the following statements into the appropriate impairment category. This exercise should be completed with reference to the specific tests and measures listed and defined in Chapter 2 of the *Guide to Physical Therapist Practice* (see also Box 8-1).

Impairment Statement	Impairment Category
1. R elbow flexion PROM 0-60°.	_____
2. Walks with uneven step lengths and ↑ weight-bearing time on the R side.	_____
3. Sensation intact B LEs below knee, 10/10 correct responses.	_____
4. Mini-Mental State Examination score 19/30 (cognitive assessment).	_____
5. AROM B UEs—no limitations noted.	_____
6. Right facial nerve intact.	_____
7. Circumference midpatella L knee: 10"; R knee: 9.25".	_____
8. Rates pain in low back 5/10 sitting for 10 min, pain described as aching/throbbing.	_____
9. Skin intact B LE and trunk.	_____
10. Berg Balance Scale score = 31/56 indicating high risk for falls.	_____
11. Demonstrates antalgic gait pattern.	_____
12. B patellar tendon reflexes 2+.	_____
13. B lung fields clear to auscultation.	_____
14. Incentive spirometry in sitting c maximal volume = 1750 mL.	_____
15. Pt. has forward head and flattened lumbar lordosis.	_____
16. Pt. is alert and oriented to ×2 (person and place).	_____
17. HR ↑'d to 110 beats/min p 5 min walking at 1.0 m/sec.	_____
18. Proprioception sensation impaired L ankle 2/8 correct responses.	_____
19. R hand grip strength 15 kg as measured by handheld dynamometer, avg. 3 trials.	_____
20. Eye movements, smooth pursuit, and visual fields intact (cranial nerves II, III, IV, and VI).	_____

EXERCISE 8-2

Identify the errors in the following statements documenting impairments. Write a more appropriate statement in the space provided. Use the Case Examples at the end of this chapter for guidance.

Statement	Rewrite Statement
EXAMPLE: Demonstrates poor standing balance.	Pt. unable to stand in place >10 sec s̄ LOB.
1. Sensation is impaired.	
2. ROM is moderately limited.	
3. Pt. c/o excruciating pain.	
4. Pt. has L leg edema.	
5. Pt. demonstrates a significant ↑ in HR c̄ stair climbing.	
6. Pt.'s reflexes are hyperactive.	
7. Pt. doesn't know what's going on.	
8. Pt. has abnormal gait pattern.	
9. Pt. has poor endurance.	
10. Pt. walks c̄ L knee pain.	

CHAPTER 9

Documenting the Assessment: Summary and Diagnosis

LEARNING OBJECTIVES

After reading this chapter and completing the exercises, the reader will be able to:

1. Describe the role of physical therapists in establishing and documenting a diagnosis.

2. Describe the characteristics of the Assessment section of an evaluation report.

3. Appropriately document an Assessment for different case scenarios.

This chapter presents the Assessment section of the initial evaluation documentation by the PT. The assessment is a pivotal section of the initial evaluation. In it, the PT draws on information presented in the previous sections to arrive at a decision regarding the main problems to be addressed and the probable causes of those problems. The sections of the initial evaluation that follow the Assessment are used to propose goals and a plan for achieving those goals.

The Assessment section has three purposes: (1) to provide a summary of the evaluation and the PT's clinical judgments about the case; (2) to confirm, extend or, if necessary, question the referral diagnosis; and (3) to justify the necessity of physical therapy intervention.

The notion that PTs make a diagnosis is an important one and has become more readily accepted within the physical therapy and medical communities. Therefore this chapter begins with an explanation of diagnosis and a consideration of the rationale for diagnosis by PTs. The case examples at the end of this chapter provide sample documentation of the Assessment section in various clinical settings.

Diagnosis by Physical Therapists

DEFINITION OF DIAGNOSIS

The term *diagnosis* refers to both a process and the product of that process. In a general sense, diagnosis as a process is an investigation or analysis of the cause or nature of a condition, situation, or problem. Diagnosis as a product is a statement or conclusion from such an analysis, typically a recognizable label that identifies the nature or the cause of the problem. Thus an auto mechanic can diagnose what is wrong with a car, or an electronics technician can arrive at a diagnosis as to what is wrong with a computer. In medicine, diagnosis has traditionally referred to the act of identifying a disease from its signs and symptoms as well to the decision reached by that process. In medicine the diagnostic label often identifies the pathology or disease process presumed to be the underlying cause of the patient's signs and symptoms.

Diagnosis in physical therapy has been considered controversial because some believe that it should be the sole prerogative of physicians. Indeed, some would argue that PTs do not have the training to make a correct diagnosis of a patient's condition, nor are they able to order and interpret the myriad of tests available to the modern physician. However, this perspective is based on a strict definition of diagnosis—that it is the act of determining the nature and location of a pathologic condition. If a broader view is used—that diagnosis is the process by which any professional, not just a physician, determines the cause of a problem—then the term can be used to describe the process that PTs use to determine the causes of the problems faced by their patients.

DIAGNOSTIC PROCESS

The term *diagnosis* refers to a process that all PTs engage in: the act of evaluating the physical and subjective findings to make a decision about whether physical therapy will be helpful to a patient and, if so, what kind of therapy the patient should receive. The diagnostic process involves making a clinical judgment based on information obtained from history, signs, symptoms, examination, and tests that the therapist performs or requests. Different methods of diagnosis have been advocated; a few are discussed briefly in Figure 9-1 (also see References).

The American Physical Therapy Association's House of Delegates has shifted its position from one that recognizes the right of a PT to make a diagnosis ("may establish" in 1984; APTA HOD, 1984) to one that requires a diagnosis for each patient ("shall establish" in 2007; APTAHOD, 2007) (Box 9-1). However, any diagnosis or classification should be within the legal realm of physical therapy, as defined by state practice acts (Jette, 1990).

Thus the PT has a professional responsibility to engage in the diagnostic process even when the patient has been referred with a diagnosis by a physician. First and foremost, the PT must determine whether the patient's condition is appropriate for physical therapy intervention. Going through the process of determining that a patient's condition is appropriate for physical therapy by ruling out medical conditions that would be inappropriate requires, in effect, that the therapist make a diagnostic decision regarding the nature of the pathology and its severity. Deciding that the pathology causing a patient's pain is not cancer, not myocardial infarction, and not an infection in the kidney requires a diagnostic process in which the nature of the pathology is investigated. (Some use the term *screening* to refer to this process.)

Diagnosis – The Process

Inductive methods

- *Inductive reasoning* – the process of deriving general principles from specific facts or instances

- Clinician infers diagnosis from specific signs and symptoms

Hypothetico-deductive methods

- *Deductive reasoning* – a conclusion follows necessarily from stated premises, inferring specific instances from general principles

- *Hypothesis* – a tentative explanation, a conclusion taken to be true for the sake of argument or investigation, an assumption

- Clinician generates hypothesis – *tentative diagnosis*

- Clinician uses deduction to determine the specific signs or symptoms that should be present

- Clinician tests whether deduced signs or symptoms are actually present

Pattern recognition methods

- *Associative memory* — learned knowledge and experience with other patients: a "mental database" of diagnostic labels and associated signs and symptoms

- Clinician matches a specific pattern of signs and symptoms with patterns in associative memory

FIGURE 9-1 Different methods can be used in the process of formulating a diagnosis.

Resolutions of the American Physical Therapy Association House of Delegates Relevant to Diagnosis

DIAGNOSIS BY PHYSICAL THERAPISTS HOD P06-08-06-07 (Program 32) [Amended HOD P06-97-06-19 HOD 06-95-12-07; HOD 06-94-22-35, Initial HOD 06-84-19-78] [Position]

Physical therapists shall establish a diagnosis for each patient/client. Prior to making a patient/client management decision, physical therapists shall utilize the diagnostic process in order to establish a diagnosis for the specific conditions in need of the physical therapist's attention.

A diagnosis is a label encompassing a cluster of signs and symptoms commonly associated with a disorder or syndrome or category of impairment, functional limitation, or disability. It is the decision reached as a result of the diagnostic process, which is the evaluation of information obtained from the patient/client examination. The purpose of the diagnosis is to guide the physical therapist in determining the most appropriate intervention strategy for each patient/client. In the event the diagnostic process does not yield an identifiable cluster, disorder, syndrome, or category, intervention may be directed toward the alleviation of symptoms and remediation of impairment, functional limitation, or disability.

The diagnostic process includes obtaining relevant history, performing systems review, selecting and administering specific tests and measures, and may include the ordering of tests that are performed and interpreted by other health professionals. The physical therapist's responsibility in the diagnostic process is to organize and interpret all relevant data.

In performing the diagnostic process, physical therapists may need to obtain additional information (including diagnostic labels) from other health professionals. In addition, as the diagnostic process continues, physical therapists may identify findings that should be shared with other health professionals, including referral sources, to ensure optimal patient/client care. When the patient/client is referred with a previously established diagnosis, the physical therapist should determine that the clinical findings are consistent with that diagnosis. If the diagnostic process reveals findings that are outside the scope of the physical therapist's knowledge, experience, or expertise, the physical therapist should then refer the patient/client to an appropriate practitioner.

Thus in all cases the PT is making a diagnostic decision, even though he or she is not actually making the final determination of the diagnostic label.

In addition, in the course of assessing the patient or in review when a patient does not respond to treatment, information is often uncovered that may necessitate modification or rethinking of the original diagnosis. In this case, it is the legal and professional responsibility of the PT to bring this information to the attention of the referring practitioner. This does not mean that the PT is responsible for making the definitive determination of the diagnosis. This will, for the most part, remain the responsibility of the physician, even in direct-access environments. In modern health care environments, where the PT is often one of several specialists seeing a patient, he or she participates in the process and helps the physician reach the correct diagnosis.

DIAGNOSTIC LABELS

Although there is widespread agreement among PTs about the importance of the diagnostic process, real questions exist regarding the form of the result (the diagnostic label). Some have argued that the PT should establish a physical therapy diagnosis separate from the medical diagnosis; we adopted that framework in the first edition of this text. We now believe that such an approach creates confusion. The diagnostic label should be used by PTs as it is ordinarily understood by other health care professionals, that is, as identifying the underlying disease or pathologic process presumed to be responsible for the patient's condition. This is the common understanding of the term used by all health professionals. There are certainly instances in which not enough is known about a condition to specify its cause so precisely. In these cases the diagnostic label will necessarily be descriptive (e.g., a syndrome). Because the diagnostic label often lacks pathologic specificity, Sackett and Haynes (2002) proposed considering the label as identifying the "target disorder," which he defined as "the anatomical, biochemical, physiologic, or psychologic derangement." We refer to this target disorder, the diagnostic label usually determined by the referring physician but often confirmed or extended by the PT, as the *differential diagnosis*.

Besides the overriding concern about preventing confusion, there are also significant positive reasons for using a common diagnostic label. Perhaps most importantly, physicians and other referring professionals need to learn which diagnoses are appropriate for referral to a PT. Physicians will not learn this if PTs use an alternate and essentially exclusive system. By the same token, the reimbursement systems as well as most large outcome databases are inextricably linked to diagnoses (i.e., ICD-9 or ICD-10 codes). Finally, the database of clinical research evidence that PTs both use and contribute to is primarily organized around the pathology-based diagnostic system.

Although in many cases the diagnoses of the physician and PT remain distinct, at times these diagnostic processes overlap. For example, PTs typically perform a general screening (referred to as a *systems review* in the *Guide to Physical Therapist Practice*,

2001) to rule out serious pathologic conditions, such as tumors or heart disease, that are not appropriate for physical therapy intervention. This is sometimes referred to within the physical therapy community as *differential diagnosis*. If evidence of such a pathologic condition is found, the PT must refer the patient to an appropriate practitioner for further testing. This requires the therapist to at least consider the possible pathologic conditions, even if he or she will not verify their presence or absence. Thus specific tests and measures used in the differential diagnosis process must be documented in the evaluation, and any modifications to the medical diagnosis based on a physical therapist's findings that are within his or her legal purview to make, should be documented in the Assessment.

PHYSICAL THERAPY DIAGNOSTIC SYSTEMS

The notion of a physical therapy diagnosis, referred to earlier, arose from the belief by many PTs that the traditional medical diagnosis was not particularly helpful in directing intervention. In this view, the process of diagnosis should involve classifying or labeling the dysfunction—typically at the impairment level or, in ICF terms, at the level of body structure and function. Physical therapy, however, does not yet have generally agreed upon labels or classification systems, although much current research activity is aimed at creating and testing diagnostic systems (Scheets et al., 1999; Delitto and Snyder-Mackler, 1995). At present, two or three different types of systems are used that provide standardized labels or classifications of diagnosis for patients seen by PTs:

1. *Guide to Physical Therapist Practice*, part II: preferred practice patterns (Figure 9-2). The preferred practice patterns defined in the *Guide* are accepted as diagnoses made by physical therapists. These practice patterns encompass many possible ICD-9 diagnoses. They classify patients according to a clustering of impairments and related health conditions.

   Example: Impaired motor function and sensory integrity associated with progressive disorders of the central nervous system

Since their introduction, the preferred practice patterns have not gained widespread acceptance in clinical settings, which may be because these patterns lack specificity. Within each practice pattern, the tests and measures and interventions that can be used are

Musculoskeletal ⟺	Neuromuscular ⟺	Cardiovascular Pulmonary ⟺	Integumentary
Prevention of demineralization	Falls: Prevention	Prevention of CP disorders	Prevention of integumentary disorders
Impaired posture	Impaired neuromotor development	Deconditioning	
Impaired muscle performance	Nonprogressive CNS—congenital	Impaired airway clearance	Prevention of superficial skin disorders
Impaired connective tissue	Nonprogressive CNS—adult	Impaired CV pump	Partial-thickness scar Full-thickness star
Localized inflammation	Progressive CNS	Impaired ventilatory pump	Impaired bone, fascia, and muscle
Spinal disorders	Peripheral nerve injury	Respiratory failure—adult	
Fracture	Acute/chronic polyneuropathy	Respiratory failure—neonate	
Joint arthroplasty	Nonprogressive spinal cord	Impaired lymph	
Bone/tissue surgery			
Amputation	Coma		

FIGURE 9-2 Preferred practice patterns from the *Guide to Physical Therapist Practice* (2001).

virtually identical. Thus categorizing patients into a pattern does little to assist the therapist in treatment planning and clinical decision making.

2. Classification systems. PTs have become the practitioners who have the appropriate training to develop a proper diagnosis of the causes of movement dysfunction. Much research is currently underway to develop diagnostic classification schemes, or treatment-based classifications, for certain patient populations, including stroke (Scheets et al., 2007), low back dysfunction (Delitto et al., 1995; George & Delitto, 2005; Van Dillen et al., 1998), and neck pain (Fritz & Brennan, 2007). The primary purpose of such classification systems is that subgroups of patients can be identified from key history and examination findings, and these subgroups can then be given distinctively different interventions that are specially suited to their condition. The classification of subgroups is based not on health condition, but typically on a combination of findings at the level of impairments and activities.

A very important role of classification in diagnosis is the determination of etiology (literally, what caused the disorder). In many instances, especially when there is a musculoskeletal disorder, the PT must determine whether the patient's abnormal movement or postural patterns caused the disorder or are the result of the disorder. Many current classification systems emphasize this distinction. Other classification schemes are based on what types of treatment approach the disorder is most likely to respond to.

Use of classification systems is still relatively new in regard to research efficacy, but it can have a potentially powerful impact on clinical decision making in physical therapy. With this in mind, we encourage therapists to incorporate this research into clinical practice where appropriate; this is also an area in which continued research is warranted.

3. Disablement systems. Guccione (1991) advocated for diagnosis by PTs to be focused on the relation between impairments and functional limitations, based on the Nagi model. Indeed, we advocated for a similar definition in the first edition of this textbook. With the adoption of the ICF framework and terminology, a more global classification system for considering diagnosis is warranted. We argue that diagnoses within the ICF framework should not just link two of the levels (impairments and activities), but rather include links within all levels of the framework (health condition, body structures and functions, activities and participation, as well as personal and societal factors). Indeed,

it has been recently recommended that enablement models should inform but not constrain any diagnostic descriptors that are developed (Norton, 2007).

HOW TO DOCUMENT THE DIAGNOSIS

Given this complex and evolving landscape of diagnosis by PTs, how should the diagnosis be documented? Think of this statement as more than merely a label; it is the summary of the diagnostic process by the PT. We therefore recommend a three-part diagnostic statement:

1. Differential diagnosis: the health condition or target disorder; may be elaborated on, extended, or questioned.

2. Classification: if possible, include further classification regarding etiology, movement system impairment, or other recognized system.

3. Relation to activity limitations and participation restrictions: how the health condition is affecting or will affect the patient's abilities and roles if untreated.

Table 9-1 shows examples of diagnostic statements. In all cases the differential diagnosis should be identified. In many cases it will involve further specification regarding location or type of tissue involved. Classification is highly recommended, especially regarding etiology. The relation of the health condition to activity and participation should be explicitly stated. Indeed, this is the key component of clinical decision making by the PT.

Assessment Section

ORGANIZATION OF THE ASSESSMENT

The extended discussion of diagnosis in this chapter is necessary because the primary purpose of the Assessment section of the initial evaluation is to present a diagnosis of the patient's problems. In effect, the Assessment presents the outcome of the clinical decision-making process. If the first three sections of the initial evaluation have been developed as proposed in the preceding chapters, then the Assessment should be relatively easy to write. Figure 9-3 reviews the clinical decision-making process and indicates the key elements of the Assessment derived from this process.

It is useful to structure the Assessment as a summary statement, highlighting the key problems along with the diagnosis and adding a statement of the patient's overall prognosis or potential to benefit from physical therapy. One important reason to do this is that some professionals reading the

TABLE 9-1	EXAMPLES OF DIAGNOSES BY PHYSICAL THERAPISTS	
Diagnosis by Physician	**Diagnosis by Physical Therapist**	**Comments**
1. COPD 2° to emphysema with acute pneumonia	Acute: impaired coughing ability resulting in inadequate clearance of airway secretions with potential for fluid accumulation in lungs and infection. Chronic: impaired expiratory control resulting in poor endurance during upper extremity functional activities, esp. dressing.	Note that in the acute case the primary problem is to prevent secondary complications that might exacerbate the primary pathologic condition. In the chronic case, the problem is functional and cause is at the impairment level.
2. s/p Medial meniscus tear R knee	Acute: joint effusion, pain, and limitation in ROM of right knee resulting in potential muscle atrophy and prolongation of healing. Chronic: pain and limitation of ROM of right knee, knee extensor weakness resulting in difficulty in walking and climbing stairs.	The acute case illustrates a common characteristic of orthopedic physical therapy: in the early states of recovery, the "problem" often is how best to promote healing and prevent secondary complications, or how to return patient to previous level of activity without harming and allowing repair to heal.
3. s/p Total hip arthroplasty in RLE 2° to osteoarthritis	Acute: general weakness; poor transfer and walking skills with immediate risk of complications due to inadequate mobilization. Chronic: longstanding limitation in hip ROM and strength; habitual Trendelenburg-type gait deviation with resulting poor endurance and limited maneuverability in walking.	In the acute case, the immediate problem is how to mobilize the patient and to prevent secondary complications. The diagnosis also addresses participation by specifying when patient will be able to function in home.
4. Left middle cerebral artery stroke	Left-sided stroke with 1° impairment of residual force production deficit resulting in impaired mobility and standing balance.	This case identifies a primary impairment (force production deficit) that, in the therapist's opinion, is the primary contributor to the patient's activity limitations (impaired mobility and standing balance) (Scheets et al., 2007).
5. R shoulder pain, possible supraspinatus tendonitis	Medical diagnosis of R shoulder pain is further defined to include supraspinatus impingement leading to supraspinatus tendinosis. Pain, muscle weakness, restricted shoulder ROM, and crepitus result in limitations in performing overhead activities and difficulty sleeping.	In this case, the medical diagnosis is nonspecific. Diagnosis may be stated directly or alternatively documented as further defining the medical diagnosis.
6. Low back pain with L4-5 herniated disk	L4-5 hypermobility with hip joint hypomobility; exacerbation of pain symptoms with flexion movements; muscle spasms and pain limit patient's sitting tolerance and prevent patient from working in full capacity. Treatment-based classification: extension syndrome.	In this case, the diagnosis is further clarified by the results of the PT's examination findings. A treatment-based classification system is used to categorize the patient for treatment purposes (George & Delitto, 2005).

evaluation will skip directly to the Assessment. In addition, it is often useful to have a succinct summary statement ready to insert directly for letters to referral sources or insurance companies. For this reason, it is important to minimize the use of abbreviations and provide clear, unambiguous statements in this section.

When structured as a summary statement, the Assessment section includes three specific components, as follows.

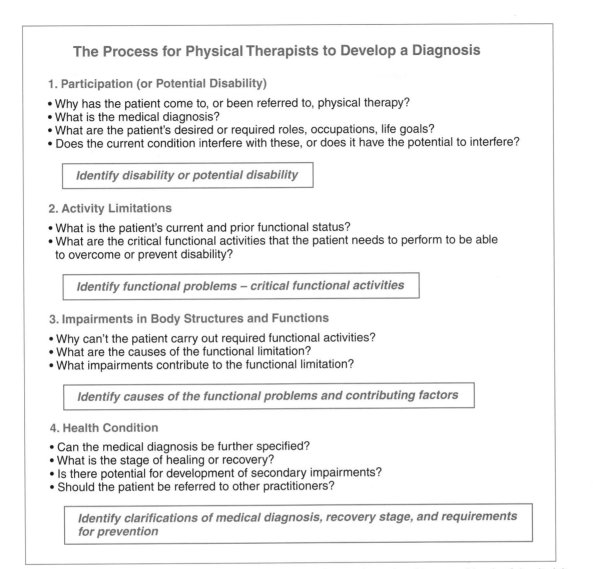

The Process for Physical Therapists to Develop a Diagnosis

1. Participation (or Potential Disability)

- Why has the patient come to, or been referred to, physical therapy?
- What is the medical diagnosis?
- What are the patient's desired or required roles, occupations, life goals?
- Does the current condition interfere with these, or does it have the potential to interfere?

> *Identify disability or potential disability*

2. Activity Limitations

- What is the patient's current and prior functional status?
- What are the critical functional activities that the patient needs to perform to be able to overcome or prevent disability?

> *Identify functional problems – critical functional activities*

3. Impairments in Body Structures and Functions

- Why can't the patient carry out required functional activities?
- What are the causes of the functional limitation?
- What impairments contribute to the functional limitation?

> *Identify causes of the functional problems and contributing factors*

4. Health Condition

- Can the medical diagnosis be further specified?
- What is the stage of healing or recovery?
- Is there potential for development of secondary impairments?
- Should the patient be referred to other practitioners?

> *Identify clarifications of medical diagnosis, recovery stage, and requirements for prevention*

FIGURE 9-3   The process of developing a physical therapy diagnosis involves analysis of problems at all levels of the disability model.

Three Components of the Assessment

1. **Summary statement:** The introductory sentence should briefly describe the patient and summarize the background information.
2. **Diagnosis:** Next, state the differential diagnosis or health condition along with further classification. It may be necessary here to present an alternative to the referring diagnosis, along with a rationale. Finally, describe the patient's activity limitations, key impairments contributing to those limitations, and participation restrictions or potential participation restrictions that will result from those limitations.
3. **Potential to benefit from physical therapy:** Conclude with a statement summarizing the patient's potential to benefit from physical therapy and the reasons why treatment is or is not indicated. This can include a summary of the types of interventions that the patient would be benefit from.

The Assessment section is the appropriate place to provide specification of the nature and location of the health condition if the PT's examination has revealed this information. The stage of recovery or healing is almost always relevant to the overall assessment. In addition, the PT must always be alert to the possibility of secondary impairments that might develop as a result of the original health condition. These secondary impairments may in turn exacerbate the health condition or produce new disorders. It is appropriate to document these risks in the Assessment section.

The Assessment section also serves an important function to summarize the medical necessity for intervention (see Chapter 15). If there is a medical necessity for physical therapy intervention, it is important to state that the patient "requires" physical therapy services rather than "would benefit" from these services. As seen in the case examples at the end of this chapter, and in Chapter 4, all Assessments end with a similar statement that addresses medical necessity.

Examples of Assessment sections documented as part of an initial evaluation are included at the end of this chapter. Keep in mind that these are presented as summary statements; in many instances it is acceptable to leave out the information that has already been presented in other sections of the initial evaluation.

Common Pitfalls in Assessment Documentation

There are several common pitfalls in writing the Assessment section. These usually result from an overly general or vague statement. For example:

> *Pt. has ↓ strength and ROM, which is leading to limitations in ADL.*

The problem here is somewhat obvious. This statement could apply to approximately 90% of all patients seen by a physical therapist. The statement should be more specific:

> *Weakness in knee and hip extensors and limitation in hip extension PROM prevent Pt. from being able to perform bed mobility and transfers independently.*

Another common example of an overly general statement is the following:

> *Pt. is a good rehab candidate.*

This does not sound so bad until we imagine the converse statement:

> *Pt. is a poor rehab candidate.*

Neither of these statements is particularly helpful. What is meant by "good" or "poor"? Both statements merely label the patient, the latter in a way that seems unfair and arbitrary. A better approach is to state more objectively what specific functional limitations might be remediated by a course of rehabilitation therapy. For example:

> *Pt. requires 6-8 sessions of strengthening exercises and functional training to become sufficiently skilled in transfers and self-care to function independently at home.*

This statement merely implies that the patient is a "good" candidate for rehabilitation because he or she will benefit from it.

If the patient will not likely benefit from further rehabilitation, a clear reason should be given. For example:

> *Pt. has insufficient voluntary movement in fingers of right hand to benefit from therapy to increase usage of right arm.*

Or:

> *Pt. is no longer showing improvement in walking velocity and will therefore not benefit from further therapy related to this functional goal.*

In general, it is probably not a good idea to make blanket statements about the rehabilitation potential of any patient. Instead, limit statements about prognosis to specific functions for which there is clear evidence one way or the other.

Summary

- The Assessment section of the initial evaluation is used to summarize the findings of the evaluation and to present the diagnosis.

- The diagnostic process by PTs has three components: (1) confirmation of the health condition or target disorder; (2) classification by etiology, movement system, or treatment response; and (3) determination of the fundamental relations among health condition, impairments, activity limitations, and participation restrictions as well as contributions of personal and societal factors.

- In addition to the diagnosis, the Assessment section is often structured as a summary statement, restating the diagnosis, highlighting key problems, and making a general statement regarding the patient's need for physical therapy.

CASE EXAMPLE 9-1

Documenting Assessment
Setting: Inpatient Rehabilitation

Name: Jose Martinez   **D.O.B.:** 8/31/85   **Date of Eval.:** 10/5/09

CURRENT CONDITION: 6 wk s/p TBI 2° to MVA

ASSESSMENT

Pt. is a 24 y.o. male 6 wk s/p TBI and has residual cognitive and motor impairments. Pt. is impulsive, confused, and becomes agitated easily. His memory deficits limit his cognitive abilities as well and learning new tasks is difficult. These cognitive impairments, in conjunction with L-sided weakness and spasticity, have led to limitations in pt.'s ability to safely and independently perform tasks related to bed mobility, self-care, transfers, and wheelchair mobility. Pt. also presents with impaired proactive and reactive standing balance, which is the primary factor limiting his ambulation ability at this time. Before injury, the patient was a full-time student, living with his family, and he enjoyed active leisure activities. His residual cognitive and motor limitations have led to safety concerns and lack of independence in functional abilities and significant limitations in social, personal, and occupational life roles. Pt. requires intensive 1:1 6 days/wk b.i.d. physical therapy to address the above-stated impairments and activity limitations in light of his cognitive and behavioral impairments.

CASE EXAMPLE 9-2

Documenting Assessment
Setting: Inpatient Acute Care

Name: Jessie Goldstein   **D.O.B.:** 2/3/47   **Date of Eval.:** 5/31/09

CURRENT CONDITION: s/p radical hysterectomy 5/29/02 2° to cervical CA

ASSESSMENT

Pt. is a 62 y.o. woman s/p radical hysterectomy 2° to cervical CA. Incision site is healing well, but pt. reports significant pain and discomfort in abdominal area. Pt. has limitations in trunk mobility and abdominal strength 2° to surgery. These impairments are limiting pt.'s independence in bed mobility, transfers, and ambulation as well as overall comfort in a sitting and supine position. Pt. requires short-duration physical therapy to improve overall strength and endurance, education regarding appropriate mobility and pain management techniques, and instruction in home program to facilitate recovery.

CASE EXAMPLE 9-3

Documenting Assessment
Setting: Health/Wellness Center

Name: Emily Ko   **D.O.B.:** 9/1/24   **Date of Eval.:** 12/2/09

CURRENT CONDITION: Pt. is 85 y.o. female self-referred for Falls Risk Assessment; hx of 2 falls in past month

ASSESSMENT

Pt. is an 85 y.o. female referred for a falls risk assessment. Pt. presents with deconditioning, generalized weakness, and poor proactive balance. In addition, pt.'s scores on Berg Balance Scale and Timed Up and Go are indicative of high risk for falls. Pt. is at risk for declining independence and limitations in functional activities and is at significant risk for falls during dynamic activities such as reaching, walking, or turning. Pt. requires PT intervention to address these specific impairments and functional limitations and to receive education about fall risk prevention.

EXERCISE 9-1

In each of the following cases a therapist's rough notes appear in the left column. Using these as a guide, formulate a plausible Assessment that includes (1) a summary statement, (2) diagnosis, and (3) potential for physical therapy. It may be necessary to refer to other diagnosis-specific resources to create the most clinically accurate assessment. Refer to Case Examples and guidelines in this chapter as needed.

CASE INFORMATION	ASSESSMENT
Case 1: Outpatient	
59 y.o. man, s/p R THR 2° to osteoarthritis, 3 wk previous. Pt. past acute stage; no significant pain or swelling; incision well healed.	
PARTICIPATION: Sales representative, travels by car, unable to work since surgery.	
ACTIVITY LIMITATIONS: Needs assist for transfers into car, walks slowly with walker, up to 100 ft at a time, needs assist on steps.	
IMPAIRMENTS: Weakness in R hip flexors, abductors, and extensors; habitual gait deviations from preop antalgic gait. R hip √ and abduction ROM limited.	

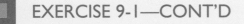 EXERCISE 9-1—CONT'D

CASE INFORMATION	ASSESSMENT

Case 2: Outpatient

43 y.o. female with MS diagnosed 3 yr previous; recovering from recent exacerbation.

PARTICIPATION: Clerical worker in major downtown office building; rides train and bus to work; resists using cane. Pt. is fearful of falling during commute and needs extra time during commute.

ACTIVITY LIMITATIONS: Requires assist to go up and down steps; walks slowly; walking difficulties exacerbated in crowded places.

IMPAIRMENTS: Only mild weakness; standing balance easily disturbed, esp. when patient is distracted.

Case 3: Inpatient*

48 y.o. woman admitted to an acute care hospital with complaints of severe abdominal pain, diminished appetite with nausea and diarrhea for 4 days. PMH, end-stage liver disease; liver transplant 4 yr ago, end-stage renal disease with hemodialysis 2×/wk hypertension and sacral pressure sore onset ×4 mo.

ACTIVITY LIMITATIONS: Mobility limited to wheelchair. Mod. to maximal assistance for all bed mobility and transfers.

IMPAIRMENTS: Posture: The supine position most frequently observed was with the head of bed elevated >6°. Muscle strength –2+/5 gross lower extremity strength, 3–/5 gross upper extremity strength. Wound: 3.7 × 3.4 cm with 2-3 cm of undermining; 85% yellow rubbery eschar; 15% red granulation.

EXERCISE 9-1—CONT'D

CASE INFORMATION	ASSESSMENT

Case 4: Outpatient

39 y.o. female $\bar{c}$ diagnosis of cervical strain. Onset of symptoms occurred 6 wk ago.

PARTICIPATION: CPA at local firm, currently unable to tolerate typical 8-10 hr work day 2° to symptoms. Majority of time typically spent on phone and computer.

ACTIVITY LIMITATIONS: Occasionally requires pain medication to assist with sleeping at night. Unable to talk on phone 2° to pain with phone cradling position. Unable to tolerate computer work >2 hr 2° to increased pain.

IMPAIRMENTS: Static sitting posture presents with a decrease in cervical lordosis and an increase in thoracic kyphosis. Limited AROM with R-side flexion and rotation at C-spine. Flexed, rotated, and sidebent left at C5 and C6. Weakness in bilateral lower trapezius: 3/5, bilateral middle trapezius/rhomboids: 4/5, and cervical extensors: 3+/5. Pain rated as 3/10 at rest and 6/10 after working 2 hr; described as throbbing and occasionally shooting.

Case 5: Inpatient Rehabilitation, Burn Center[†]

23 y.o. female college student sustained 11% TBSA full-thickness scald burn to right anterior thigh, anterior lower leg, and dorsal foot. s/p skin grafting surgery to excise burn eschar and skin graft the wound 5 days ago.

PARTICIPATION: Previously active in playing tennis weekly. Full-time graduate student; lives in apartment with 2 roommates; elevator to enter, all living on one floor.

ACTIVITY LIMITATIONS: Able to amb. independently 20 ft in 19.5 sec; step to gait; Tinetti Gait assessment 7/12. Stands independently without support; independent and safe with transfers.

IMPAIRMENTS: 11% TBSA, full-thickness burns to right anterior thigh, anterior lower leg, dorsal foot; potential for scarring after healing/surgery. Pain in right lower extremity 4/10 at rest, with movement 6/10. ROM: R knee ext/flex 0-90°; right ankle dorsiflexion 5°, plantar flexion 20°. Edema noted right lower extremity.

---

*Adapted from Hamm RL: Tissue healing and pressure ulcers. In Cameron M, Monroe LG, editors: *Physical rehabilitation: evidence-based examination, evaluation, and intervention,* Philadelphia, 2007, Saunders Elsevier.

†Adapted from Ward RS: Burns. In Cameron M, Monroe LG, editors: *Physical rehabilitation: evidence-based examination, evaluation, and intervention.* Philadelphia, 2007, Saunders Elsevier.

CHAPTER 10

Documenting Goals

LEARNING OBJECTIVES

After reading this chapter and completing the exercises, the reader will be able to:

1. Describe the important aspects of writing goals at the participation, activity, and impairment levels.

2. Distinguish between short-term and long-term goals.

3. Describe the essential components of a well-written functional goal.

4. Identify poorly written goals and make modifications to goals.

5. Appropriately document participation, activity, and impairment goals for a written report.

This chapter presents the Goals section of the initial evaluation. Establishing anticipated goals and expected outcomes is a critical part of the process of establishing a plan of care for a patient and is one of the cornerstones of physical therapy documentation. *The Guide to Physical Therapist Practice* (APTA, 2001, p. S38) defines anticipated goals and expected outcomes as

> ...intended results of patient/client management that indicate the changes in impairment, functional limitations and disabilities, and the changes in health, wellness and fitness needs that are expected as the result of implementing the plan of care. [They] also address risk reduction, prevention, impact on societal resources and patient/client satisfaction. The anticipated goals and expected outcomes in the plan should be measurable and time limited.

PTs, in collaboration with patients, set *goals* designed to measure progress toward specific *expected outcomes*. Therefore the term *goal* is used throughout this book to document this process. Through documentation of these goals, therapists express their knowledge of a patient's specific problems, formulate the prognosis, and provide the foundation for developing an intervention plan specific to the individual patient's needs.

Three important aspects about the process of setting expected outcomes should be emphasized. First, in establishing goals, the PT makes a professional judgment about the *prognosis*, that is, the likelihood of functional recovery. The prognosis is, in effect, a prediction about the future, and therefore it depends on a very high level of skill, knowledge, and experience. Nevertheless, it should not be assumed that establishing a prognosis requires years of experience. Indeed, one of the most beneficial aspects of evidence-based practice is the increased availability of information about prognosis.

Second, the process of setting goals is a collaborative effort between the therapist and the patient and often the patient's family and other professionals. Randall and McEwen (2000) have developed this point cogently. They have proposed a method for writing goals that is very similar to the one proposed in this textbook. The term *patient-centered* is especially useful because it emphasizes that successful therapy mandates that the goals be focused on what the patient wants to accomplish. As they comment, "For goals to be truly patient-centered, they should be relevant to the patient's desired outcomes, not to what the therapist thinks is 'best' for the patient" (Randall & McEwen, 2000).

Third, goals should guide the therapeutic process throughout its course. If rehabilitation is perceived as a journey, goals are a statement of the destination that the patient and the PT are attempting to reach. For goals to function effectively as a guide they should be referred to during every treatment session, and between sessions as well, as the patient implements his or her "home program." Thus the goals are not simply documented during the initial evaluation; they should be referred to or addressed in every treatment or progress note. A method for doing this using the SOAP note format is presented in Chapter 12. Case Examples 10-1, 10-2, and 10-3 at the end of this chapter provide sample documentation of goals written in initial evaluation reports in various clinical settings.

A Traditional Approach: Short-Term and Long-Term Goals

The traditional approach to documenting goals has been to distinguish between short- and long-term goals. Here the distinction is based primarily on the time course of rehabilitation. For example, a typical long-term goal might be:

> Patient will walk independently for distances up to 1000 ft outdoors without assistive devices within 1 month.

A short-term goal related to this long-term goal might be:

> Patient will walk 200 ft on level surfaces indoors with quad cane and requiring contact guarding within 1 wk.

Thus the concept of a short-term goal is that it is an intermediate step toward achieving the long-term goal. This approach can be useful, especially in rehabilitation settings where treatment may continue for an extended period (see Case Example 10-1). However, with changes in the health care system and especially in payment policy, patients are less likely to be treated over an extended period by a PT. A notable exception is pediatric school-based therapy, where children are often seen over the course of a year. In this situation, long-term goals and short-term objectives are typically written (see Chapter 14).

Writing Goals at Three Different Levels

Although in certain instances establishment of short-term intermediate goals helps to provide a guiding framework for a complex course of rehabilitation, this text advocates a different approach in which the therapist establishes expected outcomes at three different levels: participation goals, activity goals, and impairment goals.

PARTICIPATION GOALS

Participation goals express the expected outcomes in terms of the specific roles in which the patient wishes to be able to participate. These goals provide the "big picture"—what is the overall purpose of the physical therapy intervention? The participation goal for one patient may be to return to work, for another to be able to care for her children, for a third to be able to go to church.

ACTIVITY (OR FUNCTIONAL) GOALS

Activity goals express the expected outcomes in terms of the skills needed to participate in necessary or desired roles. Activity goals are the key component of any goal section and they should never be omitted. For example, an activity goal may be to walk from the bed to the bathroom, to put on a shirt, or to drink from a cup. Because of their importance, activity goals are the focus of much of this chapter.

IMPAIRMENT GOALS (OPTIONAL)

Impairment goals express the expected outcomes in terms of the specific impairments in body structures or functions that contribute to the functional limitations. Although the emphasis in this text is on writing activity or functional goals, in some situations one or more goals of therapy involve reduction or elimination of impairments. Therefore in such cases explicit setting of impairment goals is reasonable so that outcomes can be monitored. For example, an impairment goal may be to achieve 4/5 strength in the quadriceps, increase range of motion (ROM) of knee flexion to 110°, or improve symmetry of step length during gait. Impairment goals also may be viewed as short-term goals used as benchmarks on the way to attaining activity goals. These goals are particularly important for patients who may have serious activity limitations, such as immediately after a stroke or spinal cord injury. Changes in impairments, such as strength, may be the only immediate demonstration of improvement in the patient's status, and therefore they may be more sensitive indicators of progress. The goal of therapy is then for the improvements in impairments to ultimately result in improved functional activities.

Linking Impairment and Activity Goals

Impairment goals must always be linked to the activity goals in some way. This linkage should be explicitly stated in the Assessment section. Sometimes therapists link an impairment goal to a activity goal when they are writing the goal. For example, "Pt. will increase knee flex ROM from 85° to 95° so that patient can rise from a seated position" (93° of knee flexion is required for rising from a seated position; Laubenthal, 1972).

Although this is an acceptable strategy that is often recommended, it may be more concise and clear to simply write a functional goal related to reaching items in tall cabinets. The increase in shoulder flexion may or may not be an important impairment/short-term goal, depending on the factors contributing to the activitiy limitation. A primary reason that such goals often are not useful is that typically more than one impairment contributes to an activity limitation. In the previous example the patient may have a strength deficit in addition to loss of ROM in the shoulder. Thus the patient could attain the goal of improving ROM in the shoulder, but if strength was not improved, the patient would still not be able to reach items in a tall cabinet. The discussion of the often complex link between any observed limitations and impairments may therefore be more appropriate for the Assessment section.

In summary, the focus of therapy should almost always be on achieving meaningful activities, and reaching the impairment goals should be subordinate to attaining the activity goals.

Fundamentals of Well-Written Functional Goals

Skillful goal writing is deceptively difficult; the PT easily may fall victim to several pitfalls. Therefore the process of learning how to write goals begins by defining the fundamental characteristics of goals and illustrating some of the pitfalls.

GOALS ARE OUTCOMES, NOT PROCESSES

The single most important characteristic of goals is that they are outcomes, not processes. This is also the characteristic that is most often forgotten, especially by beginning students. A goal is something that the *patient*, not the PT, will do. The goal defines an end state, not the process that results in that state. The following is an example of a poorly written goal:

> *Pt. will be taught proper precautions following hip replacement surgery.*

This is not a goal, but a plan for achieving the goal. The goal is for the patient to know the precautions, which can be incorporated into a goal, such as follows:

> *Pt. will be able to state proper hip replacement precautions.*

A better, more specific goal would be as follows:

> *Pt. will be able to demonstrate proper hip replacement precautions during bed mobility, sitting, and transfer tasks.*

The use of *able to* in these statements is an excellent way to ensure that the goal is defining an end state—that is, an ability or skill. However, it is not essential in writing the goal. The previous goal could be written without those words, as in the following example:

> *Pt. will demonstrate proper hip replacement precautions during bed mobility, sitting, and transfer tasks.*

If the patient demonstrates the precautions, it can be assumed that he or she is "able to." Nevertheless, often the PT should at least mentally include the words "able to," especially if the therapist is unsure whether the goal is being properly stated.

GOALS SHOULD BE CONCRETE, NOT ABSTRACT

One of the most challenging aspects of writing goals is expressing them in concrete terms. The following goal highlights this challenge:

> *Pt. will demonstrate increased control during reaching movements…*

This statement is hopelessly general and abstract. What is meant by "control during reaching movements"? Ideally, goals should be stated in terms of an action or functional task that the individual will perform and must include a concretely stated outcome, such as:

> *Pt. will reach to pick up a cup…*

Too often goals are written in such general terms as to be almost useless. For example, the following goals, written in clinical shorthand, are poorly written:

> *Ind. ambulation*
>
> *Ind. ADL*
>
> *Functional strength in UEs*

Such goals should be avoided in favor of measuring performance on concrete, specific tasks or activities.

WELL-WRITTEN GOALS ARE MEASURABLE AND TESTABLE

A goal should be stated in such a way that the measurement or testing procedure is explicit. The following goal is neither measurable nor testable:

> *Good sitting balance*

One of (many) problems with this goal is that it is unclear how sitting balance will be tested. In particular, use of terms such as *good, fair,* and *poor* is not recommended because these terms usually imply something different for each person. A better way to write the goal is as follows:

> *Pt. will be able to sit unsupported on the edge of a mat table for up to 1 minute…*

Here the goal is stated in such a way that the test is embedded in the goal itself. One of the reasons goals are so important is that they provide a way of determining whether progress is being made in therapy. Therefore frequent testing is essential.

GOALS ARE PREDICTIVE

Setting goals requires therapists to generate a prediction. The goal states that the patient will be able to accomplish something in the future that he or she cannot accomplish now. The prediction must be feasible and at the same time challenging. The therapist must also set a specific time within which this goal will be reached. As noted earlier, this aspect is especially challenging for student PTs who have little or no previous experience. Two suggestions may help for students dealing with this problem. First, the rehabilitation literature is an excellent starting point for researching typical times required for achieving certain functional outcomes. Second, goals are not written in stone. As a patient progresses in a rehabilitation program, it is appropriate for goals to be revised to reflect the patient's current status and projected capabilities.

The predictions that therapists make in setting goals will therefore not be perfectly accurate because individual patients differ from each other and from the average results in clinical studies. In general, it is better to err on the side of being too optimistic, expecting a bit more from the patients than they may be capable of achieving. If the PT is wrong, then the consequence is that patients do not quite make it, but they are (usually) no worse than if more modest goals had been set. If, on the other hand, the PT errs on the side of being too conservative in setting a patient's goals, the consequence may be that the patient does not accomplish what he or she is capable of. This approach does not advocate unrealistic optimism in setting goals but instead reflects a preference to challenge patients.

GOALS ARE DETERMINED IN COLLABORATION WITH THE PATIENT AND THE PATIENT'S FAMILY OR CAREGIVERS

Collaboration with the patient and his or her family or caregiver is the most obvious of the fundamental characteristics of goals and yet is the most consistently violated principle. Too often the therapist develops a set of goals at the time of writing the initial evaluation, but because the patient is not present at the time, the therapist assumes that these are the goals most important to the patient. Even more

detrimental to the rehabilitation process is that the patient may not even be told what the goals are, or they are related only in the most general terms. If the goal is for the patient to be able to walk 500 feet in 2 minutes, this goal should have been determined in collaboration with the patient. When patients are aware of the specific aspects of a goal, they often are more dedicated to achieving that goal, and may even work on it on their own time.

A Formula for Writing Goals

Goals have a specific structure, and the first step in learning to write goals is to learn to apply this structure in the process. Applying the principles developed in this chapter, a goal has five necessary components:

1. Who will accomplish the goal (Actor)
2. The action that the individual will be able to perform (Behavior)
3. The circumstances under which the behavior is carried out (Condition)
4. A quantitative specification of performance (Degree)
5. The period within which the goal will be achieved (Expected Time).

These components of a goal and examples are explained further in Figure 10-1. This formula is adapted from a scheme originally developed by Kettenbach (2003).

The five components shown in Figure 10-1 are most readily applied to documentation of activity goals. Some of these components are not pertinent when writing disability or impairment goals (covered later in this chapter). Nevertheless, all properly written activity goals should include all five components. Thus the following formula can be applied to writing an activity goal:

$$Goal = A + B + C + D + E$$

Using this formula, the following goal might be constructed:

> *Mr. McCarthy* (Actor) *will walk* (Behavior) *on level surfaces with a walker* (Conditions) *and min A* (Degree) *for a distance of 100 ft in 2 min (Degree) within 1 wk* (Expected Time).

This goal can easily be modified by substituting different components as follows:

> *Mr. McCarthy will walk on level surfaces with a walker and min A for a distance of 500 ft in 5 minutes* (different Degree) *within 2 wk* (different Expected Time).

Or:

> *Mr. McCarthy will walk outdoors on uneven surfaces with a cane* (different Conditions) *and min A for a distance of 100 ft in 2 min within 1 wk.*

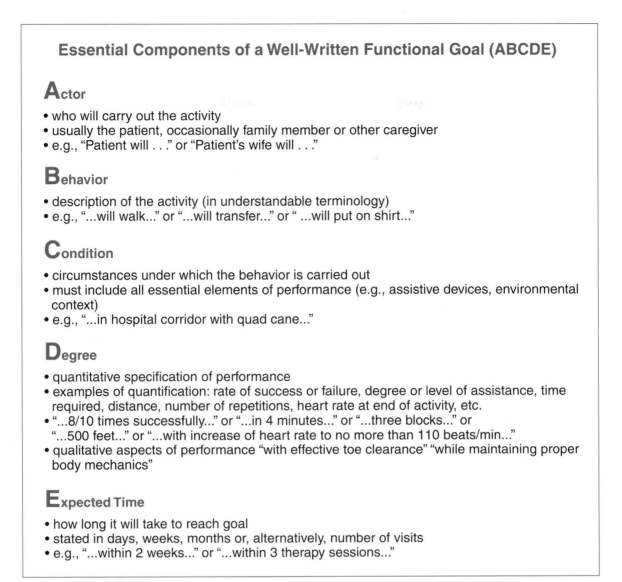

Essential Components of a Well-Written Functional Goal (ABCDE)

Actor

- who will carry out the activity
- usually the patient, occasionally family member or other caregiver
- e.g., "Patient will . . ." or "Patient's wife will . . ."

Behavior

- description of the activity (in understandable terminology)
- e.g., "...will walk..." or "...will transfer..." or " ...will put on shirt..."

Condition

- circumstances under which the behavior is carried out
- must include all essential elements of performance (e.g., assistive devices, environmental context)
- e.g., "...in hospital corridor with quad cane..."

Degree

- quantitative specification of performance
- examples of quantification: rate of success or failure, degree or level of assistance, time required, distance, number of repetitions, heart rate at end of activity, etc.
- "...8/10 times successfully..." or "...in 4 minutes..." or "...three blocks..." or "...500 feet..." or "...with increase of heart rate to no more than 110 beats/min..."
- qualitative aspects of performance "with effective toe clearance" "while maintaining proper body mechanics"

Expected Time

- how long it will take to reach goal
- stated in days, weeks, months or, alternatively, number of visits
- e.g., "...within 2 weeks..." or "...within 3 therapy sessions..."

FIGURE 10-1 Essential components of a well-written goal (ABCDE). (Modified from Kettenbach G: *Writing SOAP notes*, ed 3, Philadelphia, 2003, FA Davis.)

Thus a wide range of goals can be constructed by mixing and matching the different components. The benefits of this approach are twofold. First, goals will be properly written, that is, not missing any essential components. Second, this approach is designed to encourage functionally oriented goals because the focus is on the patient and the action or activity he or she will be performing.

TIME-SAVING STRATEGIES

Writing goals, particularly writing well-written goals, can be very time consuming. One strategy that therapists can use to write goals more efficiently is to use a table format. Table 10-1 provides an example of outcome goals listed in such a format. In this table, several shortcuts have been taken. First, the Actor is omitted (because it is assumed to be the patient).

However, each of the goals lists a Behavior, Condition, Degree, and Expected Time. In addition, a rationale is provided for each goal, providing further clarification for third-party payers. Second, by eliminating full sentences for the goals, fewer words are written, thus saving a significant amount of time. Note that in this table the goals are still patient centered and not generalized goals that could be applied to any patient.

The Art of Writing Patient-Centered Goals: Going Beyond the Formula

If the writing of good documentation can be said to be an art, then it is in the writing of goals that the artistry is expressed. The therapist must rise above the formula and create goals, in collaboration with the patient,

TABLE 10-1	A TABLE USED IN AN OUTPATIENT PHYSICAL THERAPY CLINIC TO DOCUMENT FUNCTIONAL ACTIVITY GOALS FOR A PATIENT			
Activity	Target Performance	Rationale	Method of Assessment	Due Date
Pain-free sitting	45 min	To allow for community transportation	Patient report	14 days
Pain-free side lying	Up to 8 hr	To allow for restful sleep	Patient report	7 days
Even-terrain ambulation	45 min pain-free	To allow for community and household ambulation	Patient report	14 days
Uneven-terrain ambulation	20-25 ft	To maximize safety with community amublation	Observation	21 days
Stair climbing	20 stairs ascend and descend without railing	To allow for independent household ambulation	Observation and patient report	21 days

Adapted from Fearon H, Levine SM, Lee GR: APTA Audio Conference Presentation, March 26, 2009.

that will guide the therapeutic process toward the best possible outcome. The key to creating artful goals is to make them *patient-centered*. A patient-centered goal is one expressed in terms of specific activities that are meaningful to the patient. The first step is to start with a fairly generic but still acceptable goal:

> Pt. will walk on level surfaces with a walker and min A for a distance of 100 ft in 2 min within 1 wk.

The goal can be reformulated so that it is more patient-centered as follows:

> Pt. will walk from his bedroom to his kitchen with a walker and his wife's assistance in 2 min within 1 wk.

A simple change makes the goal much more meaningful to the individual. Another example starts with a fairly generic goal:

> Pt. will feed herself independently within 1 wk.

Again, the goal can be reformulated in a way that is more patient-centered:

> Pt. will eat full bowl of dry cereal and milk c̄ a spoon using R hand in 10 min within 1 wk.

Of course, the assumption here is that Ms. Henry wants to be able to eat cereal in the morning. The patient-centered goal, in addition to being more relevant to the patient, is intrinsically more testable and measurable.

Randall and McEwen (2000) state that the main reason for writing patient-centered functional goals is that "people are likely to make the greatest gains when therapy and the related goals focus on activities that are related to them and that make a difference in their lives." The key to this is taking the time to discuss the goals with the patient so that the goals are formulated in terms that are meaningful to him or her. Then the goal is stated in as concrete a manner as possible.

Determining Expected Times for Goals

Determining the appropriate expected time frames for a goal can be particularly challenging. Inevitably, the PT makes an educated guess about how the health condition, medical history, and many other factors will affect how quickly a patient will achieve a goal. Although determining expected time frames can be highly subjective, PTs should use current research and their clinical experience and judgment to determine the most reasonable time frame.

Expected time frames are typically written in weeks. In certain settings where the length of stay is typically short, such as acute care hospital settings, goals can be set in terms of days. Time frames can also be written in terms of number of PT sessions by which they are likely to be achieved (e.g., *Pt. will walk 200 ft in hospital corridor c̄ min A within 6 sessions*).

Choosing Which Goals to Measure: Prioritizing and Benchmarking

As with documentation of activities, choosing which goals to measure can be tricky. Sometimes it is relatively straightforward. If the patient's primary functional problems are related to pain while walking, the focus of the activity goals will be on walking. However, sometimes there are many different goals that can be chosen. In these situations, two specific strategies can be implemented for choosing appropriate goals: prioritizing and benchmarking.

PRIORITIZING GOALS

Take, for example, the case of a patient who is acutely ill in the hospital who is currently dependent in all activities of daily living and requires maximal assistance for bed mobility, transfers, and standing. In such a situation, a therapist should probably not choose the task of walking down the hall as the first goal. First, the therapist must, in coordination with the patient and his or her family, prioritize the patient's needs. In this situation, establishing a goal of independent bed mobility and transition to sitting may be a more appropriate early goal.

BENCHMARKING

As discussed in Chapter 7, benchmark activities are those that are amenable to showing improvement as a result of physical therapy intervention. Therapists can thus choose benchmark goals, which will differ depending on the patient and his or her stage of learning. Simple tasks like transfers may be most useful early in rehabilitation, whereas more complex tasks like shopping or preparing meals are usually more appropriate later.

Writing Participation and Impairment Goals

In this chapter, most of the discussion has focused on techniques that are appropriate for writing activity goals. Factors that should be considered when the PT writes participation goals and impairment goals are now considered.

PARTICIPATION GOALS

Generally, participation goals can and should be written just as activity goals are written. The difference is that the activity that is the subject of the goal is stated in more general terms (overall participation in work, home, recreation, etc.) than it would be in an activity goal, where the focus is on performing specific tasks or skills. The following statements are examples of participation goals.

Example 1: *Mr. Rasheed* (A) *will return to work* (B) *as a bus driver* (C) *able to accomplish all regular duties* (D) *within 1 month* (E).

Example 2: *Ms. Loring* (A) *will take care* (B) *of her two children at home* (C) *without daytime assistance* (D) *within 2 months* (E).

Example 3: *Mr. Fox* (A) *will attend* (B) *church services* (C) *daily* (D) *within 6 wk* (E).

Example 4: *Ms. Samson* (A) *will return* (B) *to jogging for fitness and recreation* (C) *4×/wk* (D) *within 2 months* (E).

In participation goals, the Condition typically clarifies the nature of the activity or activities. These goals make little sense if they are not followed up by activity goals that detail the specific skills needed to fulfill these roles. It may not always be the case that the activity goals will directly lead to the participation goal. The participation goal may be a goal that is not attainable for several months, which may be beyond the patient's expected duration of treatment in the current setting. This is illustrated in Case Example 10-3. In this case, the patient will likely undergo two separate episodes of PT—one immediately after the accident (for which the goals are listed), which may last only a few weeks, and another episode after the fractures have healed. The participation goal, however, is still stated as a long-term outcome for the patient—to return to school in her full capacity.

IMPAIRMENT GOALS

Impairment goals are considered optional for most evaluation reports. They should be included only if specific impairment-level objectives will be worked on during therapy. In some clinical settings, these are referred to as *therapy goals*. As mentioned earlier, short-term goals can be focused on impairments and long-term goals on functional activities.

It is very important that the impairment goals are linked in some way to activity goals. The link should be clearly stated in the Assessment section of the initial evaluation. An example of an Impairment goal would be as follows:

PROM of L knee flexion (C) *will increase* (B) *to 110°* (D) *within 3 wk* (E).

In this case, the reason that increasing ROM of the left knee is important must be addressed (e.g., what activity is being limited by this ROM deficit?).

The goal stated above does meet the essential components of a well-written goal. The Condition is ROM of left knee flexion, and Degree is measured in joint ROM. Impairment goals are often not written with the Actor specified, as it is assumed that the statement is made with relation to the patient. Furthermore, it would not sound incorrect if a goal read "Pt. will increase ROM in R knee." It then appears that the *patient* is doing something specific to increase the ROM. Thus impairment goals are often stated without the actor explicitly specified, although the Behavior (B), Condition (C), Degree (D), and Expected Time (E) should be included. Some more examples include:

Example 1: *Strength R shoulder flexion* (C) *will increase* (B) *to 4/5* (D) *within 3 wk* (E).

Example 2: *Single limb stance on R leg* (C) *will improve* (B) *to 10 sec* (D) *within 2 wk* (E).

Example 3: *Pain in R shoulder* (C) *will decrease* (B) *to 2/10* (D) *within 1 wk* (E).

Example 4: *Circumference of R anterior thigh wound* (C) *will decrease* (B) *to 2 cm* (D) *within 4 wk* (E).

A common pitfall when documenting impairment goals is to not specify the Degree (D). Some examples include:

↑ *strength R biceps*

↓ *pain in L ankle*

These goals are not well written because they do not include specific measures. In the first example, if a patient's strength increased even a minimal amount, the goal could be met. This might make it difficult to justify the need for continued intervention to achieve even greater strength in the biceps. If, however, the amount of strength (e.g., manual muscle testing grade) was specified as a goal, this would allow all involved parties—patient, therapist, physician, third-party payers—to be aware of the specific expected outcomes.

Summary

- Goals should be distinguished as to whether they are participation goals, activity goals, or impairment goals.
- Well-written goals have certain fundamental characteristics. They are focused on outcomes, not processes. They are concrete, not abstract. They are measurable and testable. They are predictive and are based on collaboration between therapist and patient.
- Goals have five essential components: the Actor, the Behavior, the Condition, the Degree, and the Expected time.
- Although these components can be used to construct a goal in a mechanical way, therapists are expected to go beyond the formula to create goals that are patient-centered; that is, stated in terms of activities and environments that are meaningful to the patient.

CASE EXAMPLE 10-1

Documenting Goals
Setting: Home care

Name: Martin Jones   **D.O.B.:** 5/7/54   **Date of Eval.:** 5/10/09

CURRENT CONDITION: 55 y.o. male, hx of diabetes, s/p B transtibial amputation (left: 4 yr ago; right, 4 wk ago)

Participation Goal

Pt. will live in apartment I'ly and will return to duties as cantor in temple within 3 mo.

Long-Term Activity Goals

1. Pt. will walk through all rooms inside apartment I'ly c̄ walker and B prostheses within 8 wk.
2. Pt. will walk 3 blocks home ↔ temple c̄ crutches and B prostheses c̄ supervision of housekeeper or friend in 20 min within 12 wk.

Short-Term Activity Goals

1. Pt. will don shrinker to R residual limb c̄ correct technique whenever OOB within 2 days.
2. Pt. will demonstrate proper performance of LE preprosthetic strengthening exercises within 2 days.
3. Pt. will stand at edge of bed c̄ CG of therapist c̄ walker and L prosthesis for up to 5 min within 2 days.
4. Pt. will transfer independently bed ↔ W/C and W/C ↔ bathroom c̄ only L prosthesis within 1 wk.
5. Pt. will walk with walker from bedroom ↔ kitchen I'ly c̄ walker and L prosthesis in 2 min within 3 wk.

Impairment Goal

1. Circumferential measurement of R distal limb will decrease by ¾″ within 4 wk for permanent prosthesis fitting.

CASE EXAMPLE 10-2

Documenting Goals
Setting: Acute Care Hospital

Name: Mario Nieto	**D.O.B.:** 10/14/33	**Date of Eval.:** 11/5/09

CURRENT CONDITION: 76 y.o. male s/p R THR 1 day ago 2° degenerative joint disease; PWB R LE.

Activity Goals

1. Pt. will demonstrate proper THR precautions during transfers and dressing 3/3 trials within 1 day.
2. Pt will transfer bed ↔ chair with armrests 3/4 trials within 2 days.
3. Pt. will walk independently with walker up to 100 ft in 3 min indoors on level carpeted and tiled surfaces within 3 days.
4. Pt. will walk up and down one flight of stairs with single handrail c̄ contact guarding within 3 days.

CASE EXAMPLE 10-3

Documenting Goals
Setting: Outpatient

Name: Keisha Brown	**D.O.B.:** 1/9/93	**Date of Eval.:** 2/12/09

CURRENT CONDITION: 16 y.o. female s/p fx R distal tibia and fx R proximal humerus 1 wk ago 2° to MVA; NWB R LE.

Participation Goal

Pt. will attend regular classroom in high school and participate in all activities, including extracurricular sports, within 4 mo.

Activity Goals

1. Pt. will demonstrate proper performance of home program of active exercises within 3 days.
2. Pt. will transfer wheelchair ↔ car c̄ stand-pilot transfer c̄ min A of father or mother within 2 wk.
3. Pt. will use motorized wheelchair independently in school hallways, elevators, and outside paved areas, while effectively avoiding obstacles and keeping up with peers within 2 wk.

Impairment Goal

1. Pt will tolerate R leg in dependent position for 30 min within 1 wk.

EXERCISE 10-1

For each goal, indicate what type of goal it is (Participation, Activity, or Impairment). Write one or more letters in the column at the right to indicate the missing or problematic component (A = Actor; B = Behavior; C = Conditions; D = Degree; E = Expected Time). More than one component may be missing or problematic in a single example. Rewrite each goal in the space below, adding or changing the missing or problematic components using plausible details. Identify A, B, C, D, and E in each answer.

EXAMPLE: Patient will walk 300 ft in 4 min c̄ walker and require contact guarding.

Type: Activity

Answer: Patient (A) will walk (B) on level hallway surface (C) 300 ft (D) in 4 min (D) using walker (C) and requiring contact guarding (D) within 5 days (E).

Problem: C, E

1. Independent in transfers in 2 wk.

Type:

Problem:

2. Patient will be functional in ADL within 3 wk.

Type:

Problem:

3. Return to work in 3 mo.

Type:

Problem:

4. Increased strength in quadriceps to 5/5 bilaterally.

Type:

Problem:

5. Pt. will ↕1 flight of stairs in 1 min.

Type:

Problem:

6. Pt. will demonstrate increased R hip ROM.

Type:

Problem:

7. Pt. will return to school.

Type:

Problem:

8. Pt. will get from his room to therapy.

Type:

Problem:

EXERCISE 10-2

Identify the errors in the following statements documenting Activity Goals. Rewrite a more appropriate statement in the space provided.

Statement	Rewrite Statement
EXAMPLE: Transfers will improve.	Pt. will transfer from bed ↔ w/c c̄ min A, within 1 wk.
1. Pt. will experience less pain.	
2. Pt. will progress from a walker to a cane within 3 wk.	
3. Educate pt. on hip precautions within 2 sessions.	
4. Pt. will walk with a normal gait pattern within 4 wk.	
5. Ⓘ ADLS in 2 wk.	
6. Pt. will ascend and descend stairs within 3 days.	
7. Pt. will not have pain when reaching.	
8. Pt. will sit for 5 min.	
9. Pt. will improve standing balance.	
10. Pt. will transfer from sit → stand in 2 wk.	

CHAPTER 11

Documenting the Plan of Care

LEARNING OBJECTIVES

After reading this chapter and completing the exercises,
the reader will be able to:

1. Identify and describe the components of documentation of the Plan of Care.

2. Appropriately document a Plan of Care as part of an initial evaluation.

3. Discuss the importance of documenting informed consent.

The Plan of Care documentation section details the physical therapy techniques and procedures that will be used to accomplish the stated activity goals. In this section of the report, the PT documents the Plan of Care to be followed in future sessions until the goals are reached and records any interventions that may have already been completed during the examination process.

In documenting the Plan of Care the PT usually states the proposed frequency and duration of physical therapy visits in addition to a tentative date for reevaluation. The PT then describes the interventions, preferably prioritizing them in descending order. Categorizing the interventions into the three distinct areas outlined by the *Guide to Physical Therapist Practice* (American Physical Therapy Association, 2001) can help organize this section (Figure 11-1). These three categories are (1) coordination, communication, and documentation, (2) patient-related instruction, and (3) interventions. This categorization, while not required, is useful because therapists often focus exclusively on describing the procedural interventions and minimize or even omit interventions involving coordination of care, communication with individuals involved in the patient's care, and patient-related instruction. Thus listing each of these three categories helps to ensure that all aspects of physical therapy interventions are addressed.

Components of the Plan of Care

Before documenting the components of the Plan of Care, the PT should first indicate the recommended frequency and duration of this plan. For example: *Pt. will be seen 2×/wk, 30 min sessions for 6 wk.*

COORDINATION/COMMUNICATION

The therapist should document the coordination of care that occurs directly with a patient, his or her family members, or any individuals directly involved in the patient's care. Such individuals may include PTAs, other medical personnel, caregivers, or teachers:

> *Diagnosis and plan of care were discussed with PTA, who met pt. and pt.'s family at the completion of the evaluation.*

In an initial evaluation report the PT also reports his or her plan for any anticipated coordination or communication that is relevant to physical therapy:

> *Pt.'s HHA will be instructed in appropriate guarding during standing activities and ambulation to maximize pt.'s safety while facilitating active participation by pt.*
>
> *(PT will) coordinate with John's SLP re: strategies to maintain upright positioning in W/C, and possible use of adaptive equipment during mealtimes.*

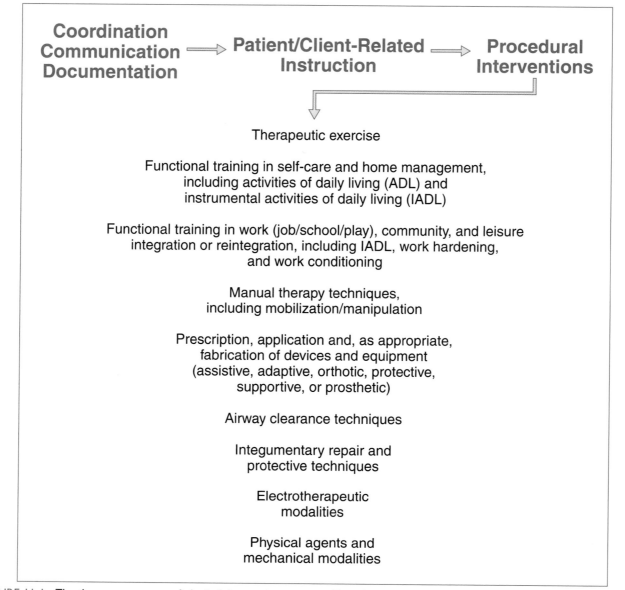

FIGURE 11-1   **The three components of physical therapy intervention.** (From American Physical Therapy Association: *The guide to physical therapist practice*, ed 2, Alexandria, VA, 2001, American Physical Therapy Association.)

PATIENT-RELATED INSTRUCTION

All physical therapy intervention involves some aspect of patient education or instruction. This section should include a general description of the nature of the instruction. For example, the therapist can report:

Pt. will be instructed in care of wound.

Although the specific details of this instruction may not need to be documented in the evaluation report, inclusion of any educational materials given to the patient to be kept in the medical record or chart is helpful. Another example that could be included in a report is:

Pt. will be educated on proper positioning in bed.

It could be argued that this statement does not provide enough detail about specifically what is meant by "proper positioning" or why positioning is important for this patient. An alternative documentation might be:

Pt. will be educated on positioning self in side-lying position with pillow between knees to maintain back alignment and improve comfort while sleeping.

INTERVENTIONS

The Interventions section of the Plan of Care can include a wide variety of interventions ranging from therapeutic exercise to training in self-care skills to airway clearance techniques (see Figure 11-1). First, documentation of interventions should flow logically and systematically from other aspects of the report. For example, if stair climbing is identified as an activity limitation and improved speed and efficiency in stair climbing is listed as an activity goal, then part of the intervention would logically entail training in stair-climbing skills (Case Examples 11-1 and 11-2). Sometimes, however, the justification for physical therapy interventions is not so readily apparent. For example, therapists use electrotherapeutic modalities for many different reasons, including muscle reeducation and reduction of swelling. When the purpose for using a particular intervention is not clear, the therapist must take the time to document in the report a concise rationale for the intervention chosen. For example:

NMES to R quads for muscle reeducation.

US to proximal extensor carpi radialis to promote tissue healing.

As with other sections of the physical therapy report, documentation of interventions should be detailed appropriately. For example, simply stating "gait training" is too vague. Specification of more detail about the gait training—such as to improve safety during outdoor ambulation or to improve endurance, speed, or efficiency of gait pattern—is essential. Alternatively, providing too much detail in this section wastes the therapist's time and clouds the report with extraneous information. For example, if progressive resistive strengthening exercise for the right quadriceps and hamstrings is one of the procedural interventions for a particular patient, the PT need not document the specific number of repetitions, sets, positioning, or exact types of exercises that will be performed. Similarly, documentation of modalities in the initial evaluation need not include specific parameters. This information is more appropriately conveyed in each treatment note documentation, as the parameters are likely to change over the course of the episode of care.

Therapists should document only those interventions that are within the scope of physical therapy practice. This section should not include reports of interventions performed by other medical professionals. Rather, this information should be described either in the Coordination/Communication heading or in the Reason for Referral section.

Documenting Skilled Intervention

An important component of documenting the Plan of Care is to demonstrate to third-party payers that the intervention proposed for the patient requires the skilled services of a PT. The interventions listed in the Plan of Care therefore need to encompass those interventions that are within the PT's scope of practice (based on state law).

Therapists may have difficulty justifying the need for their services if the intervention plan includes a statement similar to the following:

Practice walking on variety of surfaces

It is unclear from this statement *why* the skilled services of a PT are needed. Instead, terms such as *gait training* are useful. Therapists should also consider further justification of the need for a therapist's skilled intervention, such as:

Gait training to improve effective foot clearance and maximize safety.

Documenting Informed Consent

The principle of informed consent is integral to health care. Whereas traditionally such consent was taken for granted, the modern approach is to verify informed consent in writing. Documenting informed consent has two benefits: It serves as evidence that informed consent was obtained, if there is a dispute at a later date; and (perhaps more importantly) it reminds practitioners to take this crucial last step before beginning treatment.

Informed consent can be documented either by (1) having the patient (or responsible family member) sign a standard form or (2) by reporting that consent was obtained at the end of the written initial evaluation. In the absence of a standard form, an appropriate variant of the following statement should be inserted at the end of the Plan of Care section:

The findings of this evaluation were discussed with [insert name of patient or responsible party] and he [or she] consented to the above plan of care.

If the patient is a minor or not competent to give informed consent, then the evaluation and plan of care should be discussed with a responsible person (e.g., parent, guardian, or spouse). If other persons are present during the discussion of informed consent, the PT should indicate who they were.

Finally, the concept of informed consent implies that the patient or responsible party has the right to *not* consent to the recommended plan of care, either in whole or in part. If that occurs, the PT should indicate in detail those parts of the Plan of Care with which the patient disagrees and briefly summarize the reasons given.

Summary

- The therapist documents the details of the patient's activity limitations and impairments throughout the functional outcome report; these details should logically lead to specific goals and an appropriate Plan of Care designed to achieve those goals.

- The Plan of Care is typically the last section in a physical therapy report. It reflects the compiling of information from all other aspects of the report and can be the most highly scrutinized section.

- The Plan of Care includes three types of interventions: coordination/communication, patient-related instructions, and interventions.

- Although the Plan of Care of an initial evaluation report can be short and concise, it should provide sufficient detail so that the justifications for the chosen interventions are clear.

- Following the Plan of Care, a statement indicating that informed consent was obtained should be included.

CASE EXAMPLE 11-1

Documenting Plan of Care
Setting: Outpatient Cardiac Rehabilitation

Name: Jason Press   **D.O.B.:** 3/15/53   **Date of Eval.:** 9/10/09

CURRENT CONDITION: s/p percutaneous transluminal coronary angioplasty 8/27/09

PLAN OF CARE

Pt. will be seen for PT 3×/wk for cardiac rehabilitation, 45-min sessions.

Coordination/Communication

Review cardiac guidelines with patient and wife; discuss strategies for exercising at home. Review Rate of Perceived Exertion (RPE) scale and warning signs.

Patient-Related Instruction

Pt. will be instructed in HEP to include progressive walking routine and use of heart rate monitor and home blood pressure monitor. Discussed lifestyle modifications (activity level; weight loss).

Interventions

- Phase II cardiac rehabilitation including monitored activity (treadmill walking, stationary bike, and UE ergometry), performed at 70% of maximal heart rate and <11-13 RPE, HR no greater than 30 bpm above resting.
- Warm-up and cool-down prior to aerobic activity, with emphasis on total body flexibility routine.
- Introduction to UE strength training with handheld weights (2 kg to start).

CASE EXAMPLE 11-2

Documenting Plan of Care
Setting: Acute Care Hospital

Name: Joseph Jacobs   **D.O.B.:** 6/17/39   **Date of Eval.:** 11/1/09

CURRENT CONDITION: 1 day s/p right total hip replacement.

PLAN OF CARE

Pt. will receive PT 2×/day, 30-min session; anticipated D/C 11/4/09.

Coordination/Communication

F/u with hospital SW re: d/c plan and necessary adaptive equipment—raised toilet seat, tub bench, walker.

Patient-Related Instruction

Pt. instructed in total hip precautions and exercises (hip isometrics, ankle pumps, glut sets, quad sets) preoperatively on 10/20/09 (handout given). Will continue reviewing precautions and exercises each session. Exercises to be performed 3×/day.

Interventions

- AROM exercises B LEs—progression from ankle pumps, glut sets, and quad sets to active knee flexion/extension, hip flexion, abduction, and extension following THR precautions.
- Bed mobility and transfer trng while maintaining hip precautions, maximizing independence.
- Balance training in standing to improve standing tolerance during functional activities.
- Gait training for short distances (10-20 ft) with standard walker, progressively increasing distance and decreasing VCs for safety and foot placement.
- Elevation trng: curbs and stairs to promote independence and safety.

CASE EXAMPLE 11-3

Documenting Plan of Care
Setting: Outpatient

Name: Brian Jones   **D.O.B.:** 9/23/92   **Date of Eval.:** 10/15/09

CURRENT CONDITION: 1 wk s/p R ACL reconstruction

PLAN OF CARE

Pt. will be seen for PT 3 days/wk for 4 wk, 45-min sessions. Re-eval in 2 wk.

Coordination/Communication

Consult with athletic trainer at school who will be working with Brian within 2 wk.
Follow-up phone call in 5 days with MD to coordinate progression of exercise program.

Patient-Related Instruction

Brian will be instructed in the following:

- PROM exercises for knee flexion and extension for use both in the clinic and at home
- Proper use of CPM machine for passive knee ROM
- Use of ice and elevation to reduce swelling and pain
- Patellofemoral self-mobilization to increase joint mobility
- Isometric quad sets
- Instruction in safe use of crutches in all environments

Intervention

- US and soft tissue massage to improve circulation and decrease LE edema
- NMES to R quads for muscle reeducation
- AROM and progressive resistive strengthening exercises to increase strength of R quadriceps, hamstrings, and gastroc/soleus
- Gait trng to improve safety and endurance during ambulation, including uneven surfaces, ramps, and stairs
- Balance activities in standing to improve RLE stability
- Progressive trng, once appropriate, on stationary bike, NordicTrack, and treadmill to increase cardiovascular and muscular endurance
- Plyometric trng in preparation for return to sport

EXERCISE 11-1

Indicate in which component of the Plan of Care each statement should be classified: Coordination/Communication (CC), Patient-Related Instruction (PI), Intervention (I), or Not Pertinent (NP). Statements that either do not belong in this section or are not relevant to be reported in an evaluation should be classified as NP.

1. Pt. will be instructed in self-stretching of right wrist and elbow. _____

2. Past medical hx is significant for HTN. _____

3. Referral to orthotist to evaluate for specific AFO. _____

4. Functional training to address balance and coordination during morning bathroom routine. _____

5. RLE strengthening exercises such as squats, stair stepping, and obstacle negotiation to improve standing and walking ability. _____

6. Pt. will be able to negotiate walking over 6-inch-high obstacles. _____

7. Discuss with pt. options for long-distance mobility, including use of wheelchair. _____

8. Strength of right hip abductors will increase to 4/5. _____

9. Trng with appropriate assistive device (straight cane or quad cane) during ambulation indoors and outdoors and transfers to improve safety, speed, and distance. _____

10. Pt. will view video modeling strategies for improved UE function in patients who have had a stroke. _____

11. Pt. will be instructed in home walking program to improve speed and endurance; walking daily beginning with 10 min and progressing to 20 min over 4 wk. _____

12. Instruct pt.'s wife in soft tissue massage for right upper extremity and guarding techniques for outdoor ambulation. _____

EXERCISE 11-2

Identify the errors in the following statements documenting the Plan of Care. Rewrite a more appropriate statement in the space provided.

Statement	Rewrite Statement
EXAMPLE: Gait training.	Gait trng within home with manual and verbal cues to improve gait symmetry and speed.
1. Practice walking.	
2. Apply hot packs.	
3. Pt. will be able to walk 10 ft to the bathroom.	
4. Pt. will be given strengthening exercises.	
5. Coordinate care with all nursing personnel.	
6. Assess work environment.	
7. Pt. will increase right hamstring strength.	
8. Balance training.	
9. Pt. will receive ultrasound at 1.0 W/cm², 1 MHz to R quadriceps (VMO), in a 10-cm area just proximal and slightly medial to R knee, moving ultrasound head slowly in circular fashion for 10 min, each session.	
10. Pt. will take pain relief medication as needed.	

Statement	Rewrite Statement
11. Home evaluation.	_____
	_____
12. Reduce R ankle edema.	_____
	_____
13. Teach family to care for pt.	_____
	_____
14. Practice pressure-relief techniques.	_____
	_____
15. E-stim to anterior tibialis.	_____
	_____

CHAPTER 12

Treatment Notes and Progress Notes Using a Modified SOAP Format

LEARNING OBJECTIVES

After reading this chapter and completing the exercises, the reader will be able to:

1. Identify and describe the key components of a treatment note.

2. Identify and describe the key components of a progress note.

3. Appropriately document components of treatment notes and progress notes using a modified SOAP format.

Treatment notes and progress notes are a key component of physical therapy documentation. In fact, many therapists spend a majority of their documentation time writing these types of notes. Although the focus of this book thus far has been on documenting the initial evaluation, all elements included in treatment or progress notes are essentially components of the initial evaluation. The concepts discussed in the previous chapters all apply here.

Although there are no formal guidelines from either APTA or CMS regarding the structure of treatment or progress notes, such documentation can become unwieldy without some organization. The SOAP note is a commonly used format and is one with which most medical personnel are familiar (see Chapter 2 for the history and development of the SOAP note). The SOAP format is relatively easy to master and provides a quick format for writing a treatment note. This chapter presents a format for writing both treatment notes and progress notes using a modified SOAP format.

Modified SOAP Format

The acronym SOAP stands for *s*ubjective, *o*bjective, *a*ssessment, and *p*lan. This format was discussed briefly in Chapter 2 and is presented here as a framework for treatment and progress note documentation. However, the original design for use of the SOAP note is not how it is currently used by most medical professionals. The SOAP note was designed to promote a sequential rather than an integrative approach to clinical decision making and was linked to the problem-oriented medical record, which is no longer routinely used. However, with some modifications the SOAP note can provide the foundation for efficient, effective functional outcomes documentation in rehabilitation.

The figures and tables in this chapter outline key components of these notes to meet criteria necessary for optimal clinical decision making, third-party payment, and legal purposes. Because treatment notes must serve such diverse purposes, there may be a tendency for therapists to write excessively long notes. Strategies for simplifying documentation are provided in Box 12-1. Furthermore, the case examples at the end of the chapter demonstrate how such notes are modified for different patients in different practice settings.

Treatment Notes

Treatment notes are written for each encounter a PT or PTA has with a patient (Case Examples 12-1, 12-2,

BOX 12-1

Time-Saving Tips for Writing Session Notes

- Keep printout of patient's goals readily visible in the front of the patient's chart.
- Use tables and flowcharts whenever possible (Case Example 12-5) for documenting both interventions and outcomes.
- When documenting tests and measures, focus on *changes* to patient's status.
- Use electronic documentation whenever possible. Even if your facility has not yet implemented a complete system, use a word processor and write your own documentation template.

and 12-3). Although APTA documentation guidelines and most third-party payers require documentation for each physical therapy encounter, the format of treatment note documentation is at the discretion of each institution.

Treatment notes are written for four distinct reasons:

1. *Legal documentation.* A treatment note importantly provides a legal record of what was done in a therapy session and why. For this reason, documentation of the specifics of the interventions performed and the patient's reaction to those interventions is critical.

2. *Third-party payment.* Third-party payers typically request that treatment notes be provided as proof of service. Medicare, for example, requires documentation to create a record of all treatments and skilled interventions to justify the use of billing codes.

3. *To facilitate functional outcomes and clinical decision making.* Writing a treatment note that focuses on functional outcomes helps to maintain a therapist's attention on patient-specific goals. Each treatment note allows the therapist the time to reevaluate the patient's progress and goals and to consider changes to the plan of care.

4. *As a record for other therapists in case of absence.* In the event that a therapist is absent, it is important for any covering therapist to have a complete record of the specific interventions that were performed with a patient.

FRAMEWORK FOR TREATMENT NOTE DOCUMENTATION

The framework for treatment note documentation includes goals (G), subjective (S), objective (O), assessment (A), and plan (P) (Figure 12-1).

Goals

From a functional outcomes perspective, the focus of treatment notes should be on the specific goals that are being addressed. Thus the goals should be readily visible to the therapist as he or she writes the treatment note. This can be accomplished by adding a statement at the beginning of the SOAP note that identifies the goals, possibly including only those that were the focus of that treatment (restatement of the goals that were set at the time of the intial evaluation or last progress note). Alternatively, therapists can easily have the patient's goals reproduced at the beginning of the SOAP note. This can be more easily accomplished using computerized documentation.

Common Pitfall

Goals are not included. Restating the goal(s) forces the therapist to maintain a focus on the outcomes toward which therapeutic intervention is directed.

Subjective (S)

In the Subjective section of the treatment note, the therapist documents the patient's subjective responses to interventions and any changes in participation or activity limitations. This section could include any relevant statements or reports made by the patient, patient's family members, and/or caregivers. The purpose of this section is to detail the patient's own perception of his or her condition, which can relate to impairments (e.g., pain), activities (e.g., ability to walk), or participation (e.g., ability to work). Box 12-2 provides more information on documenting pain in treatment notes.

This section of the note does *not* include direct observations made by the therapist. Therapists can report a patient's or caregiver's remarks in quotation marks if the exact phrasing is somehow pertinent. Documentation of subjective information should incorporate information that is relevant to the patient's progress in rehabilitation and specifically related to changes in functional performance or quality of life. It should not include extraneous information that is not directly related to the patient's current condition.

Common Pitfall

Documentation is not specific enough (e.g., *Pt. reports pain is getting better*). Such a statement needs to be more specific:

> *Pt. reports pain in left hip during walking has improved from 6/10 to 4/10.*

The therapist could also document nonpertinent information. For example, a therapist might write *Pt. reports she didn't like her last PT.* This statement is not pertinent.

	Framework for Writing Treatment Notes Using a Modified SOAP Format
Goal	• List goals for the patient.
S—Subjective	• Patient's subjective response to interventions (including any adverse reactions). • Patient's report of changes in participation or activity limitations.
O—Objective	• *Status update*—Indicate any objective, measurable changes in patient's status with regard to activity limitations or impairments. • *Intervention* (Rx)—Outline interventions that were performed, including communication and/or education with health care providers, patient, family, or significant others. Include frequency, duration, and intensity, if appropriate, as well as any equipment provided.
A—Assessment	• Indicate the progress being made toward patient's goals, including adherence to patient-related instructions. • Discuss factors that modify frequency or intensity of intervention and progression toward anticipated goals. • Modify or set new goals if necessary.
P—Plan	• Specific intervention plan for upcoming sessions. • Report what patient will be doing between sessions (e.g., home program, other interventions/tests).

FIGURE 12-1   Framework for treatment note documentation using a modified SOAP format. Recommendations from APTA Documentation (Appendix A) and current CMS requirements for treatment note documentation are incorporated into this framework.

Pt. reports she was "unsatisfied with her previous treatment results" and is hoping for more significant improvement in her walking ability.

This statement is more specific to the patient's concern.

Objective (O)

The focus of the Objective section is twofold: (1) to document the results of any tests and measures performed, specifically those that relate to achievement of the stated goal(s) (Status Update), and (2) to provide details of the interventions performed (Rx) (see Case Examples 12-1, 12-2, and 12-3). The Status Update should include any examination findings that were performed or observed (e.g., range of motion, walking speed). Documentation of the interventions (Rx) should include the procedural interventions that were performed, including location, frequency, intensity, duration, and/or repetitions, as appropriate. Some of this information can be recorded in table or flowchart form. However, the documentation must clearly show evidence of skilled intervention and the interaction between the patient and therapist (see Chapter 15).

Common Pitfall

Not enough detail is provided regarding specific interventions. Therapists may generalize the interventions performed in a treatment note, such as "E-stim" or "MH" or "Ther ex." Instead, specific details should be provided for each intervention performed:

Ther ex. seated knee ext through full range, 30 lb, 8 reps ×3; prone knee flex through full range, 20 lb, 10 reps ×3.

Assessment (A)

In the Assessment section, the therapist indicates the progress being made toward the patient's goals (including adherence to patient-related instructions), discusses factors that would modify frequency or intensity of intervention, and reports progression toward anticipated goals. The therapist should essentially summarize the patient's progress and discuss those factors contributing to or hindering progress. Therapists should report modification of goals or document any new goals in this section.

BOX 12-2

Documenting Pain in Treatment Notes and Progress Notes

In the initial evaluation, a detailed description of pain is recommended, including location, quality, severity, timing, and factors that make it better or worse (see Box 8-1). The setting in which pain occurs and any associated manifestations may also be included.

In the session note or progress note documentation, a change in any component of pain is worthy of documentation. Decrease in pain severity (e.g., "Pt. reports pain has decreased to 2/10") or quality (e.g., "Pt reports pain has gone from a burning, stabbing pain to an aching pain") can be indicators of patient improvement. It is not essential in the treatment note or progress note to completely redocument the detailed pain assessment provided in an initial note. Rather, changes in the patient's report of pain should be specifically documented.

Reports of pain (because they are inherently subjective) should typically be documented in the subjective section of a treatment note or a progress note. However, if report of pain is incidental to an objective statement, then it can be included in the objective section, e.g., "Pt. performed 10 reps ×3 sets SLR with no increase in pain." This statement's focus is on the intervention being performed.

Common Pitfall

The Assessment is too vague and not meaningful. Avoid vague terms like "Pt. tol Rx well" or "Pt. is improving." Such statements provide little insight into the effectiveness of the intervention. A better example would be:

> *Pt. has demonstrated improved tolerance to performing ther ex. regimen and has reported an increase in sitting tolerance time at work.*

Plan (P)

The final section of the treatment note outlines the Plan. Any specific interventions for upcoming sessions should be documented, including any changes in the intervention strategy.

Common Pitfall

The upcoming plan is not documented. Documentation such as "Cont Rx," while sometimes appropriate, provides no information about how the therapist plans to continue to help the patient's progress. A better example would be:

> *Increase number of repetitions in squatting and wall slide exercises to 20.*

As the therapist reviews the patient's record at the next visit, this statement will serve as a reminder of the intended plan.

LEGAL ISSUES FOR TREATMENT NOTES

Treatment note documentation is critical for legal purposes. If issues or conflicts arise, the treatment notes will be highly scrutinized. Thus therapists should dedicate appropriate time to clear and effective documentation on a daily basis. "A poorly documented patient/client record can serve as powerful evidence in support of a suit, even when the accusations are frivolous" (Lewis, 2002).

Some important documentation guidelines for treatment notes follow (Lewis, 2002; Scott, 2005):

1. *Timeliness.* Therapists should write treatment notes as soon as possible after a session. This helps keep information fresh in their minds and minimizes the chance of errors.

2. *Decision-making rationale.* Each section should flow logically from the next, and the therapist's decisions about assessment, goals, and intervention should be supported by concrete data.

3. *Patient/client behavior.* Missed or canceled appointments must be documented in the patient's medical record. For example, *Pt. called at 9:00 AM to cancel 1:30 PM appt. Pt. reports his L shoulder was sore from doing too much lifting yesterday. Next appt scheduled in 2 days.* This provides the time the appointment was canceled, detailed information as to the reason the appointment was canceled, and information about future appointments. A patient's noncompliance with recommendations or instructions given by a therapist must also be carefully and objectively documented.

4. *Prior and concurrent treatment.* Therapists should document any other interventions a patient is currently undergoing or has undergone in the past. For example, *Pt. reports he has begun acupuncture 2×/week to facilitate back pain relief.*

5. *Communications.* Any conversations (oral or written) pertinent to the patient and the rehabilitation program should be documented. Such documentation should include the name, time, issues discussed, and the resolution or action. For example: *PT called pt.'s orthopedic surgeon, Dr. Smith, to discuss pt.'s report of increased pain in L ankle at fracture site. MD stated to D/C PT immediately and refer pt. back to him for evaluation.*

6. *Informed consent and referral.* Documentation of informed consent in an initial evaluation is discussed in Chapter 3. In a treatment note, informed consent should be documented if changes to the plan of care are being

implemented. For example, the following could be documented relative to the above example: *Pt. was informed of phone conversation and MD's orders and was instructed to call MD immediately for an appt. Pt. agreed to this and stated he would call MD upon returning home.*

7. *Adverse incidents.* Therapists should follow their institutions' guidelines for documentation of an adverse incident. Typically, this is done on an incident report. Therapists should document in the medical record only pertinent clinical findings, and it is not necessary to indicate that an incident report has been filed separately (Scott, 2005).

PROGRESS NOTES

Progress notes are written to provide an update of a patient's status; these notes often are based on a reexamination (Case Examples 12-4, 12-5, and 12-6). The progress note typically covers multiple visits and therefore provides a summary of the patient's progress to date. A progress note can have a format similar to an initial evaluation, and the functional outcomes framework presented in earlier chapters can be used. However, the SOAP format can also be used.

Figure 12-2 outlines the key elements of each section of the progress note based on a SOAP format. Progress notes should be succinct and easy to read because they often are used by third-party payers to justify the need for skilled therapeutic intervention (see Chapter 15). Comparisons of preintervention and postintervention functional performance are especially useful. Therapists should document any interventions that were performed during the reevaluation period and provide justification for the need for continued therapy.

Framework for Writing Progress Notes Using a Modified SOAP Format	
Goal	• List goals for the patient.
S—Subjective	• Patient's subjective response to interventions (including any adverse reactions). • Patient's report of changes in participation or activity limitations.
O—Objective	• *Status update*—Indicate any objective, measurable changes in patient's status with regard to activity limitations or impairments. • *Intervention* (Rx)—Provide summary of interventions that were performed, including communication and/or education with health care providers, patient, family, or significant others. Include frequency, duration, and intensity, if appropriate, as well as any equipment provided. Evidence should be provided that **skilled intervention** was required to achieve the stated goals (particularly important for Medicare documentation).
A—Assessment	• Indicate the progress being made toward patient's goals, including adherence to patient-related instructions. • Discuss factors that modify frequency or intensity of intervention and progression toward anticipated goals. • Justification of continuation of therapy (state **medical necessity**) • Modify or set new goals if necessary.
P—Plan	• Specific intervention plan for upcoming sessions, with revision of original plan of care if needed. • Report what patient will be doing between sessions (e.g., home program, other interventions/tests).

FIGURE 12-2   Framework for progress note documentation using a modified SOAP format. Recommendations from APTA Documentation (Appendix A) and current CMS requirements for progress note documentation are incorporated into this framework.

Summary

- Treatment notes and progress notes can be organized as a functional outcomes report using a modified SOAP format.

- Documentation is required for every physical therapy encounter and should include information about the interventions provided and progress toward stated goals.

- Treatment notes are important legal records. Therapists should carefully document all aspects directly pertinent to a patient's current physical therapy intervention and his or her current condition.

- Progress notes provide an update of a patient's status. Progress toward the stated goals is discussed and justification for continued therapy is provided.

CASE EXAMPLE 12-1

Treatment Note
Setting: Outpatient

Name: Emily Rodriguez   **D.O.B.:** 2/3/77   **Date of Eval.:** 1/5/09

CURRENT CONDITION: 31 y.o. female 12 wk postpartum $\bar{c}$ onset of stress incontinence $\bar{p}$ vaginal delivery of first child.

Goal: Decrease urine losses from 2× daily to 1×/wk.

S: Pt. reports urinary losses of 1 tablespoon have decreased to 1×/day over past 3 days. Occurs primarily when coughing or during physical activities, such as lifting baskets of laundry, running, and jumping. Pt. continues to wear 2 panty-liners daily as continued precaution to protect clothing.

O: Status update: Biofeedback reassessment was completed in supine with noted improvement in EMG activity levels for pelvic muscle contractions. Fair strength of pelvic floor muscle contraction, held 5 sec ×7 reps.

Rx: Pt. performed pelvic floor muscle contractions $\bar{c}$ biofeedback program in the standing position. Pt. performed pelvic floor muscle contractions during a lunge to floor and back to standing, 3 reps each LE (practicing the movement for lifting a laundry basket). Practiced pelvic muscle contractions prior to a cough, 5 reps. Pt. ed: pelvic muscle contraction before cough or lifting heavy objects to prevent incontinence. Revised HEP to ↑ pelvic muscle contractions in sitting for 20 1-sec contractions; followed by 20 min of 10-sec contractions in sitting.

A: Pt. reports decrease in urinary losses over past 3 days, which correlates with observed improvements in EMG activity levels for pelvic floor muscle contractions.

P: Continue PT 1×/wk. Progress with pelvic muscle strength trng and muscle reeducation during functional tasks, with instruction in progressive HEP to improve pt.'s level of ADLs.

CASE EXAMPLE 12-2

Treatment Note
Setting: Inpatient

Name: Wally Narcessian   **D.O.B.:** 3/7/37   **Date of Eval.:** 6/20/09 (10:26:00 AM)

CURRENT CONDITION: COPD/pneumonia

Goals

1. Pt. will demonstrate productive cough in a seated position, 3/4 trials.
2. Pt. will ambulate 150 ft with supervision, no A device, on level indoor surfaces, within 45 sec (to enable in-home ambulation).

S: Pt. reports not feeling well today, "I'm very tired."

O: Status update: Auscultation findings: scattered rhonchi all lung fields.

Rx: Chest PT was performed in sitting (ant and post). Techniques included percussion, vibration, and shaking. Pt. performed a weak combined abdominal and upper costal cough that was non-bronchospastic, congested, and nonproductive. The cough/huff was performed with verbal cues. Pectoral stretch/thoracic cage mobilizations performed in seated position. Pt. given towel roll placed in back of seat to open up ant chest wall. Strengthening exercises in standing—pt. performed hip flexion, extension, and abduction; knee flexion 10 reps ×1 set B. Pt. performs HEP with supervision (in evenings with wife). Pt. instructed to hold tissue over trach when speaking to prevent infection and explained importance of drinking enough water.

A: Pt. continues to present with congestion and limitations in coughing productivity. Pt. has been compliant with evening exercise program, which has resulted in increased tol. to ther ex. regimen and an increase in LE strength. Amb. not attempted today 2° to pt. report of fatigue. Pt. should be able to tolerate short-distance amb. within next few days.

P: Cont. current treatment plan including CPT; emphasize productive coughing techniques; increase strengthening exer reps to 15; attempt amb. again tomorrow.

CASE EXAMPLE 12-3

Treatment Note
Setting: Outpatient

Name: Julie Jones   **D.O.B.:** 10/1/63   **Date of Eval.:** 6/20/09

CURRENT CONDITION: chronic left shoulder capsulitis

Goal

1. To return to playing tennis, pain-free in 4 wk.

S: Patient reports L shoulder pain localized over lateral brachial region when serving during a tennis game.

O: Status update: Patient performs tennis "serving" techniques with tennis racket on the tennis courts outside the PT gym, and reports being able to successfully complete 7 serves before the onset of pain. **Rx:** US to L inferior anterior shoulder, 1 MHz/1.0 W/cm², continuous for 5 min with patient in supine and L UE supported with pillows in abduction and external rotation. Followed by shoulder joint mob, inferior glide grade 4. Strengthening exercises with yellow Theraband for int. rotation, ext. rotation, flex and ext of L shoulder. Pt. education: practice tennis serves and review proper motion and technique.

A: Patient has been making slow gains in reducing L shoulder pain during her recreational activities of tennis. She has been able to increase the time of her tennis games from 20 min to 40 min as she is able to manage her pain more effectively.

P: Continue c̄ US, joint mobs, and stretching to increase shoulder abduction. Pt. will be given HEP to increase ROM and function of L UE next session.

CASE EXAMPLE 12-4

Progress Note
Setting: Outpatient

Name: Linda Smith   **D.O.B.:** 5/12/73   **Date of Eval.:** 8/01/09

CURRENT CONDITION: Lumbosacral strain, 2-wk reevaluation

Goals

1. Change 3-month-old's diapers on changing table without pain.
2. Carry 3-month-old for 20 min pain-free.

S: Pt. reports: "I am able to get out of bed without pain."

O: Status update: Neutral pubic bone, ASIS and iliac crest levels B. R on L backward sacral torsion remains corrected. Strength of upper abdominals: 3+/5 and lower abdominals: 2/5. Pain rated as 2/10 with diaper changing and able to carry child in carrier for 15 min, 2/10 pain. **Rx:** Rx consists of iliosacral, sacroliliac, and lumbosacral adjustments; pt. education for proper standing posture and carrying techniques; instruction in LE and trunk-stretching routine.

A: Pt. is exhibiting steady progress with trunk strength and endurance. This is needed for patient to achieve above-stated goals and to tolerate baby's continued weight gain.

P: Continue current exercise regimen with progression of lumbar stabilization exercises as tolerated. Patient independent with HEP. Physical therapy sessions will continue 3 ×/wk for 2 more wk.

CASE EXAMPLE 12-5

Progress Note
Setting: Outpatient

Name: Melissa Chau   **D.O.B.:** 12/26/83   **Date of Eval.:** 10/01/09

CURRENT CONDITION: Patellofemoral dysfunction, 1 wk reevaluation

Goals

1. Ascend and descend 2 flights of stairs, pain-free.
2. Run on level surfaces 2 miles in 20 min, 2 ×/wk, pain-free.

S: "My knee no longer hurts when I'm not walking." (rated as 0/10)

O: Rx: See flow sheet. **Status update:** *Ambulation/stair climbing:* Pt. able to walk ½ mile at comfortable speed (65 m/min). Able to ascend 2 flights of stairs pain-free. Pain rated as 4/10 (sharp pain) descending 1 flight of stairs. *Running:* Pt. has not yet engaged in running activity. *Strength*: L quadriceps: 4/5 L hamstrings: 5/5; R quads and hamstrings: 5/5. L unilateral stance time, static: 20 sec. R unilateral stance time, static: 60 sec.

A: Pt. is exhibiting a steady improvement in eccentric control of L quadriceps when descending stairs, indicated by an increase in control of descent and a decrease in reported pain. Patellar taping techniques are being used to recruit L vastus medialis. Balance deficits are still apparent as indicated by limited unilateral stance time on the left. Steady progress is being made toward the goal of pain-free stairs negotiation. Continued strength and balance gains are necessary for patient to achieve the second goal related to running. Cross-training has been emphasized as well, with cycling being introduced to the pt.'s routine.

P: Continue current exercise regimen, with progression in reps and weight as tolerated. Home program, which consists of SLRs, squats, step-ups, and patellar taping techniques, is to be completed daily. PT sessions will continue 2×/wk to include low-impact activities (e.g., jogging on trampoline). Eval. for orthotics next session.

EXERCISE FLOW SHEET

Modality/Procedure	9-27-09	9-28-09	10-1-09
Eval./treatment number	1	2	3
Evaluation	✓		
Patellar taping (L)		Medial glide	Medial glide
Patellar mobilizations (L)		Medial glide	Medial glide
Ice (at end of Rx)		10 min	10 min
EXERCISES			
Lateral step-ups		4 inch, 2 × 10	4 inch, 3 × 10
Chair squats		0# 3 × 10	0# 3 × 15
SLRs	0# 3 × 10	0# 3 × 15	1# 3 × 10
Left unilateral stance		L: 25 sec	L: 30 sec
Leg press		B: 80# L: 40# 3 × 10	B: 80# L: 40# 3 × 15
Stretching (ITB, quad/hamstrings/calf)	3 × 30 sec	3 × 30 sec	3 × 30 sec

CASE EXAMPLE 12-6

Progress Note
Setting: Outpatient Neurology Clinic

Name: Ralph Fisher	D.O.B.: 12/19/63	Date of Eval.: 7/8/09

CURRENT CONDITION: Huntington's disease (HD) × 11 yr; 1 mo reevaluation

Goals (12 wk)

1. Pt. will experience no falls during indoor or outdoor ambulation over 12-wk period.
2. Pt. will increase average outdoor walking speed on sidewalk with use of cane to 50 m/min, for distances >400 m.
3. Pt. will be independent in performing HEP.

S: Pt. reports that his balance "is getting better" and that he has had no falls in past 4 wk (since initial evaluation). He reports that he is not yet comfortable using the cane for outdoor ambulation. He reports having some difficulty keeping up with walking and turning exercises on exercise videotape.

O: Rx: Pt. has been seen 1×/wk for 4 wk to address balance impairments and ambulation difficulties related to HD. Intervention has consisted of (1) gait training on indoor and outdoor surfaces, including safety instruction and strategies to improve gait speed; (2) balance exercises and balance training in standing, emphasizing improving proactive balance; instruction in home program with exercise videotape (35 min in length)—exercises include ROM/flexibility, strengthening, and cardiovascular; discussion of home safety and recommendations made for grab bars in bathroom, removal of rugs, and supportive chair for mealtimes. **Status update:** *Activities:* Pt. is able to walk indoors s A device; avg. walking speed 42 m/min. Pt. ambulates outdoors on sidewalk with slower gait speed (35 m/min) and is very cautious. Pt. avoids stairs and uneven surfaces whenever possible due to fear of falling; these activities have not yet been assessed in therapy. *Activities of Balance Confidence* (indicative of balance confidence during various functional tasks) remains at 80% (100% = complete confidence). Continues to demonstrate LOB (to the R and posteriorly) during indoor and outdoor ambulation but has I recovery. *Dystonia:* Unchanged; mod. trunk dystonia resulting in posturing into extension and R lateral flexion. *Chorea:* unchanged; mod. chorea × 4 extremities. *Balance:* Berg Balance Scale score increased from 39 to 44; pt. improved in tandem stance, turning in place, and picking up object from floor. Single-limb stance unchanged; limited to <2 sec B.

A: Pt. has demonstrated improvements in balance as measured by the Berg Balance Scale and has not had any falls in a 4-wk period. Pt. is able to perform HEP program independently with modifications. Pt. requires continued PT to address slow walking speed (Goal 2) and standing balance impairments, focusing on single-limb stance to continue to minimize falls risk (Goal 1).

P: (1) Gait training indoors and outdoors to address safety, speed, and balance (proactive and reactive). (2) Balance training exercises, emphasizing single-limb stance activities. (3) Revision of home program to modify walking and turning activities so pt. can keep up with tape. (4) Cont. education re: use of straight cane during outdoor ambulation. (5) Evaluate stair climbing, curb negotiation, uneven surface ambulation, and initiate training for functional benefit, balance improvement, and strengthening.

EXERCISE 12-1

Identify whether the following statements belong in the Subjective (S) or Objective (O) section of either a treatment or progress SOAP note. Write a more appropriate statement in the space provided.

Statement	S or O	Rewrite
EXAMPLE: Mr. Jones reports that he has been unable to do anything.	S	Mr. Jones reports that he is unable to play the organ at church and give music lessons due to the pain in his L elbow.
1. Pt. states he hates using his walker.	_____	_____
2. Pt. has an awkward gait.	_____	_____
3. PROM at the knee is getting better.	_____	_____
4. Pt. is very confused.	_____	_____
5. Pt. reports that his son is concerned.	_____	_____
6. Pt. c/o fatigue after walking for 5 min.	_____	_____
7. Pt. complains of pain in left shoulder.	_____	_____
8. Pt. performed 10 reps of knee exercises.	_____	_____

EXERCISE 12-2

The following statements could be written as part of session SOAP notes. Using Figure 12-1, classify each of the following statements into their appropriate category based on the SOAP format: G = Goal; S = Subjective; O = Objective; A = Assessment; P = Plan.

Statement	G, S, O, A, or P
1. Performed 10 reps SLR B.	_____
2. Pt. reports she was able to walk with her daughter to get the mail yesterday and did not experience any dizziness.	_____

Statement	G, S, O, A, or P
3. Treatment next session will include progression to stationary bike ×10 min.	_____
4. Pt. walked 15 ft from bed to bathroom without SOB in 30 sec.	_____
5. Pt. states that she "felt sore" after last treatment session.	_____
6. Pt. is progressing well with increasing repetitions of LE strengthening exercises and has achieved goal 1.	_____
7. Pitting edema noted in R ankle.	_____
8. Pt. was instructed to continue to maintain R leg in elevated position while sitting at desk during the day.	_____
9. Pt. will transfer from bed to wheelchair independently, 4/5 trials within 2 wk.	_____
10. Pt. states she is anxious to return to work.	_____
11. Pt. will continue with daily walking program at home during off-therapy days, progressing to 20 min each day by next wk.	_____
12. Pt. will stand $\overline{s}$ A for up to 1 min within 1 wk.	_____
13. Pt. reports pain in low back while walking as 5/10 and 8/10 while sitting at desk at work.	_____
14. Pt's. fear of falling is limiting his progress in improving his ability to ambulate in crowded environments and outdoors.	_____
15. Pt. reports that she is going back to work on a trial basis next week.	_____

■ EXERCISE 12-3*

You are a therapist in an outpatient practice and are working with a patient who has a diagnosis of lateral epicondylitis. Write a treatment SOAP note for your patient based on the case information provided below. You should create a plausible situation, including goals, subjective, objective, assessment, and plan. (NOTE: To complete this exercise accurately, it may be necessary to consult additional resources.)

S. G. is a 40-year-old female office worker. She has been referred to therapy with a diagnosis of lateral epicondylitis. S. G. complains of constant moderate to severe pain at her R lateral elbow that prevents her from playing tennis. The pain started about 1 month ago, the morning after she spent a whole day pulling weeds, and remained unchanged in severity or frequency until 3 days ago. She reports a slight decrease in pain severity over the last 3 days, which she associates with starting to take an NSAID prescribed by her physician. She has had similar symptoms previously after gardening or playing tennis, but these have always resolved within a couple of days without any medical intervention. Objective examination reveals tenderness and mild swelling at the right lateral epicondyle and pain without weakness with resisted wrist extension. All other tests, including upper extremity sensation, range of motion, and strength, are normal.

Goals:

_____

_____

_____

_____

_____

*There is no answer for this exercise in Appendix C.

S:

_____

_____

_____

O:

_____

_____

_____

_____

_____

_____

A:

_____

_____

_____

_____

_____

P:

_____

_____

_____

_____

EXERCISE 12-4*

You are a therapist in an outpatient rehabilitation center, and you are working with a patient who has rheumatoid arthritis, primarily affecting her hands. Write a progress note (based on a 2-week time period, using a SOAP note format) for your patient based on the case information provided below. You should create a plausible situation, including goals, subjective, objective, assessment, and plan. (NOTE: To complete this exercise accurately, it may be necessary to consult additional resources.)

M. P. is a 62-year-old female with a diagnosis of rheumatoid arthritis of the hands. M. P. complains of stiffness and aching in all her finger joints, causing difficulties in gripping cooking utensils and performing other household tasks and pain with writing. The objective exam reveals stiffness and restricted flexion range of motion of the proximal interphalangeals to approximately 90° and mild ulnar drift at the carpometacarpal joints bilaterally. The joints are not warm or edematous, and sensation is intact in both hands.

Goals:

_____

_____

_____

_____

S:

_____

_____

_____

_____

O:

_____

_____

_____

_____

_____

_____

_____

_____

_____

---

*There is no answer for this exercise in Appendix C.

A:

_____

_____

_____

_____

_____

_____

P:

_____

_____

_____

_____

_____

Additional Documentation Formats

CHAPTER 13

Specialized Documentation

LEARNING OBJECTIVES

After reading this chapter, the reader will be able to:

1. List the key components of a discharge summary.

2. List the essential features of letters to third-party payers to justify need for equipment or equipment purchases.

3. Identify the key features of letters seeking to appeal denials or requesting continuation of services.

4. Discuss the considerations for providing written patient education materials.

Physical therapy documentation can take many different forms. This book has focused on documentation of the initial evaluation, as well as progress notes and treatment notes. However, PTs are involved in many other types of documentation, including discharge summaries, which are completed at the end of an episode of care, and letters to third-party payers. This chapter discusses specific issues related to some of the most common forms of specialized documentation and presents a framework for easy integration of a functional outcomes approach into each form.

DISCHARGE SUMMARIES

At the completion of an episode of care, therapists are required to write a discharge summary. The American Physical Therapy Association *Guidelines for Physical Therapy Documentation* (2008) state that "documentation is required following conclusion of the current episode in the physical therapy intervention sequence, to summarize progression toward goals and discharge plans." The main purpose of a discharge summary is to document the status of the patient at the time he or she is discharged. A discharge summary does not require a complete reevaluation. However, therapists

should report changes in the patient's participation, activities, and any limitations or impairments that are pertinent to the stated goals. These can be provided in a summary statement or in a table.

The following are essential components of a discharge summary:

- **Patient description.** This should include a description of the patient's diagnosis and background information and can also include description of current plan of care.

- **Summary of physical therapy intervention.** It should be stated for what length of time and how many sessions the patient received physical therapy services. A brief summary of the interventions that were provided can be provided.

- **Current status.** Summarize the patient's current status. This can include any impairments but should focus on the patient's functional abilities and any participation restrictions as appropriate.

- **Goals.** It should be indicated whether the goals were achieved, partially achieved, or not achieved. If goals were not achieved or partially achieved, a brief explanation or justification is warranted.

Discharge Summary

Name: Suzie Sears
D.O.B.: 5/20/50
Date: 9/26/09

Suzie Sears was initially evaluated on 7/24/08 in our Outpatient Physical Therapy Department due to a long-standing diagnosis of multiple sclerosis, with recent exacerbation of symptoms. She has been treated 3x/week for a total of 27 sessions over a period of 9 weeks. She presented with lower extremity weakness and demonstrated deficits in sitting and standing balance, transfers and bed mobility, and ambulation and stair-climbing ability.

Ms. Sears has demonstrated the following specific improvements in her functional ability:

	Initial Evaluation	Final Evaluation
Kurtze EDSS	7.5 (unable to take more than a few steps)	6.0 (intermittent assistance to walk 100 m)
MS Impact Scale (MSIS) -29 (Range 0-145)	98	65
Standing ability	Stands for 10 seconds with minimal assistance and walker	Stands for up to 5 minutes with walker independently
Transfers	Transfers with moderate assistance from walker to wheelchair	Transfers independently from walker to wheelchair within 10 seconds
Bed mobility	Minimal assistance to position self in bed, including rolling bilaterally and coming to sit	Independent in all bed mobility
Ambulation	Able to ambulate approx. 5 steps with walker and minimal assistance before fatiguing; heart rate change from 78 to 104 bpm.	Able to walk 100-150 m with walker and supervision on level surface in therapy gym; heart rate change from 82 to 96 bpm.

Ms. Sears was able to make progress with her home exercise program tolerance and is independent in performing a 30-minute video-based routine aimed at improving flexibility, balance and strength (summary of program is attached). Ms. Sears has surpassed all goals set for this therapy period, and discharge from therapy is thus warranted. The patient stated on 9/27/07 that she was happy to finally see some progress, and she is very pleased with her improved mobility. Ms. Sears continues to struggle with muscle spasms and overall fatigue, and she has received education and written literature on managing her spasms and her fatigue levels.

Ms. Sears has also been seen in consultation with the Outpatient Occupational Therapy Department for a custom wheelchair evaluation on 8/1/08. At the time of the evaluation Ms. Sears was using a scooter that was broken beyond repair. After trials of several types of chairs, a mid-wheel power wheelchair was recommended and the patient is currently awaiting its arrival. This chair will ultimately improve her safety and independence at home.

The recommendation is to discharge the patient from therapy at this time. Continue with video-based home program for continued improvement of flexibility, balance, strengthening, and home walking program. I recommend reevaluation in 4 months.

Thank You,

Sandy Bower, PT, MS
Outpatient Services
Soundshore Hospital

FIGURE 13-1   Discharge summary for outpatient setting.

- **Recommendations**. The PT should list any recommendations for the patient at this point. This plan should include home-based instructions and follow-up or reevaluation instructions. If the patient has moved to another facility (e.g., discharged from acute care to a skilled nursing facility), then any recommendations for continued therapy or other services should be provided.

Figure 13-1 is an example of a discharge summary written in an outpatient hospital setting.

LETTERS TO THIRD-PARTY PAYERS TO JUSTIFY SERVICES OR EQUIPMENT

Letters to third-party payers are frequently written by PTs. These letters are needed to provide justification for either continued services or equipment purchases. When writing such letters, it is important to consider that the reader may not be familiar with all medical terminology, and thus it is essential to avoid medical jargon and abbreviations. The tone should be kept professional, without oversimplification. Therapists should not avoid using medical terminology; however, any uncommon words or terminology should be defined.

EQUIPMENT PURCHASES

Therapists are frequently required to provide justification for the equipment that they plan to provide or wish to obtain for patients. Letters of medical necessity are often required by third-party payers for purchases of expensive medical equipment, such as customized wheelchairs, particularly those purchased through the Medicaid system. The purpose of these letters is to provide medical justification regarding the necessity of the equipment. It is also important to justify the cost. For example, the purchase of a certain piece of equipment now may reduce the need for surgery and/or extended hospital stays in the future. It is also important, whenever possible, to cite examples of research to back up your request.

The following list provides the essential components of a letter of medical necessity:

- **Patient description**. This should include a description of the patient's diagnosis and background information and can also include a description of the current plan of care.
- **Current status**. Summarize the patient's current status. This can include any impairments but should focus on the patient's level of participation and performance of activities as appropriate.

- **Equipment description**. Describe the requested equipment in detail (provide picture or other information if possible). If special components or additions above and beyond standard equipment are required, each item should be separately and explicitly justified.
- **Medical necessity of equipment**. This is the most important component of the letter. The focus here should be on medical necessity. It should include the medical need for the equipment, specify benefits to the patient, and describe the patient's ability to use the equipment. It is important, whenever possible, to include evidence from the literature to support the need for the equipment. In addition, the inability of any alternatives (particularly cheaper ones) to meet the patient's medical needs should be discussed if appropriate. Cost benefits can be explained in detail as well. For example, as seen in Figure 13-2, the use of a stander can help prevent skin breakdown and prevent osteoporosis, which are costly medical conditions.

APPEALING DENIALS OR REQUESTING CONTINUED SERVICES

Therapists also frequently write letters to request approval for additional PT visits or payment for services after a claim has been denied. In these situations, therapists should include specific objective data outlining (1) the specific progress the patient has made in therapy to date, using objective and standardized test results whenever possible, and (2) an overview of the specific skilled therapy intervention that the patient received (or will receive) and the rationale for each intervention. Tables, charts, grids, or bulleted lists are useful in demonstrating progress in therapy and are more readable for reviewers who see many files each day. Figure 13-3 provides a sample letter to a third-party payer requesting approval for additional visits for physical therapy intervention. Figure 13-4 provides a sample letter written in response to a denial for payment of services.

When available, therapists should provide reviewers and insurance companies with current literature or research reports to support the use of a particular intervention for a patient or patient population (see Figure 13-3). This can be in the form of an entire article, which is sent with a detailed letter, or a citation or summary of a research article in the body of the letter.

Therapists must take care to ensure the letters are easy to read, use correct spelling and grammar, are readable, and avoid the use of jargon. Although

Attention:
Any Insurance Co.
PO Box 5032
Norwalk, CT 06856-5032

To whom it may concern,

I am the physical therapist for Jennifer Goodstone, and I am writing this letter of medical necessity for justification for a standing frame for her home.

Description of patient
Ms Goodstone is a 62-year-old woman with a diagnosis of multiple sclerosis (MS) referred for admission to The County Rehabilitation Hospital 07/23/09 by Dr. Jones. The patient is currently under the care of Dr. Smith. Ms Goodstone was originally diagnosed with relapsing remitting multiple sclerosis in 1999. She has recently been admitted for MS exacerbation with a change in the type of MS to progressive MS. Her PMH is significant for myocardial infarction, hypertension, hypercholesterolemia, optic neuritis, and RA.

Ms. Goodstone is currently receiving multi-disciplinary rehabilitative services at County Rehab of occupational and physical therapy services. In physical therapy, she is receiving daily range of motion, therapeutic exercise, functional mobility training (transfers, bed mobility, standing, etc.), functional endurance training, and wheelchair mobility training. She has been fitted with bilateral leg braces (day and night time) to assist in maintaining lower extremity ROM. In addition to these treatments, she is standing in a standing frame for 30 minutes.

Current status
Impairments
- Decreased passive range of motion in both lower extremities, with hip extension, hip abduction, and ankle dorsiflexion being most limiting
- Increased bilateral lower extremity tone (spasticity) resulting in decreased ability to perform bowel-bladder routine, transfers, bed mobility, decreased balance in sitting on bed and in wheelchair, and an increase in leg and back pain
- Continence of bowel and bladder with longstanding history of urinary retention
- High risk for osteoporosis of spine and lower extremities secondary to her inability to weight bear through bilateral lower extremities
- Skin is intact but remains at high risk for skin breakdown and pressure sores secondary to inactivity, dependency on wheelchair for mobility, and inability to perform effective but independent pressure relief
- Limited functional endurance with significant cardiac history with continued risk for decline secondary to immobility

Functional activities
- Depression lift transfer wheelchair to/from level mat with supervision
- Sliding board transfer (SBT) wheelchair to/from bed with minimal assistance
- Sit to stand from wheelchair to bed with moderate/maximal assistance
- Stand pivot transfer using rolling walker with moderate to maximal assistance to stand and manage right lower extremity during pivot
- Ambulation: Ms. Goodstone is currently nonambulatory. She is independent in using a power wheelchair for mobility in a hospital environment.
- Upright tolerance: Ms. Goodstone tolerates standing table in County Rehab for 30 minutes with appropriate vital signs.

Equipment requested
It is recommended that Ms. Goodstone receive a standing frame for use in her home (see attached pamphlet for details on the standing frame).

Medical necessity of equipment
The standing table is used to counteract the numerous deleterious effects of immobility on major organ systems in the body: musculoskeletal, renal and urinary tract, skin and underlying tissue, respiratory system, cardiovascular system, and the digestive system. Specifically with Ms Goodstone, the benefits of this treatment are numerous, including: decreased tone/spasticity, decreased pain, improved lower extremity range of motion, improved upright tolerance, improved respiratory status, improvements in cardiovascular status and conditioning, and decreased risk for skin breakdown/pressure sores and osteoporosis, which are costly medical conditions. Before this exacerbation, Ms Goodstone was ambulating short household distances with a rolling walker and assistance of her home health aide. With the current diagnosis of progressive MS and her current physical and medical status, she will likely no longer be able to ambulate. The standing allotted by the standing table is essential in providing an effective program for addressing the risks of immobility for this patient in her home.

Thank you for your time and consideration in this matter. Please do not hesitate to contact us directly for any other questions or concerns.

Sincerely,
Jerry Garcia, PT
Superior Physical Therapy Group Inc.

FIGURE 13-2 Sample letter to third-party payer requesting specialized equipment. A brief synopsis of the patient's status is included, and the specific benefits to the patient are clearly delineated in the second-to-last paragraph.

In reply to: CBA Healthcare Inc.
Attention: Northeast Region Managed Care Division

To whom it may concern:
Subject: Request for additional physical therapy visits for Rupal Patel

Ms. Patel was referred for physical therapy evaluation and treatment 6/15/09, 2 weeks s/p left ankle fracture with ORIF. On initial evaluation this patient presented with pain, edema, decreased LE ROM and strength, as well as limitations in transfers and ambulation. She has received 6/8 authorized physical therapy sessions to date, consisting of ultrasound, stretching/strengthening, standing balance training, gait training, and patient education in safety precautions and home exercise program activities. The patient has achieved the following progress:

Measurement	Initial Evaluation	Current Status
Activities		
Lower Extremity Functional Scale (Range 0-80; 80 = no functional limitations; clinically significant change = 9 points)	35	48
Ambulation	Amb. 250 ft using toe-touch weight bearing on left leg, with bilateral axillary crutches, on level surfaces and stairs	Amb. with straight cane weight bearing as tolerated within home and outside up to 500 ft. Unable to amb. longer distances (for recreational walking, walking in shopping mall)
Transfers	Transfers independently with B axillary crutches using toe-touch WB L LE	Transfers independently with straight cane and weight bearing as tolerated LLE
Impairments		
Pain	Subjective reports left ankle pain as 8/10 on all standing/ambulatory activities	Pt. reports pain has subsided to 4/10 on standing/ambulatory activities
Anthropometric measurements Figure 8	L: 41 cm R: 35 cm	L: 37.5 R: 35 cm; indicating decrease in L ankle edema
AROM (L)	PF: 0-10° DF: 0° Inversion: 0-7° Eversion: 0°	PF: 0-20° DF: 0-5° Inversion: 0-15° Eversion: 0-7°
Strength (L)	PF: 2/5 DF: 2/5 Supination: 2/5 Pronation: 2/5	PF: 3+/5 DF: 4/5 Supination: 4-/5 Pronation:4-/5

Although significant progress has been achieved, this patient continues to present with the aforementioned impairments and activity limitations regarding her ability to perform her work duties as a retail clothing store manager as well as household duties (including carrying laundry and cleaning house). To date, manual therapy has not been not initiated due to the patient's level of pain and discomfort. However, the patient's pain levels have decreased substantially, and she would benefit from a more progressive treatment program including manual therapy. Current research has demonstrated that manual therapy can improve ankle range of motion and mobility following ankle fracture,* which can have a significant impact on facilitating return to work and full functioning within the home.

Ms. Patel requires continued PT treatment 2 ×/wk for 4 weeks (8 sessions) as described to achieve the following updated PT goals:
1. Patient will return to work full time within 2 weeks without restricted duties.
2. Patient will transfer independently without assistive device in 4 weeks/8 sessions.
3. Patient will ambulate on level surfaces, ramps (to 15° incline), and stairs up to 1000 ft (distance need to walk to work from transportation) without assistive device independently in 4 weeks/8 sessions.
4. Decreased pain to <2/10 in order to comfortably perform household chores in 4 weeks/8 sessions.

Please do not hesitate to contact me if you have any questions. Thank you for your consideration.

Sincerely,
Jean Smythe, PT
Superior Physical Therapy Group Inc.

*Lin CW, Moseley AM, Refshauge KM: Rehabilitation for ankle fractures in adults, *Cochrane Database Syst Rev* Jul 16(3):CD005595, 2008.

FIGURE 13-3 Sample letter to a third-party payer requesting approval for additional visits. The letter highlights the patient's quantitative improvements in functional performance, details the skilled intervention that was required to achieve these improvements, and provides evidence to support the benefit of physical therapy and the specific procedures used in this patient population.

June 25, 2008

ABC Insurance Co.
Re: Alicia Bremmer
Period: November 2007-March 2008

To Whom It May Concern,

This letter is being offered to provide basis for support of medical necessity for restorative outpatient physical therapy services for Alicia Bremmer for the period in question as well as continued care.

Ms. Bremmer has been treated at our facility for s/p Lumbar Fusion surgery from 7/10/08 to the present. The patient's progress was slow in a large part due to a foot drop that occurred during the above noted surgical procedure. Until recently, the patient continued to wear a Jewitt TLSO and is still using a cane for ambulation as well as an orthotic brace to compensate for left ankle weakness/instability.

Prior to injury/surgery, the patient was independent with all activities of daily living without need for an assistance device. At the present time, the patient has not achieved her prior functional status, which has adversely affected her participation as a full-time working mother of two. During the period in question, Mrs. Bremmer demonstrated an increase in her active trunk ROM, a ½ to full grade increase in left LE strength (depending on the muscle group), and an improvement in her functional test score from 19/21 to 21/21.

Ms. Bremmer responds well to manual therapy techniques as well as specific, guided exercise prescription to help her to achieve adequate hip/knee strength and to optimize neural recruitment of the left ankle musculature.

It is my professional opinion that with continued skilled physical therapy services the patient has good potential to ambulate community distances without an assistive device, improve standing tolerance >30 minutes, and to improve strength of left lower extremity in an effort to restore the patient's prior level of function. Ms. Bremmer has found the therapy to be indispensible toward restoring her prior level of function, and has continued to attend therapy on a self-pay basis.

Enclosed is a copy of the patient's record that includes evaluation/re-evaluation findings, daily notes, and the treatment plan. If you have further questions regarding this case, please feel free to contact me at 555-555-5555.

Thank You,

Joe Jones, DPT
Community Hospital

FIGURE 13-4   Sample letter to an insurance company in response to denial of payment for services. The letter highlights the patient's functional improvements, provides justification for the slow progress, and provides specific achievable functional goals for continued services.

these factors apply to all forms of documentation, they are particularly important for letters to third-party payers. Therapists should not oversimplify their documentation, but they should use terminology that can be relatively easily understood and should define any terminology that is unlikely to be known.

PATIENT EDUCATION MATERIALS

Patient education materials and home programs are one of the key components of most physical therapy plans of care. These materials are used in all types of settings and patient populations. If home exercise programs are to be used by a patient after discharge, then written handouts should be issued to patients individually (Scott, 2005). Instructions must be written carefully, with specific attention directed to the patient's educational level, language capabilities, and learning style. Whenever possible, pictures or graphical information can be very helpful to provide a visual representation of the information being conveyed.

Many different types of patient education materials are available for purchase through various organizations. Many can be tailored to individual patient needs. For example, materials are available with exercise prescription "boxes" containing hundreds of exercises that can be photocopied. The number of computer software packages designed with this same purpose has increased. Therapists should also be sure to indicate in the patient's medical record when patient education materials are given to the patient as well as any additional verbal instructions provided.

Summary

- This chapter provides an overview of various kinds of specialized documentation in physical therapy, including letters to third-party payers, discharge notes, and patient education materials.

- All forms of patient documentation should be concise, free of jargon, and focus on the important aspects related to the patient's plan of care and improving the functional outcomes.

- Although formats and requirements change frequently, the principles related to functional outcomes approach provide a consistent framework for all types of documentation.

CHAPTER 14

Documentation in Pediatrics

Lori Quinn and Agnes McConlogue

LEARNING OBJECTIVES

After reading this chapter and completing the exercises, the reader will be able to:

1. Describe the laws governing early intervention and school-based therapy in the United States.

2. Identify the key components of documentation in early intervention and school-based settings.

3. Create goals for the pediatric population based on best practice standards.

As a child progresses through the pediatric spectrum of service delivery, the documentation, evaluation, and implementation involved require a unique set of standards. The "pediatric patient" can refer to an individual from birth to 21 years of age. Consideration of the needs of the child and the family is paramount and must be incorporated into the evaluation and documentation process. Furthermore, pediatrics often involves multidisciplinary collaboration, perhaps even more so than in other patient populations. Pediatric documentation is read by a wide range of health and non-health professionals, thus requiring specific skills from the PT.

Purpose of Pediatric Evaluation

As with evaluations in other patient populations, PTs working with pediatric clients need to understand the primary purpose of their assessment to determine an overall assessment strategy. Four purposes of performing evaluations were presented in Chapter 2: descriptive, discriminative, predictive, and evaluative. A *descriptive* measure describes the child's current state of functioning, problems, and needs (e.g., activities and impairments). This is typically done through documentation of the therapist's observations and the results of any examination findings (e.g., range of motion, tone assessment), which is done for virtually every client. In addition to descriptive measures,

therapists frequently incorporate standardized testing into their initial evaluation and documentation for a pediatric client, either for *discriminative* (e.g., does the child have a developmental delay?) or *predictive* (is the child at risk for developing a certain disability?) purposes. Finally, *evaluative measures*, which are measures used to show change over time, are used for children participating in ongoing intervention or to assess changes over a certain period.

The structure of an evaluation report for a pediatric client can look quite similar to other general physical therapy evaluations, including the reason for referral, description of participation, activities and any impairments, an assessment, goals, and plan of care. However, there are some important considerations for report writing and documentation for this population. These issues are discussed as they pertain to two broad categories of pediatric clients: early intervention (typically from birth to 3 years) and school-aged (3 to 21 years).

Early Intervention

IDEA

The Program for Infants and Toddlers with Disabilities, also commonly known as Part C of the Individuals with Disabilities Education Act (IDEA 2004), is a federal program offering assistance to states to "maintain and implement a statewide, comprehensive, coordinated, multidisciplinary, interagency system of early intervention services for infants and toddlers with disabilities and their families" (IDEA 2004, section 303.1 (a)). There is a clear focus on family involvement in the wording of IDEA 2004, throughout all phases of service delivery, most notably during the early intervention program (EIP). Part C of IDEA 2004 requires that children who meet the criteria receive services from birth until the child no longer requires them or when, typically, they reach their third birthday (Box 14-1).

DETERMINING ELIGIBILITY

Aspects of eligibility for services, including physical therapy, differ from state to state because each state can use its discretion in determining the EIP. The provision of physical therapy is included among the related services to promote function and adaptation to the child's natural environment, typically in the home. Individual states govern the specific eligibility criteria for developmental delay and at-risk children. Although the criteria for eligibility vary among states, most states require scores from standardized tests as the determinant of service implementation.

For example, a therapist may be called upon to report his or her findings in terms of percent delay or as standard deviations from the norm. For example, in certain states for a child to receive services there must be a 33% delay or 2 standard deviations from the mean in one functional area or 25% delay or 1.5 standard deviations from the mean in each of two functional areas. The percentage and standard deviations may differ according to individual state requirements. Therapists working in states that require specific criteria must therefore provide the results of standardized tests in their evaluation report, which will then be used to determine a child's eligibility for early intervention services. Hawaii is currently an example of a state that does not require score reporting, relying

instead on the recommendation of the multidisciplinary team (MDT), which typically includes a speech therapist, special educator, or an occupational therapist. In addition, individual states may provide their own definition of "developmental delay," typically referring to the child who has not attained expected developmental milestones in one or more areas of development: cognitive, physical, communication, social/emotional, or adaptive.

FAMILY-CENTERED PLANNING

The focus on family-centered planning is an important component of the EIP. The ability to incorporate the family into a collaborative, team-based, problem-solving approach offers the maximal potential for success versus viewing the family and child as passive recipients of individual services. Based on current research and best practice standards, the early intervention therapist should include the following as part of the initial discussion with the family: their concerns, their expectations, the child's strengths, and the family's daily routine (Farrell et al., 2009). If the therapist is able to obtain this information before the assessment, he or she has a greater chance of capturing the child's true abilities beyond the scope of standardized testing. In addition, each infant/toddler has uniquely different needs. By incorporating the family into the assessment process, the PT offers the child the security he or she needs to allow the PT to perform the best possible evaluation that is truly representative of the child and family.

DOCUMENTATION OF EARLY INTERVENTION EVALUATIONS

Evaluations serve "dual, sometimes competing functions: providing ecologically valid, functionally relevant information and evaluating eligibility for services through normative references" (Farrell et al., 2009). Early intervention evaluation reports are primarily read by individuals who are not health care professionals—most importantly, the child's parents. *Best practice* in early intervention report writing involves several key components. The report should be free of jargon and easily interpreted by individuals outside the medical field (see Box 14-2 for more details on optimal report writing). If medical terminology is required, it should be defined whenever possible. Case Example 14-1 provides an example of a physical therapy evaluation for a young child being evaluated for early intervention services. As shown in this example, the headings for an early intervention evaluation can differ slightly from that typically written in a hospital or clinic setting but have the same general structure.

BOX 14-1

IDEA, Part C

Under Part C of IDEA, states must provide services to any child who:

"(i) is experiencing developmental delays, as measured by appropriate diagnostic instruments and procedures in 1 or more of the areas of cognitive development, physical development, communication development, social or emotional development, and adaptive development; or (ii) has a diagnosed physical or mental condition which has a high probability of resulting in developmental delay."

IDEA 2004, §632(5)(A)

BOX 14-2

Strategies for Optimal Report Writing in Early Intervention

1. Provide parenthetical definitions.

   Joey was unable to maintain quadruped (on hands and knees) when placed there. While attempting to roll supine (on his back) to prone (on his stomach) he was observed to use an extensor pattern (use of primarily one muscle group) to complete the transition.

2. Explain test results in plain language.

   The scores on the standardized test of motor development indicate that Jane is currently performing at the 3rd percentile. This means that the majority of her age-related peers are functioning at a higher level and, based on parent report, scores, age equivalents, and discipline-specific assessment, Jane is eligible for early intervention services.

3. Describe concepts functionally.

Poor example	Optimal example
Annie presented with moderate hypotonia of the trunk.	*Annie has a lower resting level of muscle stiffness than what is expected. This affects her posture and her ability to move against gravity with independence and efficiency.*

4. Eliminate negative reporting.

Poor example	Optimal example
Nikki was resistant to handling and refused to participate in the evaluation process.	*Nikki was self-directed in her play, preferring to follow her own agenda more exclusively than is typical for her age.*

5. Avoid deficit-focused language.

Poor example	Optimal example
Mark has only fair strength of his abdominals and is unable to get into sitting independently.	*Mark is able to maintain sitting when placed there. Strengthening his abdominal muscles to assist him in completing the transitions into and out of sitting will be a primary focus of physical therapy intervention.*

6. Lead with the child's competencies.

Poor example	Optimal example
Sarina does not ascend/descend the stairs reciprocally.	*Sarina is able to climb a flight of stairs. She is emergent in her ability to climb up and down the stairs using the mature pattern (step-over-step) expected of her age.*

7. Avoid "but/however" constructions.

Poor example	Optimal example
Roberto can transition sit to stand but is unable to do it without help from his mother or holding onto the couch.	*Roberto is able to transition from sit to stand when he is provided with external support from an adult or a stable surface.*

Adapted from Towle PO, Farrel AF, Vitalone-Raccaro N: Report writing in early intervention: guidelines for user-friendly, strength-based writing, *Zero to Three*, 28:53-60, 2008.

As seen in Case Example 14-1 and Box 14-2, evaluations in early intervention should focus not only on the problems or activities that the child *cannot* do, but also on what he or she is *able* to do (otherwise known as *strength-based*). Deficiencies can, and should, be highlighted in the report, but the overall tone of the evaluation should be centered on the child's abilities at the present time. Strength-based report writing is not to be interpreted as curtailing the PT from using the terminology pertinent to the profession. It is imperative, however, that the parents, as part of the family-centered planning, be able to understand and hopefully feel empowered by the therapist's assessment.

Individual family service plans (IFSPs) are required documentation for any child receiving early intervention services. This plan serves as the "contract" between the state governing agency and the family to outline the goals of early intervention for a child (McEwen, 2000). PTs are typically required to document a summary of a child's gross motor skills and goals for their continued development. These goals must be written in collaboration with the family and thus should be clearly written with specific measurable activities and time frames. IDEA mandates a review of the IFSP every 6 months. Sample IFSP goals (long-term) and objectives (short-term) are shown in Case Example 14-2.

School-Based Intervention

Although early intervention services are generally provided in the child's home, children with disabilities who are older than age 3 years typically receive services in a school setting. Physical therapy is provided when the child is eligible as mandated under Part B of IDEA. Eligibility for physical therapy requires that the child is categorized under 1 of the 13 handicapping conditions defined by IDEA 2004 and that physical therapy intervention is required to "assist a child with a disability to benefit from special education" (IDEA 2004, section 300.34). The PT is now a part of a team that can include anyone who has interaction with that child, including but not limited to, the teacher, paraprofessional, occupational therapist, and speech-language pathologist. This multidisciplinary team (MDT) collaborates to create a framework of service evaluation and implementation referred to as the individualized education plan (IEP). Each student who receives physical therapy must have an IEP in place before initiation of services. The therapist may be required to complete a full and appropriate evaluation to determine status and goals. However, eligibility does not require scores from standardized outcome measures as the determining factor.

These education plans are multidisciplinary and are completed by the personnel involved with the child's education. IEPs are designed differently by each state. In most states, therapists are required to write "a statement of the child's **present levels of academic achievement and functional performance**" as they affect his or her performance in the school setting and "a statement of **measurable annual goals, including academic and functional goals**, designed to meet the child's needs that result from the child's disability to enable the child to be involved in and make progress in the general education curriculum" (IDEA 2004). The focus of IDEA 2004 within the school setting is on goals; therapists must provide goals that are functional, relevant to the educational setting, and measurable.

IDEA mandates review of the IEP on a yearly basis. Thus therapists, educators, and other providers must write a new IEP with new goals for the upcoming year. Case Example 14-3 provides an example of an IEP written for child with cerebral palsy in a school-based setting.

In addition to the IEP, providers must assess goal achievement on a quarterly basis and provide a statement of how their goals will be measured. Another unique component of formulating the IEP is that the child becomes a crucial member of the team and has a voice in creating his or her own goals.

Functional outcomes documentation is very important in the school setting. The purpose of a PT's evaluation and intervention within the school setting is to help the child function better in the school (e.g., in the lunchroom, classroom, playground). In addition to writing summary information and goals on the IEP, therapists may complete a full evaluation or may provide justification to obtain appropriate equipment required for the child to access the educational environment (Case Example 14-4). The focus of this documentation should be on how limitations in physical functioning and gross motor skills affect the child's ability to function in the school setting. This could relate to a child's ability to move within a classroom or between classrooms, to participate in gym class or on the playground, to climb stairs in the school, to get on and off the bus, or to participate in self-care skills such as dressing and toileting. The School Function Assessment (Coster et al., 1998) provides a standardized format for therapists to evaluate such limitations.

Use of Standardized Testing

Standardized testing is frequently used in both early intervention and school-based evaluations. Case Example 14-1 provides an example of an early intervention evaluation that incorporates standardized testing documentation. As mentioned earlier, the results of standardized tests are frequently used in combination with a therapist's descriptive assessment to determine eligibility for services. The results of these tests should be documented in the evaluation report; however, the evaluation report should not focus *solely* on the results of the test and the child's performance on specific items.

Table 14-1 provides a list of some commonly used standardized tests for young children, although by no means is this list exhaustive. Each test was designed with a specific purpose, and each has its own set of strengths and weakness, discussion of which is beyond the scope of this text. The pediatric therapist is required to have sufficient knowledge of multiple standardized assessments to choose the most appropriate for each individual patient (Long & Toscano, 2002). However, some important considerations for choosing an appropriate measure are highlighted here.

DISCRIMINATIVE MEASURES

It is imperative for the therapist to know which standardized test is the most appropriate choice for a particular child. Discriminative measures "distinguish between children who have and do not have a particular characteristic" (McEwen, 2000). Such measures are necessary in early intervention to distinguish between children who are developing typically and those who have delays in development. The ability to use the appropriate test for a child's diagnosis and/or stage of development allows the therapist to make recommendations and produce goals that will offer the most accurate assessment of the individual child's abilities.

TABLE 14-1	COMMONLY USED PEDIATRIC STANDARDIZED TESTS		
Test	**Target Population**	**Age Range**	**Purpose**
Alberta Infant Motor Scale (AIMS) (Piper & Darrah, 1994)	All infants except those with significant abnormal movement patterns	Birth to 18 months or walking	Identify infants with motor delay (discriminative) and evaluate motor development over time
Bruininks-Oseretsky Test of Motor Proficiency, 2nd edition (BOT-2) (Bruininks & Bruininks, 2005)	All school-aged children	4.5 to 14.5 years	Norm-referenced discriminative measure designed to assess the motor proficiency of all students (typically developing to those with moderate motor skill deficits)
Gross Motor Function Measure (GMFM) (Russell et al., 1989)	Children with cerebral palsy; also reliable for children with Down syndrome	6 months to 16 years	Designed to evaluate change in gross motor function in children with cerebral palsy
Peabody Developmental Motor Scales-2 (PDMS-2) (Folio & Fewell, 2000)	Typically developing, suspected developmental delay	Birth to 5 years	Norm-referenced discriminative measure designed to assess gross and fine motor abilities of children from birth through age 5 years
Pediatric Evaluation of Disability Inventory (PEDI; PEDI-MCAT) (Haley et al., 1992)	Children with expected delays in functional performance	6 months to 7 years; PEDI-MCAT 6 months to 14 years	Norm-referenced discriminative and evaluative measure; designed to evaluate functional capabilities and degree of caregiver burden performance in children with disabilities 8 months to 6 years.
School Functional Assessment (SFA) (Coster et al., 1998)	Children with disabling conditions	5 to 12 years	Criterion-referenced measure that evaluates a student's performance of functional tasks and activities within the school environment
Test of Infant Motor Performance (TIMP) (Campbell et al., 2002)	Infants born prematurely	34 weeks' postconceptual age to 4 months postterm	Predictive test design to predict long-term disability in infants

Two main types of discriminative standardized tests are useful for determining a delay in motor or functional skills: criterion-referenced and norm-referenced. Criterion-referenced tests are those that use specific criteria based on observations of typical development or motor abilities. Norm-referenced tests are those that have been conducted with a large population of children, so that any one child's performance can be compared with a normative distribution. Norm-referenced tests allow for age-based comparisons.

A standardized test commonly used to measure gross motor ability in young children is the Peabody Developmental Motor Scales-edition 2 (PDMS-2) (Folio & Fewell, 2000). The Peabody is norm referenced and it provides representative test items to evaluate general motor function comparing a child with other children of his or her age. It does not presume to evaluate every area of gross motor function. Thus therapists must use clinical judgment to determine other areas of motor functioning and impairments that should be tested.

The Pediatric Evaluation of Disability Inventory (PEDI) is a standardized test that was the first norm-referenced pediatric evaluation tool designed to measure functional abilities (not developmental skills) and caregiver assistance. The PEDI can be a useful tool for identifying limitations in functional activities that are meaningful to a child and for potentially measuring change over time as a result of intervention.

PREDICTIVE MEASURES

When evaluating very young children, therapists may not be able to demonstrate delay in motor skills because the child is to too young to demonstrate active movement. Instead, therapists are often trying to determine or predict whether the child is at risk for some future disability or delay. Such tests are designed to be *predictive*. Several tests in recent years have been designed with such a purpose in mind, particularly for premature infants. The Test of Infant Motor Performance (TIMP), for example, has been found to have predictive validity in identifying premature infants at high risk for delayed motor development (Campbell et al., 2002; Kolobe et al., 2004).

EVALUATIVE MEASURES

Finally, disease-specific measures can be very useful so that children can be measured on a scale that is pertinent to their specific disabilities. For example, the Gross Motor Function Measure (GMFM) has been validated in children with cerebral palsy and is also valid for children with Down syndrome. The GMFM was designed to specifically evaluate change in gross motor function in children with cerebral palsy. In addition, the Gross Motor Function Classification System (GMFCS) allows a therapist to use five levels of classification to chart changes in motor function during intervention and as the child grows or motor abilities develop.

WHEN IS STANDARDIZED TESTING NOT APPROPRIATE?

Standardized testing is not appropriate in some cases. A child may not be able to follow directions to perform a specific test, or no test may be developed to measure the child's specific problems. In these cases, informed clinical opinion is warranted. Sometimes when children have severe motor impairments, the norms developed for a specific test may no longer be valid. Therapists therefore must provide compelling documentation to explain the nature of the child's problem and why and how it does (or may) result in delayed development. The therapist may find that combining sections of specific standardized tests allows for a baseline of information, which is commonly referred to as an *ecological assessment*. This type of assessment allows the therapist to report findings that reflect *aspects* of standardization, either criterion-referenced or norm-referenced, outside the parameters for true standardization.

Goal Writing for the Pediatric Client

FUNCTIONAL GOALS

In the school-based setting, therapists are typically involved in writing components of the IEP that are related to the specific services they are providing. Arguably, the most important component of the IEP is the goals. The annual goals provide the foundation for the type of activities that should be addressed during the upcoming year. According to McEwen (2000), annual goals should "be functional, discipline-free, chronologically age-appropriate, and meaningful to the students and the students' family. They should also include activities that the student can perform frequently and they should address both the present and the future needs of the student" (p. 54). Goal writing on the IEP is mandated to address specific goals related to functioning in the school (see Case Example 14-3 for sample IEP goals). Therefore writing strictly impairment-related goals in this setting is not meaningful. Goals are read by parents and school personnel, who are often not familiar with medical terminology. Therapists should avoid jargon and define terms when necessary (see Chapter 2 for more detail on avoiding jargon).

In addition, it is important to discuss the relevance of *function* as it pertains to the child throughout his or her development. During early intervention services, *function* for the child refers to accessing his or her natural environments. The scope of this term includes all aspects of the typical routine expected for that age. The therapist needs to clarify what that entails for the individual child and family; it is not simply assuming that the child must be assessed and treated within the home environment only. For instance, take the example of a mother who reports that her child is not accessing the playground to the extent that she should. The therapist needs to assess the child within the playground environment and where appropriate, formulate goals that address her participation at the playground and her ability to access the particular pieces of equipment within it.

Many standardized tests used by PTs focus on performance of gross motor tasks versus functional performance. It is important to clarify the difference because assessments should be viewed as a source of subsequent goals. *Gross motor tasks* can be comprised of tasks such as ball manipulation, jumping, skipping, hopping, or standing on one leg. These tasks are expected at certain stages of development and may indicate areas of treatment intervention for the therapist. For example, a child who is not jumping by the age of 3 years may have issues related to strength, balance, or motor planning/coordination. These areas would be the focus of intervention strategies during treatment but should not be considered the *functional* goal for the child. A *functional goal* must address specific components or activities required to access or function efficiently within the child's environment (refer to Chapter 8 for additional discussion). Using the example of the 3-year-old child who is unable to jump: If we hypothesize that, in addition to the inability to jump, the child is only able to climb the stairs with a step-to-step pattern using the handrail and hand-hold, then it is clear that working to have the child use a more mature pattern to move independently from the ground floor to his or her bedroom on the second floor should be the functional goal for the therapist. Focusing on the child's ability to jump independently is *not* the functional goal but may be a treatment intervention that the therapist works on to carry over to the goal of stair climbing.

WRITING COLLABORATIVE GOALS

IEP goals should be formulated with the child, teacher, family, and faculty directly involved in the child's daily routine: paraprofessional, bus driver, cafeteria attendant, and so on. This collaborative approach allows the therapist the ability to create optimal goals within the school setting that address all aspects of expected function within the school, such as transfers onto/off of the bus; ability to feed, dress, and safely complete transfers during toileting; and carry a cafeteria tray in an open environment.

FORMAT FOR WRITING GOALS: ABCDE

To assist therapists in creating goals for the school setting, they should follow the goal formulation format of ABCDE (see Chapter 11). For this population, the *A*ctor, *B*ehavior, *C*ondition, and *D*egree are required elements; the *E*xpected Time is typically inherent because each IEP is for 1 year and the IFSP is for 6 months. (The short-term goals or benchmarks may require a statement of expected time.) The Condition is crucial for school-based therapists because they are expected to write goals that are educationally relevant. This would indicate that as part of the functional routine within the school environment, the therapist should assess the academic tasks pertinent to the individual child and create goals accordingly. For example, accessing the educational curriculum for the individual child may include tasks such as retrieving books in the library, using computers within the classroom, and participating in science labs and art class.

CONTEXT SPECIFICITY AND USE OF MEASUREMENT CRITERIA

Writing goals within the school setting has two critical components. First, goals need to be context specific, ideally defined by a relevant task that would enable the child to be involved in and make progress in the school setting. Second, goals need to be measurable so that goal attainment is quantified (McConlogue & Quinn, 2009). School-based PTs must familiarize themselves with the routine of the children with whom they are working. Goals that are formulated should be particular to the individual child's needs, take into account the child's environment, enhance performance of their daily routine, and assess the comparison to the routine of the typically developing peers within the same environment.

A goal analysis form can help therapists analyze their goals (annual, short-term, or benchmarks) to ensure that the goals are, in fact, functional and measurable as required by IDEA (McConlogue & Quinn, 2009) (Figure 14-1). Such a form can be useful in guiding therapists to write goals that are context specific and use specific measurement criteria.

Objective measurement criteria are required according to IDEA. Therapists should use measurements that evaluate the degree of skill in performing functional tasks: consistency, efficiency, and flexibility. *Consistency* can be measured in the number of days per week or the number of consecutive observations.

This can include the teacher, caregiver, parent, and/or other professionals. *Efficiency* in the simplest form can be reported as the amount of time for a task to be completed. *Flexibility* refers to the child's ability to perform the task in a variety of settings/environments. The following example includes all three optimal measurement criteria (see also Figure 14-1 for examples of IEP goals).

> Example: *Sarah will climb the stairs during transition from class to cafeteria (a total of 12 steps) and during the transition from cafeteria to outdoor recess (flexibility) (a total of 10 steps) within 3 minutes each (efficiency), as reported by her paraprofessional, a minimum of 3 days/week (consistency).*

GOAL ATTAINMENT SCALING

Goal Attainment Scaling (GAS) is another useful tool in creating and analyzing IEP goals. The GAS is a 5-point scale used to quantify individual goal achievement. It can be particularly useful when creating goals for a child with multiple handicapping conditions. In such a case, it may be difficult for the PT to define functional tasks for the child if the child is dependent for all activities of daily living (ADLs). Furthermore, the evaluation may be limited due to lack of available standardized assessments to address the unique performance levels of a child with severe limitations in function. The GAS allows the therapist to identify the most basic components of a task and to chart the progress of the child as he or she works toward achieving the task one component at a time. The use of the GAS is not limited to patients with severe limitations and can be used to chart intervention efficacy for any child. Case Example 14-5 provides an example of GAS used for a pediatric client.

Summary

- This chapter provides an overview of the specialized documentation involved for the pediatric client. Sample evaluations, letters of justification, IFSPs, and IEPs are provided to assist therapists in incorporating functional outcomes assessment with this population.

- All documentation in pediatrics should be concise, free of jargon, and focus on improving functional outcomes.

- Standardized assessment measures are an important component of pediatric documentation and can be used for discriminative, evaluative, and predictive purposes.

- Goal writing for the pediatric patient must be done in collaboaration with the child whenever possible and with other team members. Goals should be functional in nature, context specific, and include measurement criteria.

GOAL # (see below)	1	2	3	4	5	6	7	8
A. ANALYSIS OF GOALS RELATED TO CONTEXT								
Goals in which context WAS NOT specified								
Goal is defined by remediation of an impairment. Task is not specified. (e.g., ROM, strength, alignment)			X					
Goal is defined by a developmental skill. Context is not specified. (e.g., stand through 1/2 kneeling, balance on one foot)		X						
Goal is defined by an isolated task. Context is not specified. (e.g., crawl, sit with trunk erect)	X							
Goals in which context WAS specified								
Goal is defined in the context of a life skill. (e.g., mobility, feeding, dressing, toileting)					X	X	X	
Goal is defined in the context of an academic task. (e.g., classroom activities)				X				
Goal is directed at training other personnel to supervise/reinforce activity. (e.g., teacher, paraprofessional)								X
B. ANALYSIS OF GOALS RELATED TO MEASUREMENT CRITERIA								
Independence (e.g., amount of assistance, progression of equipment)				X	X	X		
Endurance (e.g., distance)				X			X	
Movement patterns (quality descriptors)		X					X	
Efficiency (e.g., time)				X	X		X	
Consistency (e.g., # trials)						X	X	X
Flexibility (e.g., environment changes)						X		X
No measurement criteria	X		X					X

GOAL 1: N.B. will sit with an erect trunk.*

GOAL 2: N.R. will kick a stationary ball toward a target by stepping up and kicking with her right foot.

GOAL 3: R.C. will normalize her base of support by increasing the width of her base of support.

GOAL 4: J.L. will walk from his desk to the blackboard, a distance of approximately 15 feet, utilizing Lofstrand crutches and minimal assistance, within 1 minute.

GOAL 5: Z.X. will propel his wheelchair from his classroom to the cafeteria, given stand-by assistance, in 5 minutes.

GOAL 6: W.O. will negotiate open environments (playground, classroom, hallway), given supervision from his paraprofessional during the school day, 5/5 days/wk.

GOAL 7: K.A. will ascend 1 flight of stairs (14 steps), utilizing a reciprocal pattern without external support, within 3 minutes, 4/5 days/wk.

GOAL 8: The paraprofessional will safely transfer S.R. from wheelchair to classroom seating system, toilet, and cafeteria table, 3/5 days/wk.

*Although "erect trunk" is related to a movement pattern, it is not specifically measurable and was therefore classified as "no measurement criteria."

FIGURE 14-1   A goal analysis form developed to analyze physical therapy–related IEP goals in a school setting. Eight different goals are analyzed here, considering the type of task and context specificity as well as the use of different types of measurement criteria (McConlogue & Quinn, 2009).

CASE EXAMPLE 14-1

Early Intervention Evaluation
Suzanne Jones, DPT Jones Pediatric Therapy (555) 555-5555

Name: Jane Johnson   **D.O.B.:** 4/5/08   **Date of Eval.:** 10/15/09

Reason for Referral

(Typically includes reason for referral, location and time of evaluation and information about the child—who was present, behavior, and communication.)

Jane is an 18-month-old girl diagnosed with developmental delay. She has been referred for physical therapy evaluation secondary to concerns regarding her ability to access her environment independently. Her mother has made additional requests for evaluations in speech and occupational therapies.

Communication with the mother occurred prior to evaluation to determine Jane's schedule and to plan the optimal time for evaluation, in addition to discussing Jane's strengths/interests and the overall concerns of her family. Birth history was typical: Jane was born at term with no complications. Jane was evaluated in her home after her nap at 3 PM. Her mother and older brother, age 5, were present.

Behavior/Communication

She readily interacted with the therapist throughout the evaluation. Jane is able to communicate primarily with vocalizations and inflections of her voice. She has a vocabulary of approximately 4-6 words and enjoys identifying her favorite toy: "baby." She was able to respond to 1-step requests: "give me the ball." In addition, she was able to identify her mother and brother by looking at and calling out to them. She was frustrated when not understood or unable to complete a physical task and would begin to cry. She was consoled quickly and was motivated to continue to play.

Activity/Participation

(Typically includes assessment of child's ability to function within his or her natural environment.)

DEVELOPMENTAL POSITIONS/MOBILITY: Jane is able to sit independently and manipulate (play with) toys on her lap. She will lean on one of her extended arms when reaching outside her base of support (contact with the ground or seating surface) and is able to successfully retrieve what she needs. She is able to keep her balance if challenged to the front or side but has difficulty when challenged to the back. Throughout the evaluation, Jane preferred ring sitting (knees bent with soles of the feet facing each other) on the floor and would quickly attempt to get back into that position. She achieves this by flexing (leaning) her trunk forward and pushing herself back over her pelvis (hips) with her upper extremities (arms).

Jane sleeps in a crib and has begun pulling to stand on the rails when she wakes up in the morning. She enjoys being carried around. Jane is able to creep on hands and knees for 2-3 consecutive cross-pattern advancements and with coaxing from her family. She prefers to scoot across the floor in a ring-sit position, utilizing her legs to pull herself, with her trunk flexed forward and her arms out for balance. She is able to get around quickly and was observed to move throughout the main floor of her home utilizing this pattern. She has difficulty climbing the stair; her mother reports Jane has a fear of falling and she prefers to carry her up and down.

Jane was observed to pull up to stand utilizing the couch for support. She is able to stand with upper extremity support and will hold on with alternating (right or left) upper extremities to reach for a toy but is resistant to standing independently. She enjoys taking 4-5 steps with her push toy and is recently able to take a few steps when an adult holds her hands out to the sides.

Continued

Early Intervention Evaluation—*cont'd*

ACTIVITIES OF DAILY LIVING:

1. *Feeding.* Jane utilizes a bottle, which she is able to hold independently when propped into a reclining position. She is able to eat small finger foods and is reported to be a "fussy eater"—eating only certain pureed foods. She enjoys being with her family at mealtime and is starting to attempt to feed herself with a spoon. She utilizes a highchair during mealtime and certain play activities. Her seated posture is an area of concern for the family as she consistently "slumps" to the side and is unable to stay upright despite attempts at supporting her position.

2. *Bathing.* This is reported as an area of difficulty for the family as she does not enjoy the bath and requires support to maintain safe positioning.

3. *Dressing.* Jane enjoys removing her socks and attempts to remove her shoes by pulling at the Velcro straps. She is compliant in allowing her mother to dress and undress her.

4. *Play.* She is involved in an organized playgroup and her mother reports that she has great difficulty keeping up with her peers. She enjoys the songs and will attempt to pop bubbles, roll the ball, and will clap at the end of each class. She is currently the only one in her class who is not walking yet. In the playground, Jane enjoys the infant swing as her primary mode of play. She enjoys playing with her brother and despite the age difference, they are reported to play well together. She enjoys looking at books and will attempt to do simple shape puzzles. Her favorite doll, which is also a small blanket, is generally required as a comforting object.

5. *Transitions.* Jane is carried throughout the day for all transitions. She utilizes a stroller during family walks/outdoor transportation. Her mother reports that when she is food shopping, she has a difficult time keeping her daughter upright in the seat of the shopping cart and has devised a plan where she props her up in the cart itself, with Jane looking forward, and that this seems to work best for them.

Impairments (Musculoskeletal Assessment)

1. *Strength.* There is sufficient strength of the upper and lower extremities to support her body weight in stance (standing) and while maintaining a sitting posture over an extended arm. She is able to complete a pull to sit with head lag noted (she has difficulty keeping her head in the center, with her chin tucked during an assisted sit-up; children of her age are expected to complete this activity without a head lag). She is able to roll independently to alternate sides. She is able to lift toys of moderate load (estimated to weigh 10% of her body weight) and is able to bang, throw, and squeeze a variety of toys and balls. There is evidence of emergent strength of the lower extremities as she pulls to stand through half-kneel (one leg with the foot flat, the other on the knee) and is able to take some steps when given support.

2. *Range of Motion.* There is full range of motion throughout the joints of the upper and lower extremities.

3. *Tone.* (Tone refers to the resting level of muscle stiffness that allows our bodies to efficiently initiate movements and to support those movements against gravity with ease.) Jane exhibits generalized hypotonia (lower resting level of muscle stiffness than is expected at this age). This is notable for the trunk musculature, primarily the abdominal (stomach) muscles.

4. *Balance.* Static (stationary) balance is categorized as follows: She is able to maintain her balance in positions where her base of support is wide (body contact to surface support is large). When static balance is tested in positions against gravity (kneeling, standing), she has greater difficulty and frequent loss of balance. Dynamic balance (with movement) is an area of difficulty for Jane at this time with loss of balance noted when challenged outside her base of support.

CASE EXAMPLE 14-1

Early Intervention Evaluation—*cont'd*

5. *Alignment/Posture.* Jane has difficulty in utilizing a variety of efficient postures to access her environment. While seated in ring-sit, Jane exhibits rounded shoulders, a forward head posture (head not in line with shoulders), and a rounded back. While standing, Jane's legs are in a wide base of support and her feet are significantly pronated (flat), more than what is expected at her age.

Standardized Assessments

(These are tests that measure a child's performance on certain tasks to that of their peers or as specific levels for individual task performance)

The following standardized assessments were used:

1. *Alberta Infant Motor Scale.* The scores indicate that Jane is currently performing below the 5th percentile. This means that, currently, the majority of her age-related peers are functioning at a higher level.

2. *Pediatric Evaluation of Disability Inventory.* Scored as follows: Self Care: 40.4, Mobility: 20.3, and Social Function: 50.8. (Reported as Normative Standard Scores for Functional Skills, which allows comparison to peers with the mean (average) score set at 50 and a standard deviation of 10. Children are expected to function within 2 standard deviations of the mean. Therefore, a range of functional skill scores between 30 and 70 is expected.) This indicates that Jane has delays in development compared with her peers and, in particular, exhibits the greatest difficulty in the category of Mobility.

Assessment/Plan of Care

Based on the scores from the standardized assessments, therapist observation/evaluation, and in agreement with the parental concerns, Jane is eligible to receive physical therapy early intervention services. It is recommended that Jane receive physical therapy 2 times per week for 45-minute sessions. Areas of concern for the family, such as bathing, feeding, and outdoor play, will be discussed and addressed.

Goals

Goals for intervention will focus on assisting Jane to achieve her expected motor milestones: independent ambulation; stair climbing and readily accessing her environment. Specifically, within the next 6 months:

1. Jane will be able to transition from sitting on the floor to stand, without utilizing a support surface, as reported by her mother, a minimum of 5 times per day.

2. Jane will walk self-directed throughout the ground floor of her home, without upper extremity support, on a daily basis to access the bathroom, kitchen, or family area as reported by her mother.

3. Jane will ascend or descend the stairs, holding onto the rail, with a step-to-step pattern within 3 minutes and given standby assistance for safety a minimum of 2 times per day, as reported by mother or therapist.

If you have any questions, please don't hesitate to contact me.

Sincerely,

Suzanne Jones, DPT, License #53093484

CASE EXAMPLE 14-2

Sample IFSP Summary and Goals
Individualized Family Service Plan

Child's Name: Jane Johnson   **D.O.B.:** 4/5/08   **EIID#:** 12345   **Developmental Area:** Motor
Service Provider: Suzanne Jones, DPT

Child's Present Level of Physical Development, Cognitive Development, Communication Development, Social/Emotional Development, and Adaptive Equipment:

Jane is able to communicate her needs with a variety of vocalizations and 4- to 5-word vocabulary. She is able to respond to requests made of her and is able to recognize and point out her family members. She is motivated to interact with those around her and appears to get frustrated with more difficult tasks such as creeping on all fours, standing, or walking. She likes to hold toys that are within her base of support and has some difficulty with manipulation during fine motor play.

Jane's family reports that she has difficulty staying upright when positioned in a sitting posture, such as during mealtimes, at the playground in the swing, or in the supermarket cart.

This is a great area of concern for her mother during bathtime and mealtime. Jane is not yet walking and prefers to be carried.

Statement of Outcomes Expected for Both Child and Family, Along With Criteria and Timelines to Determine Progress:

1. Jane will be able to maintain sitting postures during mealtime and bathtime so that her mother is able complete both activities without fear and with success by using adaptive equipment as needed, throughout their daily routine within 3 months.

2. Jane will be able to access the playground equipment, including the swing, with minimal assistance or prompts to maintain herself upright, as reported by the mother, within 3 months.

3. Jane will be able to ambulate as her primary means of mobility to access her home environment, the playground, and the organized playgroup environment, as reported by her mother, within 6 months.

Services, Frequency, and Duration Required to Meet the Needs of the Child and Family:

Physical therapy: 45 minutes 3×/week

Occupational therapy: 45 minutes 2×/week

Speech therapy: 45 minutes 3×/week

Natural Environments in Which the Supports and Services Will Be Provided:

Home, playground, organized playgroup, shopping center

CASE EXAMPLE 14-3

Sample IEP Used in a School Setting
Individualized Education Program: Present Level of Academic Achievement and Functional Performance

School District #1	Name of student: Liam Johnson

Describe the Student's Strengths and Ability to Participate in the Educational Program:

Liam is determined to participate in all class activities and insists on peer interaction throughout the school day. He requires assistance only when he is physically unable to achieve a task, such as during transfers into or out of his wheelchair or when he is required to lift objects such as textbooks. He is extremely motivated and eager to learn. Liam is performing at or above grade level in all subject areas.

Describe the Student's Present Level of Academic Achievement or Functional Performance:

Liam is able to manipulate many aspects of the school environment with independence. He is able to operate his power wheelchair independently in open spaces, requiring only verbal reminders for navigation and safety awareness. Liam describes his greatest frustration as not being able to get the books from his backpack, which is kept on the back of his wheelchair, relying on assistance to retrieve or return specific items required during each class, such as books and laptop. He is able to independently manipulate his laptop and produce work that is required of him. Liam is currently learning to use a posterior rolling walker for indoor mobility, requiring assistance to maintain a direct course and taking self-directed rest periods for distances greater than 150 feet. He would like to use his walker during all classroom transitions and be able to sit at a desk or cafeteria table with independence.

Measurable Annual or Functional Goal to Enable the Student to Be Involved in and Progress in the General Education Curriculum:

1. Liam will use his walker to transition from his classroom to the cafeteria (distance of 200 feet) without rest periods or assistance, within 3 minutes, 5×/week.

2. Liam will retrieve his laptop from the back of his chair, given standby assistance, 2×/day.

Short-Term Objectives or Benchmarks for Achieving Each Goal:

1a. Liam will transfer from wheelchair to walker, performing set-up (swing-away footplates and unbuckling seatbelt and scooting to edge of chair with feet flat on floor) independently, requiring assist at pelvis to shift weight forward over feet to stand up with upper extremity support, 2/2 trials per day.

1b. Liam will use his walker to transition from the classroom to the cafeteria (200 feet) given standby assist and one rest period (30 seconds or less), within 5 minutes, 5×/week.

2. Liam will scoot to the edge of his chair independently and, using hand rests, rotate toward the back of his chair given assist at the trunk to maintain balance to retrieve his laptop from his backpack within 3 minutes, 3/3 attempts per day.

Procedures for Measuring the Student's Progress Toward Meeting the Annual Goal:

PT, teacher, paraprofessional report, and daily progress chart.

Schedule of Reports of Student's Progress Toward Annual Goal to Be Provided:

Quarterly along with report card.

CASE EXAMPLE 14-4

Letter of Medical Justification for Equipment
Jump Ahead Physical Therapy
Stockton, Florida
Martin Smith, MS, PT
(555) 555-5555

Name: Katy McKenna	**D.O.B.:** 5/16/03	**Diagnosis:** Cerebral palsy	**Date:** 9/15/09

To whom it may concern,

This letter is to request a posterior walker for Katy McKenna. Katy is a 6-year-old girl currently enrolled in a kindergarten class at her local school. She has cerebral palsy, classified as spastic diplegia and categorized on the Gross Motor Function Classification as a Level III. This indicates that she has the potential to be an independent ambulator with an assistive device.

Katy is motivated to participate in activities with her peers. She is currently receiving physical therapy 3 times a week, 45 minutes each session, to assist her to maximize her ability to participate throughout the school day.

Katy's overall strength and endurance are sufficient to allow her the ability to transfer from sit to stand from her classroom chair or adapted stroller with standby assistance only. Her stride length and cadence have improved over the past year and allow her the opportunity to transition from her class to the cafeteria, gym, library, or recess without having to use the adapted stroller. Her gait pattern is typical for a child with her diagnosis: without an assistive device her center of mass is forward (trunk flexed), she is plantegrade (on her toes) with bilateral lower extremities (both legs) in a flexed, internally rotated, and adducted alignment (bent and turned in posture). Currently, she exhibits limited postural control, frequent loss of balance, and is not safe when ambulating without an assistive device. She uses bilateral hinged ankle-foot orthotics to assist with maintaining alignment during activities in stance (standing). She has no significant functional deficits involving the trunk or upper extremities.

Katy has been trained 3 times a week, 20 minutes each session, for the past 3 months utilizing a program-based (belonging to the school) gait trainer to ambulate. She requires frequent assistance to navigate in situations where the gait trainer is too cumbersome to turn or propel without external assistance. A loaner posterior walker was obtained for 1 month for the purpose of trial and training. Katy is able to navigate the posterior walker throughout her classroom with independence. She requires intermittent assistance when navigating in open environments, such as the halls or at recess. Katy is learning to stand up from the ground utilizing her walker and is independently able to transfer from her classroom chair to the posterior walker. She is now able to participate in gym class and is able to perform the classroom job of going to the main office for messages, as well as keeping pace with her peers during classroom transitions.

We are, therefore, requesting approval for the purchase of a posterior walker to address the following goals: independent ambulation utilizing the posterior walker, given distant supervision, to achieve the full independence she needs to participate safely and without external support or assistance during her school activities.

Katy's ability to improve her independence and her ability to function within her school environment require her to use a posterior walker. Goals for physical therapy will include ambulation on different surfaces and in a variety of contexts. If you have any questions, please do not hesitate to contact me.

Sincerely,

Martin Smith, MS, PT

CASE EXAMPLE 14-5

Use of Goal Attainment Scaling for a Pediatric Client

Goal Attainment Scale for Mitch Hansen: Mitch will participate during transfers into and out of his wheelchair

−2 Dependent throughout transfer.	X 9/15/09			
−1 Lifts head away from headrest for >3 seconds.		X 12/22/09		
0 Maintains upper trunk erect for >3 seconds when supported at the pelvis/lower trunk.			X 3/29/10	
+1 Maintains trunk erect when given support at the pelvis for >5 seconds.				X 6/10/10
+2 Actively brings trunk forward in order to scoot forward in wheelchair given assist at the pelvis.				

EXERCISE 14-1

Identify the errors in the following statements that could be found in an early intervention evaluation report, which will be read by other service providers and the child's parents. Rewrite a more appropriate statement in the space provided.

Statement	Rewrite Statement
1. The child was uncooperative.	
2. John has poor strength.	
3. Lucy has spasticity of B hamstrings and gastrocs.	
4. Kelly cannot walk and is currently wheelchair bound.	
5. Tommy can climb stairs but can only do so with one hand held by his mother.	
6. ROM R knee ✓ 100°.	
7. Samantha sits in W-sitting with excessive kyphotic posture.	
8. Timmy performed very poorly on the PEDI with a standard score of 20.	

EXERCISE 14-2

Based on the following case scenario, write three plausible IEP goals that would be appropriate for this child.

Tim is an 8 y.o. boy with diagnosis of spina bifida. *Activity/Participation*: He is able to walk in school, on flat tile surface, with Lofstrand crutches. He is slower then his peers (avg. gait speed 0.8 m/sec) and is having difficulty managing his books to travel between classes this year. He prefers taking the elevator in the school over using the stairs, and uses a wheelchair for long-distance mobility, including any outdoor activities at school. *Impairments*: Mild L thoracic C-Curve scoliosis; PROM limited R ankle dorsiflexion $-5°$; weakness knee flexion R 2+/5; L 3–/5; ankle dorsiflexion R 2/5, L 2+/5; ankle PF R 0/5, L 1/5; hip extension 0/5 B. Impaired sensation L4-S2 dermatomes.

GOALS

1. _____

_____

2. _____

_____

3. _____

_____

CHAPTER 15

Payment Policy and Coding

Helene M. Fearon, Stephen M. Levine, and Lori Quinn

LEARNING OBJECTIVES

After reading this chapter and completing the exercises, the reader will be able to:

1. Define third-party payers.

2. Describe Medicare policies and the key elements of documentation for Medicare and other third-party payers.

3. Outline Medicare guidelines for documenting skilled therapy services.

4. List the components of documenting initial evaluations, progress notes, treatment notes, reevaluations, and discharge summaries for Medicare.

5. Understand use of ICD-9 (diagnosis) coding and CPT (procedure) coding for billing and payment purposes.

6. Summarize guidelines for CPT coding that may enhance payment for services and minimize denials.

The topic of health care reform in the United States includes a change in the way health care services are financed. Current reform initiatives include legislative provisions that may have a significant impact on how health care insurance is structured and therefore have an inevitable effect on what is required for medical record documentation. The purpose of this chapter is to provide an overview of current payment policy in the United States and understand its effect on documentation by therapists. Of note, the information presented here is likely to change, so readers are encouraged to use this chapter as an overview of payment policy but to consult current health care policy manuals, Web sites, and other related resources for the most up-to-date information.

Third-Party Payers

A *third-party payer* is an organization or entity that finances health care services for a patient or client. The patient is considered the first party and the health care provider is considered the second party. In the United States third-party payers are typically either insurance companies or third-party administrators, which are private entities, or Medicare or Medicaid, which are government-run agencies.

For all third-party payers, it is necessary from the outset for therapists to justify the necessity of the services they are providing. The principal way this is achieved is through appropriate documentation of therapy services because this is the key method for payers to obtain information about the legitimacy of the services for which they are providing payment. One of the primary roles of third-party payers is cost containment. The United States currently has the highest per-capita health care expenditure in the world (Kaiser Family Foundation, 2007). This is due in part to the rising and unsustainable costs of health care. Reviews and audits of rehab services commonly demonstrate that services are provided without the evidence to support their effectiveness or relation to positive health and functional outcomes. Documentation often does not justify the necessity of services based on the patient's clinical presentation. Both government agencies and insurance companies are under pressure to find methods to reduce health care costs, especially for services that may not be necessary. Therefore the medical necessity for services, as defined by the third party responsible for payment of health care claims, is more likely to be scrutinized.

Third-party payers set standards or policies regarding the method and amount of payment for health care services they cover. These policies affect physical therapy and other providers of rehabilitation services, and moreover are often developed specifically for rehab services because of concerns of overutilization and unwarranted variation in treatment provided. For example, an insurance company may set a limit on the number of physical therapy visits in a calendar year or may determine that only certain types of interventions will be covered for a particular diagnosis. Each third-party payer typically also has its own requirements for billing and documentation. As discussed in Chapter 2, physical therapy documentation has many different purposes—one of which is to provide justification for payment by third-party payers. Although therapists must become familiar with the policies and requirements of each of their patient's third-party payers, many—if not most—payers look to Medicare to set the standard for payment policy, including documentation requirements. Therefore the focus of much of this chapter is on current Medicare requirements because therapists who are familiar with and incorporate these guidelines for documentation and coding will, in most instances, meet the requirements of most other third-party payers.

MEDICAID

Medicaid provides health care benefits to people (1) who meet certain financial requirements or (2) have a permanent disability. Medicaid is administered by individual states, which set guidelines regarding individual eligibility and services. The Centers for Medicare and Medicaid Services (CMS), a government agency, provides recommended guidelines for documentation purposes related to patients who receive Medicare or Medicaid benefits (CMS, 2008). Because Medicaid guidelines are updated frequently and are state driven, an in-depth discussion is beyond the scope of this book. For additional information, see http://www.cms.hhs.gov/home/medicaid.asp.

MEDICARE

Because Medicare is the largest source of funding for medical and health services for people in the United States without private health insurance, its guidelines and regulatory features are of particular concern to PTs and rehabilitation professionals. Furthermore, Medicare is often looked to as a standard from which other companies design their own coverage and payment decisions. Many policies adopted by Medicare have been incorporated by other private third-party payers.

Medicare is the federal health insurance plan for individuals aged 65 years and older. Individuals with a permanent disability are also eligible to receive Medicare benefits. Medicare Part A is hospital insurance provided by Medicare; it applies to payment for services rendered in a hospital setting, skilled nursing facility, inpatient rehab, or home health agency after discharge from the hospital. Medicare Part B is medical insurance to pay for medically necessary services and supplies provided in an outpatient setting. Individuals pay a premium to receive this coverage. Part B covers outpatient care, including physician's services, physical, occupational, or speech therapy, and services provided in the home when the patient is no longer considered homebound. The discussion in this text focuses on Medicare Part B requirements for documentation because outpatient practice comprises the majority of physical therapy practice. Although some components and requirements for documentation of Medicare Part A and B differ, the general principles are the same. Efforts continue to eliminate discrepancies in documentation requirements between inpatient and outpatient settings. Medicare requirements related to documentation in the inpatient setting should be reviewed as you proceed with the process of improving documentation skills because this area is currently under review.

For Medicare services, the CMS contracts with different insurance companies (previously called *Medicare carriers* or *intermediaries* and now called *Medicare Administrative Contractors* [MACs]) to manage and implement Medicare benefits. Medicare Contracting Reform (section 911 of the Medicare Prescription Drug, Improvement, and Modernization Act of 2003) mandated that the Secretary for Health & Human Services replace intermediators and carriers to administer the Medicare Part A and Part B fee for service (FFS) programs, contained under Sections 1816 and 1842 of the Social Security Act, with the new MAC authority. There are 15 new MACs processing Part A and Part B claims. These MACs require specific documentation to justify payment under the Medicare benefit. Title XVIII of the Social Security Act, section 1833(e), prohibits Medicare payment for any claim that lacks the necessary information to process the claim. Section 1862(a)(1)(A) of the Act allows payment to be made only for those services considered *medically reasonable and necessary*.

The *Program Integrity Manual* (CMS), Chapter 3, Section 3.11.1, states:

For Medicare to consider coverage and payment for any item or service, the information submitted by the provider or supplier…must be corroborated by the documentation in the patient's medical records that Medicare coverage criteria have been met.… This documentation must be maintained by the physician and/or provider and available to the contractor upon request.

KEY FEATURES OF MEDICARE DOCUMENTATION

Failure to submit requested documentation will result in complete or partial denial of payment for services. For a service to be covered under the Medicare program, all the following must be true:

- It must have a benefit category in the statute (therapy services are a benefit under section 1861 of the Social Security Act).
- It must not be excluded.
- It must be reasonable and necessary.

In addition to the coverage requirements listed above, the following additional Conditions of Payment must exist for therapy services to be paid under Medicare:

- The individual "needs" therapy services.
- A plan for furnishing such services has been established by a physician or nonphysician provider or by the therapist providing such services and is periodically reviewed by a physician or nonphysician provider.
- Services are or were furnished while the individual is or was under the care of a physician.
- Services must be furnished on an outpatient basis.

Medicare provides guidance to its requirements in its Benefit Policy Manual (BPM), 100–02, Chapter 15, Section 220. Following are the key elements of Medicare documentation excerpted from the BPM, that must exist to support payment for therapy services under Medicare and that must be evident in the documentation throughout the therapy episode of care:

1. **Medical necessity.** Medicare refers to the concept of medical necessity using the terms "reasonable and necessary" in its benefit policy language. Many physical therapists wrongly believe the physician's order or referral establishes medical necessity for physical therapy services. Although a physician's order or referral (which some refer to as a *prescription,* although this is not the professionally accepted or appropriate term) is not required by Medicare, the Medicare benefit for therapy services does require that the patient be under the care of a physician for some diagnosis (which may or may not be related to the diagnosis for which

the therapist is treating the patient) for therapy services to meet coverage guidelines. However, simply because the patient is under a physician's care and a referral to physical therapy has been made does not automatically justify the medical necessity of therapy services. Medical necessity for therapy services is determined by the evaluating physical therapist, and there must be clear evidence of this medical necessity demonstrated in the physical therapist's documentation. It is critical for therapists to understand that documentation of the initial evaluation is the baseline from which medical necessity for therapy services is established, progress toward identified functional goals will be measured, and payment for services can be justified.

2. **Reasonable and necessary.** The BPM clarifies that to be considered reasonable and necessary, the following conditions must each be met:

- The services shall be considered under accepted standards of medical practice to be a specific and effective treatment for the patient's condition. Acceptable practices for therapy services are found in:
  - Medicare manuals (such as Publications 100-02, 100-03, and 100-04)
  - Contractors Local Coverage Determinations (LCDs and NCDs are available on the Medicare Coverage Database at http://www.cms.hhs.gov/mcd)
  - Guidelines and literature of the professions of physical therapy, occupational therapy, and speech-language pathology
- The services shall be of such a level of complexity and sophistication or the condition of the patient shall be such that the services required can be safely and effectively performed only by a therapist or under the supervision of a therapist.
- There must be an expectation that the patient's condition will improve significantly in a reasonable (and generally predictable) period, or the services must be necessary for the establishment of a safe and effective maintenance program required in connection with a specific disease state.
- The amount, frequency, and duration of the services must be reasonable under accepted standards of practice. The contractor shall consult local professionals or the state or national therapy associations in the development of any utilization guidelines.

Although the BPM provides a broad identification of the requirements for coverage under Medicare, CMS provides significant discretion in determining the specific services to be considered "reasonable and necessary" to its MACs. The MACs do this through establishment of LCDs, which are published decisions by an MAC indicating whether particular services are covered on a MAC-wide basis, in accordance with Section 1862(a)(1)(A) of the Social Security Act (i.e., a determination as to whether the service is reasonable and necessary)" (CMS, *Program Integrity Manual*).

3. **Skilled services.** For therapy services to be considered medically necessary or "reasonable and necessary" under the Medicare benefit (as well as most other third-party payers), they must also be of a skilled nature. The BPM identifies that services are considered to be skilled when the knowledge, abilities, and clinical judgment of a therapist are necessary to safely and effectively furnish a recognized therapy service whose goal is improvement of an impairment or functional limitation. Services must not only be provided by the "qualified professional" (the therapist) or "qualified personnel" (the therapy assistant), they must also "require the expertise, knowledge, clinical judgment, decision making and abilities of a therapist that assistants, qualified personnel, caretakers, or the patient cannot provide independently." Also, a therapist may not merely supervise any care being provided by a therapy assistant, but must also apply his or her skills regularly during the episode of care by actively participating in the treatment of the patient. This involvement must be evident in the documentation.

A therapist's skill may also be required for safety reasons if a particular condition or status of the patient requires the skill of a therapist to perform an activity that might otherwise be done independently by the patient at home. Once the patient is judged safe for independent performance of the activity, the skill of a therapist is not required and reasonable and necessary requirements are not met under Medicare.

Services provided by professionals or personnel who do not meet CMS qualification standards, and services provided by qualified people that are not appropriate to the setting or conditions, are not considered skilled services. In addition, services that are repetitive or reinforce previously learned skills or maintain function after a maintenance program has been developed, are considered unskilled services and do not meet the requirements for covered therapy services in Medicare manuals. They are therefore not payable using codes and descriptions for therapy services.

In the BPM, CMS provides examples of how a therapist's skills may be documented in the medical record, such as the following:

- By the clinician's descriptions of the skilled treatment
- By identifying the changes made to the treatment from a clinician's assessment of the patient's needs on a particular treatment day
- By identifying the changes attributable to progress the clinician judged sufficient to modify the treatment toward the next more complex or difficult task

In summary, the deciding factors regarding whether services are considered skilled and "medically necessary" are always whether the services are considered reasonable, effective treatments for the patient's condition and require the skills of a therapist, or whether they can be safely and effectively carried out by nonskilled personnel without the supervision of qualified professionals. If at any point in the therapy treatment it is determined by the treating therapist, *or through review of the documentation* by an MAC (or other third party) that the treatment does not legitimately require the services of a qualified professional, the services will no longer be considered reasonable and necessary and therefore are not considered for payment under the Medicare benefit.

INITIAL EVALUATION

Medicare identifies specific documentation components necessary to meet minimal documentation requirements, which include the initial evaluation and plan of care, certification (and recertification) of the plan of care, treatment notes, progress notes, and a discharge report. The initial evaluation is the most critical component of documentation because it establishes the medical necessity for therapy interventions, identifying the necessity for a course of therapy through documented objective findings and subjective patient self-reporting. In addition to clearly identifying these findings, documentation of the evaluation should list any complexities that are present and, where not obvious, describe the impact of these complexities on the prognosis and/or the plan for treatment such that it is clear on reviewing the documentation that the services planned are appropriate for the individual.

Medicare provides guidance for including areas that should be evident in the documentation of the initial evaluation, including but not limited to the following:

- A diagnosis (where allowed by state and local law) and description of the specific problem(s) to be evaluated and/or treated
- Documentation supporting illness severity or complexity

- Documentation identifying any medical care before the current episode, if any
- Documentation indicating the patient's social support, including where the patient lives (e.g., private home, private apartment, rented room, group home, board and care apartment, assisted living, skilled nursing facility), who they live with (e.g., lives alone, spouse or significant other, child or children, other relative, unrelated person(s), personal care attendant)
- Documentation indicating objective, measurable, beneficiary physical function, including the following:
  - Functional assessment scores from commercially available therapy outcomes instruments
  - Functional assessment scores from tests and measurements validated in the professional literature that are appropriate for the condition/function being measured
  - Other measurable progress toward identified goals for functioning in the home environment at the conclusion of the therapy episode of care

As indicated in the beginning of this chapter, many, if not most, third-party payers look to Medicare to set the standard for documentation of therapy services. Therefore therapists are strongly encouraged to develop consistent documentation standards based on an understanding of these Medicare requirements. In addition to the above concepts, Medicare identifies the following elements as key factors that should be documented by the PT for the initial evaluation. Each of the following elements has been explained in detail in other chapters:

- Demographic information, such as patient's age, date of birth, primary diagnosis (*International Classification of Diseases,* Ninth Revision [ICD]-9 code, or ICD-10), facility and patient identification numbers
- Date of onset of symptoms or any exacerbation of a chronic condition that warrants a new episode of care
- Medical history, which should include the likely impact of any unrelated conditions on the anticipated plan of care
- Reason for therapy intervention
- Current status—subjective and objective evaluation of impairments and functional activities, including the relation between impairments and functional activities
- Signature (including professional designation) and date

Furthermore, Medicare requires that therapy services must relate directly and specifically to a written treatment plan (plan of care), which shall contain, at minimum, the following:

- The diagnoses for which therapy is being provided
- Long-term treatment goals, which should be measurable, pertain to identified activity limitations, and be developed for the entire episode of care (any impairment goals should be linked to a functional activity)
- Type of treatment (e.g. physical therapy, occupational therapy) and the anticipated frequency and duration of therapy services

CERTIFICATION AND RECERTIFICATION OF THE PLAN OF CARE

Medicare requires certification of the Plan of Care (POC) for each interval of treatment. In the outpatient setting, this initial certification period can typically be up to but cannot exceed 90 calendar days from the initial therapy evaluation and treatment. Certification requires that the POC, including the minimally required elements, be signed and dated by the physician or non-physician provider (MD, DO, NP, CNS, PA, and OPM and OD as appropriate), and provides evidence in the medical record that the patient is under the care of a physician. Certification of the POC by the physician must occur within 30 days of the initial evaluation.

Medicare payment and coverage conditions require that the POC be recertified every 90 days if medically necessary treatment continues to be required for an extended period or whenever a significant change in the patient status or POC occurs. Examples provided by Medicare of a "significant change" include a change in diagnosis, an extension of the duration of care previously certified, or a change in the long-term functional goals. Changes in the interventions provided or frequency of treatment appropriate to a change in the patient status as therapy progresses are not considered significant changes and would not require recertification of the POC. It is not required that the same physician or non-physician provider who participated initially in recommending or planning the patient's care certify or recertify the plans.

TREATMENT NOTES

Third-party payment (including Medicare) relies on documentation as its primary (if not only) source of determining whether a claim is paid or denied. Therefore although therapists may be providing excellent patient care and obtaining clinical results reflecting positive functional outcomes, if this information is not evident in the medical record the care provided may go uncompensated by third-party payers. Thus therapists must be diligent in making sure that their documentation appropriately reflects the skilled care the patient is receiving as well as the patient's current objective functional status.

Therapists have historically focused their documentation on recording the specific activities or exercises that the patient is performing, typically listing exercises on flow sheets or within the treatment notes that appear to be of a repetitive nature or reinforcing previously learned activities, without focusing on the *interaction* between the therapist and patient. Typically, exercise documented solely in this fashion will not be considered for payment. Skilled care is best documented in the medical record by focusing documentation on what expertise, knowledge, clinical judgment, or decision making abilities the therapist or assistant is providing to the patient during the visit, in addition to recording the specific procedural interventions or techniques being performed by, or provided to, the patient.

With the exception of a few areas in which Medicare requirements are different than other third-party requirements, such as the requirement of the physician certification of the POC, therapists are best served if they are "payer blind" with regard to ensuring documentation adequately justifies payment for therapy services and focus on documenting consistently for all patients regardless of third-party payer. All the issues discussed in Chapter 12 related to treatment notes are also applicable for Medicare documentation. Current Medicare guidelines state that the purpose of the treatment note is to serve as a record of the skilled interventions that were provided to the patient and document the time of the services to justify use of CPT codes used to bill therapy services (see the billing and coding section below). This is critical because in the event of an audit, a reviewer can determine whether specific interventions should be paid only if the appropriate treatment documentation is present. Reviewers look for evidence that the intervention could have been provided independently or by other nonskilled personnel, so documentation of provision of skilled intervention by the PT is a key component evaluated by Medicare and other third-party reviewers.

The exact format of the treatment notes is not specified by Medicare or its contractors. Although many therapists use a grid format or flow sheet covering several days of interventions, this format is often deficient in providing the required elements of documentation of a treatment note. The treatment note, in whatever format it takes, should include information indicating the skilled intervention that was performed, any major changes in the patient's condition, and any progress, in objective and measurable terms, toward the stated goals.

PROGRESS REPORTS

Third-party payers require that progress toward established functional goals be evident in the therapy documentation to help auditors and reviewers determine whether the services provided are payable under defined benefit categories. If progress is documented within the routine documentation of treatment notes so that such progress is clearly evident, then a separate progress report is not required as long as the key components of a progress report are included.

If the treatment notes do not identify objective and measurable progress, then Medicare Part B requires a progress note to be documented in the outpatient setting at least once every 10 treatment days, or once during each 30 calendar-day period, whichever is less (there are currently no Medicare guidelines for Part A). For Medicare payment purposes, information required in progress reports shall be written by "a clinician," that is, either the physician or non-physician provider who provides or supervises the services, or by the therapist who provides the services and supervises an assistant. It is not appropriate for therapy assistants to document progress reports, although assistants can document data that they have collected and that can be used by the therapist to document the progress report.

The progress report should contain many of the same components of the initial evaluation but should also discuss the progress (or lack of progress) and justification of the need for continued skilled therapy or discharge, if appropriate. Reports of the patient's subjective statements, if relevant, should be included as well as objective measurements or description of changes in status relative to each goal currently being addressed in treatment, if they occur. Progress reports should also include assessment of improvement and extent of progress (or lack thereof) toward each goal. Plans for continuing treatment, reference to additional evaluation results, and/or treatment plan revisions should also be documented in the progress report.

REEVALUATION

Continuous assessment of the patient's progress is a component of ongoing therapy services and is not separately payable as a reevaluation. A reevaluation is not a routine, recurring service but is focused on evaluating progress toward current goals, making a professional judgment about continued care, modifying goals and/or treatment, or terminating services. A formal reevaluation is covered only if the documentation supports the need for further tests and measurements after the initial evaluation.

Indications for a reevaluation include the following:

- New clinical findings
- A significant change in the patient's condition
- Failure to respond to the therapeutic interventions outlined in the plan of care
- Before planned discharge for the purposes of determining whether goals have been met

NOTE: Recertification and reevaluation are very different things. A reevaluation can be a billable service if the requirements for performing it are met but, as noted, it is not necessarily a routine component of an episode of care. Recertification is a paper transaction that must be performed at least every 90 days, but the recertification process does not necessarily require that a reevaluation be performed.

DISCHARGE SUMMARY

When a patient is discharged from care, it is necessary to document a discharge summary. This documentation summarizes the treatment, progress toward goals and, importantly, outlines any recommendations or plans for the patient (other treatment, services, etc.) At the discretion of the clinician, the discharge note may include additional information. For example, it may summarize the entire episode of treatment or justify services that may have extended beyond those usually expected for the patient's condition. Therapists should consider the discharge note the last opportunity to justify the medical necessity of the entire treatment episode in case the record is reviewed. See Chapter 13 for more information on writing discharge summaries.

SUGGESTIONS FOR IMPROVED DOCUMENTATION FOR MEDICARE AND OTHER THIRD-PARTY PAYERS

1. Initial evaluations should consider three important components:
   - The services are considered part of the covered benefit for therapy services.
   - Skilled intervention of a PT is required to provide those services.
   - The intervention is reasonable and necessary.
2. Focus on function and functional outcomes:
   - The initial evaluation should include measures of participation restrictions and activity limitations in addition to impairment measures.
   - Goals should be measurable and relate to patient-centered functional activities.
   - Quantifiable outcome measures should be used to evaluate progress whenever possible.
3. Avoid vague terminology:
   - Instead of "Pt. is improving," write "Pt.'s ambulation distance has improved from 250 ft to 500 ft (avg. gait speed increased from 0.6 to 0.8 m/sec)."
   - Instead of "Pt. is tolerating treatment well," write "Pt. demonstrates increased lumbar spine mobility by 20° flexion and decreased pain in sitting position after manual therapy treatment."

Prospective Payment, Billing, and Coding

PROSPECTIVE PAYMENT

Prospective payment systems are used in home health agencies, skilled nursing facilities, and rehabilitation hospitals as a means to manage escalating Medicare costs. A prospective payment system is a means of payment for health care services in which Medicare payment is made based on a predetermined, fixed amount associated with a patient's diagnosis or classification. CMS has developed different patient classification systems for different health care settings. These classifications are determined by specialized documentation completed by medical personnel to categorize the patient's condition/status according to various functional and medical factors, depending on the setting.

The Minimum Data Set, Outcome and Assessment and Information Set, and the Inpatient Rehabilitation Facility-Patient Assessment Instrument are the assessment instruments used in skilled nursing facilities, home health agencies, and inpatient rehabilitation, respectively. Table 15-1 describes each of these tools.

The primary purpose of these tools is to provide a method for patient classification for prospective payment. In addition, these standardized tools provide methods for quality control and outcomes assessment across a wide range of patient populations.

The involvement of therapists in completing these tools varies depending on the institution or agency. Some institutions require PTs to complete portions of these tools, such as the mobility section, and others require nursing staff to complete the entire assessment. These tools use numerical ratings rather than narrative reporting, and extensive training is typically provided. If computerized documentation is used in a practice setting, these forms can be completed more easily and integrated into institution-specific documentation formats (see Chapter 16 for examples of computerized documentation using these standardized assessment tools).

TABLE 15-1	EXAMPLES OF REQUIRED FORMS IN SETTINGS UNDER PERSPECTIVE PAY METHODS	
Form	Setting or Population	Description
Inpatient Rehabilitation Facility-Patient Assessment Instrument (IRF-PAI)	Inpatient rehabilitation: prospective payment system	Uses FIM scores and comorbidities to classify patients into specific case-mix groups and payment categories
Minimum Data Set-Resource Utilization Groups (MDS-RUGS)	Nursing home: skilled nursing facilities	Comprehensive assessment of patient's functional status and medical condition; used to categorize patients into resource utilization groupings to determine the amount of payment
Outcome and Assessment and Information Set (OASIS)	Home health agencies	Measures outcomes in home health care and determines reimbursement for services

BILLING AND CODING

To bill a third-party payer for services rendered, for the purposes of being reimbursed under a stated benefit, PTs need to document their clinical services and also provide two main components that reflect the reason for the need for their services (medical necessity) and describe procedures performed. Third-party payers each have their own billing requirements but most, if not all, incorporate the reporting of standard terminology for diagnosis (ICD-9) and treatment procedures (CPT-4). Providers must submit a claim form, the most common being the CMS-1500 form, used to bill charges provided to the Medicare beneficiary. This is also typically required by other third-party payers. For Medicare, most providers or facilities are required to submit their bills through an electronic payment system. Although limited, some health care providers may be exempt from this requirement and therefore

may submit their claims by printed documentation. Figure 15-1 shows the CMS-1500 claim form, which is the standard claim form used by a noninstitutional provider or supplier to bill Medicare contractors for services. As seen in the figure, the claim form typically requires therapists to document demographic information about the patient as well as diagnosis codes (#21) and CPT procedure codes (#24D).

When considering the billing and payment process, it is a reasonable goal for therapists to always strive for the most correct coding, which will then result in the most appropriate payment on the first attempt to receive payment on a claim. Following the guidelines listed below and frequently consulting with current CMS and other third-party payer guidelines can help therapists minimize denial of payment. If payment is denied, therapists typically have recourse by way of appeal. The appeals process requires further documentation by the therapist and thus can be very time consuming, with an administrative burden that increases the cost of the claims process.

Coding of Diagnosis

An important component of documentation for billing purposes involves assigning a diagnosis or diagnoses to the patient's condition. This diagnosis is a medical diagnosis, and the standard terminology for these diagnoses was developed by the *International Classification of Diseases* (Ninth Revision, Clinical Modification, ICD-9-CM). (**Note:** The diagnosis the patient is referred with is typically a medical diagnosis, but the therapist needs to identify a treatment diagnosis for billing purposes, which may often be different than the referring medical diagnosis.) In 1967 the World Health Assembly adopted the World Health Organization Nomenclature Regulations, which required member states to use the ICD in its most current form for mortality and morbidity statistics. Thus ICD is the international standard for classifying diagnoses for a variety of purposes. In the United States, the ICD-9-CM is "the official system of assigning codes to diagnoses and procedures associated with hospital utilization" (National Center for Health Statistics, 2007). ICD-10, the most recent version of ICD terminology, is currently scheduled to be implemented by CMS as of October 2013. Various other countries, including Canada and the United Kingdom, have been using ICD-10 terminology for years. Therapists in the United States must therefore familiarize themselves with these new codes well before they take effect.

Both ICD-9 and ICD-10 code sets are contained in manuals that provide numerical listings of more than 14,000 diagnoses, ranging from medical to psychiatric conditions. For billing purposes, a therapist must

1500

HEALTH INSURANCE CLAIM FORM

APPROVED BY NATIONAL UNIFORM CLAIM COMMITTEE 08/05

☐☐ PICA   PICA ☐☐☐

CARRIER →

| 1. MEDICARE ☐ (Medicare #) | MEDICAID ☐ (Medicaid #) | TRICARE CHAMPUS ☐ (Sponsor's SSN) | CHAMPVA ☐ (Member ID#) | GROUP HEALTH PLAN ☐ (SSN or ID) | FECA BLK LUNG ☐ (SSN) | OTHER ☐ (ID) | 1a. INSURED'S I.D. NUMBER | (For Program in Item 1) |

2. PATIENT'S NAME (Last Name, First Name, Middle Initial)

3. PATIENT'S BIRTH DATE MM | DD | YY   SEX   M ☐   F ☐

4. INSURED'S NAME (Last Name, First Name, Middle Initial)

5. PATIENT'S ADDRESS (No., Street)

6. PATIENT RELATIONSHIP TO INSURED   Self ☐   Spouse ☐   Child ☐   Other ☐

7. INSURED'S ADDRESS (No., Street)

CITY   STATE

8. PATIENT STATUS   Single ☐   Married ☐   Other ☐

CITY   STATE

ZIP CODE   TELEPHONE (Include Area Code)   ( )

Employed ☐   Full-Time Student ☐   Part-Time Student ☐

ZIP CODE   TELEPHONE (Include Area Code)   ( )

9. OTHER INSURED'S NAME (Last Name, First Name, Middle Initial)

10. IS PATIENT'S CONDITION RELATED TO:

11. INSURED'S POLICY GROUP OR FECA NUMBER

a. OTHER INSURED'S POLICY OR GROUP NUMBER

a. EMPLOYMENT? (Current or Previous)   YES ☐   NO ☐

a. INSURED'S DATE OF BIRTH MM | DD | YY   SEX   M ☐   F ☐

b. OTHER INSURED'S DATE OF BIRTH MM | DD | YY   SEX   M ☐   F ☐

b. AUTO ACCIDENT?   PLACE (State)   YES ☐   NO ☐

b. EMPLOYER'S NAME OR SCHOOL NAME

c. EMPLOYER'S NAME OR SCHOOL NAME

c. OTHER ACCIDENT?   YES ☐   NO ☐

c. INSURANCE PLAN NAME OR PROGRAM NAME

d. INSURANCE PLAN NAME OR PROGRAM NAME

10d. RESERVED FOR LOCAL USE

d. IS THERE ANOTHER HEALTH BENEFIT PLAN?   YES ☐   NO ☐   If yes, return to and complete item 9 a-d.

READ BACK OF FORM BEFORE COMPLETING & SIGNING THIS FORM.
12. PATIENT'S OR AUTHORIZED PERSON'S SIGNATURE I authorize the release of any medical or other information necessary to process this claim. I also request payment of government benefits either to myself or to the party who accepts assignment below.

SIGNED _____ DATE _____

13. INSURED'S OR AUTHORIZED PERSON'S SIGNATURE I authorize payment of medical benefits to the undersigned physician or supplier for services described below.

SIGNED _____

PATIENT AND INSURED INFORMATION →

14. DATE OF CURRENT: MM | DD | YY   ◄ ILLNESS (First symptom) OR INJURY (Accident) OR PREGNANCY(LMP)

15. IF PATIENT HAS HAD SAME OR SIMILAR ILLNESS. GIVE FIRST DATE MM | DD | YY

16. DATES PATIENT UNABLE TO WORK IN CURRENT OCCUPATION FROM MM | DD | YY   TO MM | DD | YY

17. NAME OF REFERRING PROVIDER OR OTHER SOURCE

17a. ___   17b. NPI

18. HOSPITALIZATION DATES RELATED TO CURRENT SERVICES FROM MM | DD | YY   TO MM | DD | YY

19. RESERVED FOR LOCAL USE

20. OUTSIDE LAB?   YES ☐   NO ☐ $ CHARGES

21. DIAGNOSIS OR NATURE OF ILLNESS OR INJURY (Relate Items 1, 2, 3 or 4 to Item 24E by Line)

1. ⌊___   3. ⌊___

2. ⌊___   4. ⌊___

22. MEDICAID RESUBMISSION CODE   ORIGINAL REF. NO.

23. PRIOR AUTHORIZATION NUMBER

24. A. DATE(S) OF SERVICE From MM DD YY — To MM DD YY	B. PLACE OF SERVICE	C. EMG	D. PROCEDURES, SERVICES, OR SUPPLIES (Explain Unusual Circumstances) CPT/HCPCS | MODIFIER	E. DIAGNOSIS POINTER	F. $ CHARGES	G. DAYS OR UNITS	H. EPSDT Family Plan	I. ID. QUAL.	J. RENDERING PROVIDER ID. #
1								NPI	
2								NPI	
3								NPI	
4								NPI	
5								NPI	
6								NPI	

PHYSICIAN OR SUPPLIER INFORMATION →

25. FEDERAL TAX I.D. NUMBER   SSN ☐ EIN ☐

26. PATIENT'S ACCOUNT NO.

27. ACCEPT ASSIGNMENT? (For govt. claims, see back)   YES ☐   NO ☐

28. TOTAL CHARGE $

29. AMOUNT PAID $

30. BALANCE DUE $

31. SIGNATURE OF PHYSICIAN OR SUPPLIER INCLUDING DEGREES OR CREDENTIALS (I certify that the statements on the reverse apply to this bill and are made a part thereof.)

SIGNED _____ DATE _____

32. SERVICE FACILITY LOCATION INFORMATION

a. NPI   b.

33. BILLING PROVIDER INFO & PH # ( )

a. NPI   b.

NUCC Instruction Manual available at: www.nucc.org   **PLEASE PRINT OR TYPE**   APPROVED OMB-0938-0999 FORM CMS-1500 (08-05)

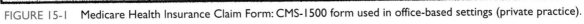

FIGURE 15-1 Medicare Health Insurance Claim Form: CMS-1500 form used in office-based settings (private practice).

decide which ICD code or codes are appropriate for each patient. Therapists should first choose a primary code—a diagnosis that best fits the reason that the patient will be receiving physical therapy services. This may be, and often is, different from the medical diagnosis that accompanies the patient to physical therapy. The therapist can also choose other diagnoses as secondary. Secondary codes are used to provide more detail in terms of the medical necessity for the interventions included as part of the POC. Secondary diagnosis codes can be descriptive of complicating diagnoses. An example would be another condition currently being treated by another provider that could affect the POC. It is important to recognize that ICD codes are a therapist's first step toward demonstrating medical necessity: What is the patient's diagnosis, and is that diagnosis amenable to physical therapy? The ICD diagnosis codes are not equivalent to a movement-system diagnosis, which is critical for treatment planning (see Chapter 9). Rather, third-party payers use ICD codes to have a common language for understanding the nature of the patient's disease, illness, disorder, or injury to make some judgments about prognosis and POC.

Structurally, ICD-9 codes are 3 to 5 digits in length with the first digit alpha (E or V) and the remaining 2 to 4 digits numeric. ICD-10 codes—3 to 7 digits in length—generally provide more detail. If appropriate, they can allow a practitioner to provide more information regarding disease specifics or location compared with ICD-9 codes. CMS recommends that providers always use the longest and most specific code available (e.g., if a 5-digit code is applicable, use that over a 4-digit code). It is still to be determined how the current reporting of ICD-9 codes will be transformed to ICD-10 reporting over the course of the next few years. We suggest therapists make a concerted effort to educate themselves about the ICD-10 system for reporting diagnosis to make this transition an easier one.

Table 15-2 lists some examples of ICD-9 and ICD-10 diagnosis codes that could be used for the same diagnosis (either medical or physical therapy). This table highlights the more descriptive nature of many of the ICD-10 codes.

In addition to these standard types of codes, V codes are codes used by therapists in facility-based settings (e.g., rehabilitation hospitals, subacute facilities, home health care). A V code is indicated if the provision of rehabilitation services (vs. a medical condition) was the primary reason for the patient's admission. If the patient has been admitted only for rehabilitation purposes, then a V code (e.g., V57.1, rehabilitation—physical therapy) is typically reported in the primary location on a claim form (UB-04).

TABLE 15-2	COMPARISON OF ICD-9 AND ICD-10 CODES
Example of ICD-9 Codes	**Example of ICD-10 Codes***
714.0 Rheumatoid arthritis	M05.769 Rheumatoid arthritis with rheumatoid factor of unspecified knee without organ or systems involvement
717.2 Derangement of posterior horn of medial meniscus	M23.321 Other meniscus derangements, posterior horn of medial meniscus, right knee
434.11 Occlusion of cerebral arteries; cerebral embolism	I69.351 Hemiplegia and hemiparesis following cerebral infarction affecting right dominant side
724.2 Lumbago (low back pain)	M9903 Segmental dysfunction, lumbar spine

*Available at: http://www.cms.hhs.gov/ICD10/02m_2009_ICD_10_CM.asp#TopOfPage.

Coding for Procedures (CPT-4 Codes)

Current Procedural Terminology (CPT-4) codes are developed by the American Medical Association for the purpose of providing a consistent and reliable reporting of procedures and service. There are three categories of CPT codes, with category I being made up of codes that describe procedures and services provided by physician and non-physician providers. Numbers are assigned to services that a medical practitioner provides to a patient. Although these codes are not specific to physical therapy, they are applicable to physical medicine and rehabilitation interventions. Therapists assign codes to the interventions they have provided as part of their plan of care for a patient, which is typically a requirement for the third-party payer. Medicare, Medicaid, and the majority of workers' compensation, local, regional, and national payers use CPT codes to adjudicate claims for payment for medical procedures. Based on the specifics of a patient's insurance policy, the payer determines the amount of payment that a qualified health care professional will receive.

As part of the billing process, and to support the procedures that include a time descriptor, therapists are required to document the total treatment time and how much of that time is spent in direct contact with the patient. The total treatment time incorporates only time spent performing skilled interventions;

time for unskilled interventions (e.g., phone calls) should be documented but is not billable. Most CPT codes include a time interval of 15 minutes, which is equivalent to 1 unit. Most third-party payers expect that at least the majority of the 15 minutes involves patient contact time to report one single unit of time. If a therapist provides more than one type of service in that time the total direct contact time should be documented with the appropriate number of units assigned. The total number of units must be a reflection of the total amount of time the therapist provided care in a direct contact manner. The total number of units that can be billed is therefore constrained by the total amount of treatment time (www.hhs.gov/therapyservices).

Determining the correct coding of interventions is critical to ensuring appropriate payment and avoiding claim denials. It is also important for legal reasons. If a therapist submits a CPT code for a procedure but it is not documented that the procedure was performed, or documentation describes a different procedure being provided, this could be a reflection of a false claim on review and audit. Such an error, although potentially innocent, may open up a therapist to additional audit, potential fines, or possibly litigation.

Table 15-3 provides a listing of the CPT codes commonly used by PTs. Each year, CPT codes can be modified, deleted, or added to accurately reflect current practice. However, simply because a procedure has a

TABLE 15-3   CPT CODES COMMONLY REPORTED BY PHYSICAL THERAPISTS*

Action	Code	Description
Evaluation		
	97001	PT evaluation
	97002	PT reevaluation
	97750	Physical performance test or measurement (e.g., musculoskeletal, functional capacity), each 15 minutes
	95851-852	Range of motion measurements*
	96000	Motion analysis, video*
	96001	Motion test with foot pressure measurement*
	96002	Dynamic surface electromyography
	96003	Dynamic fine-wire electromyography
Interventions		
Exercise, with direct (one-on-one) contact	97110	Therapeutic exercise to develop strength, ROM, flexibility, and endurance, each 15 minutes
	97112	Neuromuscular reeducation, each 15 minutes
	97113	Aquatic therapy/exercises, each 15 minutes
	97150	Group therapeutic procedures
Functional training, with direct (one-on-one) contact	97116	Gait training, each 15 minutes
	97530	Therapeutic activities, each 15 minutes
	97532	Cognitive skills development, each 15 minutes
	97535	Self-care/home management training, each 15 minutes
	97537	Community/work-reintegration training, each 15 minutes
	97542	Wheelchair management (e.g., assessment, fitting, training), each 15 minutes
	97545	Work hardening/work conditioning, each 2 hours
	97546	Work hardening/work conditioning, each additional hour
Sensory activities	97533	Sensory integration, each 15 minutes
Supervised modalities	97010	Hot/cold packs
	97012	Mechanical traction
	97014	Electrical stimulation
	97016	Vasopneumatic device therapy
	97018	Paraffin bath
	97022	Whirlpool therapy (non-Hubbard tank)
	97024	Diathermy
	97026	Infrared therapy
	97028	Ultraviolet therapy

TABLE 15-3	CPT CODES REPORTED BY PHYSICAL THERAPISTS—CONT'D	
Action	**Code**	**Description**
Attended modalities	97032	Electrical stimulation, manual, each 15 minutes
	97033	Electrical current therapy/iontophoresis, each 15 minutes
	97034	Contrast bath, each 15 minutes
	97035	Ultrasound, each 15 minutes
	97036	Hubbard tank, each 15 minutes
	64550	Application of neurostimulator
Manual therapy/massage, with direct (one-on-one) contact	97140	Manual therapy, each 15 minutes
	97124	Massage/therapeutic massage, each 15 minutes
Active wound care	97597	Selective debridement, ≤20 cm^2
	97598	Selective debridement, >20 cm^2
	97602	Nonselective debridement
Orthotics and prosthetics	97760	Orthotic(s) management and training (including assessment and fitting), each 15 minutes
	97761	Prosthetic training, upper and/or lower extremities, each 15 minutes
	97762	Checkout for orthotic/prosthetic use, each 15 minutes
Patient education in disease management	98960	Education and training for patient self-management by a qualified, nonphysician health care professional using a standardized curriculum
	98961	As above, for 2-4 patients
	98962	As above, for 5-8 patients
Biofeedback	90901	Biofeedback training
	90911	Biofeedback training, peri/uro/rect
Vestibular	95992	Canalith repositioning procedure(s) (e.g., Epley maneuver, Semont maneuver), per day
Other	98969	Online assessment and management service
	99366	Medical team conference with interdisciplinary team of health care professionals, patient, and/or family present
	99368	Medical team conference with interdisciplinary team of health care professionals, patient, and/or family not present

CPT codes are published annually and therefore are frequently modified. Please refer to American Medical Association CPT Manual for annual updates to CPT codes.
*Not as commonly reported.

valid CPT code does not mean that that service is reimbursable. That determination is made by the third-party payers, including payers contracted with Medicare as part of the MACs, Medicaid payer guidelines, or the many private-pay and managed care organizations. Therapists should be familiar with the various CPT codes applicable to physical therapy practice, even though the degree to which a therapist may be involved in the actual billing of CPT codes differs for each hospital, facility-based organization, and private practice.

The following general guidelines for CPT coding can help maximize payment for services and minimize denial of services.

Suggestions for Improving CPT Coding by Physical Therapists

- The reporting of any code must be supported by appropriate documentation of the service provided.
- The reporting of any code should be supported in the objective documentation through a clear relation to the functional activity goals included in the plan of care, and medical necessity should be evident from the documentation.
- Therapists can report codes for both group therapy and individual therapy provided on a date of

service, but documentation must support both the group treatment and the individual (one-on-one) treatment being provided as separately identifiable skilled interventions. Typically, a billing modifier is required when these two services are billed on the same date of service.

- The number of timed units that can be reported and billed for is constrained by the direct contact time.

Physician Quality Reporting Initiative

Medicare has initiated a program known as the Physician Quality Reporting Initiative (PQRI). Section 101(b) of division B of the Tax Relief and Health Care Act of 2006 (Public Law 109423; 120 Stat. 2975), which established a financial incentive for eligible health care professionals, including physical therapists, who chose to participate in the program (http://www.cms.hhs.gov/pqri/).

In 2009 provisions in the Medicare Improvements for Patients and Providers Act of 2008 (Pub. L. 110-275) that made the PQRI program permanent only authorized incentive payments through 2010. At the time of this publication there are significant efforts to further authorize PQRI with the expansion of settings that are able to report measures as well as the addition of the number and type of quality measures. Physical therapists who met the criteria for satisfactory submission of quality measures data for services furnished during the reporting period, January 1, 2009 to December 31, 2009, earned an incentive payment of 2% of their total allowed charges for physician fee schedule covered professional services furnished during that same period (the 2009 calendar year).

The 2009 PQRI in total consisted of 153 quality measures and seven measures groups. Physical therapists had a total of 11 measures that if they reported as specified would qualify the therapist for the 2% bonus incentive payment. For further information on the 2010 PQRI quality measures, click on the "Measures/Codes" link on the Web site http://www.cms.hhs.gov/pqri/.

This initiative is designed to promote and reward physicians and other qualified health care professionals for reporting on a set of quality measures on medical claims. The 11 measures applicable to PTs in 2009 included such items as documentation of pain before initiation of therapy, risk for falls, and identification of medications. Others are in development for future fee schedule implementation.

The PQRI program provides an important incentive for therapists to ensure that documentation promotes and communicates the level and outcome of the quality of health care services provided. In the future, CMS may base incentives on outcomes achieved rather than on documentation alone. (Refer to http://www.cms.hhs.gov/PQRI for up-to-date information on PQRI. CMS provides tools to assist professionals in PQRI reporting. To access these tools, click on the "PQRI Tool Kit" link on the CMS PQRI Web site.)

In an attempt to educate the Medicare beneficiary, CMS has posted a letter to Medicare beneficiaries with important information about the PQRI program. The letter is from Medicare to the patient explaining what the program is and the implications for the patient. Therapists may choose to provide a copy to their patients in support of their PQRI participation. To obtain a copy of the letter, refer to the CMS PQRI Web site.

Summary

- This chapter provides an overview of current regulations, payment policy, and guidelines in the United States as pertinent to physical therapy documentation.
- Physical therapists are required to follow policy and guidelines developed by third-party payers, including Medicare, to facilitate payment for services.
- An important component of Medicare payment is to ensure that documentation reflects that services were medically necessary and that the therapy provided represents skilled services.
- Although formats and requirements for third-party payers may change regularly, the principles related to functional outcomes documentation provide a consistent framework for all types of documentation.

Recommended Resources

- **Centers for Medicare and Medicaid Services:** http://www.cms.hhs.gov

ICD-9

- **Centers for Disease Control and Prevention:** http://www.cdc.gov/nchs/icd9.htm

ICD-10

- **Centers for Medicare and Medicaid Services:** ICD-10 Procedure Coding System

(PCS) and Clinical Modifications (CM): http://www.cms.hhs.gov/ICD10/

- **Centers for Disease Control and Prevention:** http://www.cdc.gov/nchs/icd/icd10.htm

PHYSICIAN'S QUALITY REPORTING INITIATIVE

- **Centers for Medicare and Medicaid Services:** http://www.cms.hhs.gov/PQRI/

DOCUMENTATION, CODING, BILLING, AND COMPLIANCE

- **Fearon & Levine Consulting:** http://www.FearonLevine.com/

- **American Medical Association:** http://www.ama-assn.org/ama/pub/category/3113.html

Centers for Medicare and Medicaid Services: www.cms.hhs.gov/MedHCPCSGeninfo/

American Physical Therapy Association: http://www.apta.org

CHAPTER 16

Computerized Documentation

Janet Herbold

LEARNING OBJECTIVES

After reading this chapter and completing the exercises, the reader will be able to:

1. Identify and describe the benefits of an automated documentation system.

2. Discuss the various uses of patient data obtained from computerized documentation systems.

PTs, regardless of the setting in which they work, are always key members of the patient care team. Because the PT is a member of the patient-centered team, the success of the patient encounter often depends on the communication among other multidisciplinary members. Communication between practitioners in the health care environment has often been a challenge. Health care today faces constant pressure to decrease costs, reduce waste, and provide care in a safe environment using the best-known practices of medicine. A paper-based documentation environment includes inherent barriers to improving efficiency, safety, and quality. These limitations are some of the major reasons the goal of an electronic medical record, championed by the Bush administration with continued support by President Obama, is so important. Making patient information immediately accessible and easily transferable between patient-practitioner encounters is proposed as one of the most important advances of the twenty-first century.

Evidence for Electronic Medical Records

The literature provides some evidence of the success of electronic medical records but also illustrates some of the pitfalls. In a systematic review, Wu and Straus (2006) reported improved documentation in terms of patient encounter time, more use of stand-ard variables, and improved diagnostic accuracy using a handheld electronic medical record (EMR) compared with a paper-based system in an orthopedic practice. Several nursing articles have discussed the benefits of the EMR for completeness of nursing documentation as perceived by the physician (Green & Thomas, 2008) and have reported a slight decrease in routine nursing documentation time (Hakes & Whittington, 2008), although the finding approached but did not reach significance. Clinician perception of a newly implemented EMR can play a role in its success or failure. El-Kareh et al. (2009) reported that although clinicians may perceive some initial problems with a new electronic health recording system, they are significantly more receptive to it within 1 year of its implementation.

Electronic Records in Physical Therapy Practice

A literature review in MEDLINE and CINAHL (1985-2009) yielded no results regarding the use of an EMR in physical therapy clinics or among these clinicians. Traditional physical therapy documentation has been done with pen and paper. Some clinics and institutions use only narrative notes, whereas others have migrated to preprinted forms. Preprinted forms are one way in which physical therapy documentation has become more standardized in the past few decades. But as more health care facilities adopt computer documentation systems, a gradual shift will be seen in computer use in physical therapy practices and departments. Many institutions have already made the transition to computerized documentation.

This chapter discusses some of the drawbacks to pen and paper documentation that would lead a clinic or practice to move toward computerized documentation. We further highlight the pros and cons of using computerized documentation in physical therapy practice and highlight some considerations for choosing a computer package that best meets the needs of an institution.

Drawbacks to Pen and Paper Documentation

Inherent drawbacks to the pen and paper method of documentation include the following:

- *Legibility of the notes.* Illegibly handwritten notes can lead to miscommunication, errors in practice, and denied payment.

- *Redundancy of medical and demographic information.* Therapists frequently copy information written by another health care professional into their own notes. Components such as the patient's diagnosis, date of birth, past medical history, and medications are frequently manually rewritten into therapy documentation. In addition, as the completion of regulatory forms such as the Inpatient Rehabilitation Form–Patient Assessment Instrument (IRF-PAI), the Minimum Data Set-Resource Utilization Groups (MDS-RUGS), and the Outcome and Assessment Information Set (OASIS) become necessary for reimbursement and payment, therapists and nurses must document both in the medical record as well as on the reimbursement form (Figure 15-1). Both practices result in redundancy and duplication of information at a time when efficiency of clinical practice and staff productivity are being scrutinized.

- *Difficulty with data retrieval for clinical research or outcomes analysis to promote evidence-based practice.* It has become increasingly important to demonstrate treatment effectiveness through clinical research. With handwritten documentation it is very difficult and time consuming to manually review charts and analyze notes to determine the effectiveness of treatment techniques. In many cases, the variation in note-writing style and terminology makes it impossible to extract comparative data from handwritten notes from different clinicians even for the same type of patient condition.

- *Use of abbreviations.* Abbreviations have been used for many years as a shortcut during handwritten documentation. This practice, although frequently time saving, can lead to errors in legibility and a multitude of terms meaning the same thing, thus creating confusion among clinicians.

During an age of maximizing productivity, accessing clinical data to report outcomes and a shrinking length of stay in patient days, therapists look for creative ways to streamline documentation in a method that reduces redundancy and errors and facilitates data retrieval. As a result, some facilities have sought assistance from the world of automation and have purchased or developed computerized therapy records.

Benefits of Computerized Documentation

Some benefits of computerized documentation in physical therapy practice are listed in Box 16-1.

STANDARDIZATION OF DATA ELEMENTS AND CHARTING PRACTICES

A computerized system can create a standard data collection tool format for the initial evaluation, treatment notes, reevaluations, and discharge evaluations. Therapists can use a variety of devices to access and chart in the electronic medical record. Laptops and handheld devices allow clinicians to document their services during the patient evaluation and treatment encounter with the patient present. Therapists naturally become faster and more efficient note-writers through repetition and practice. In addition, training

---

BOX 16-1

Benefits of Computerized Documentation

- Standardization of data elements and charting practices
- Elimination of redundancy and reduction of errors
- Accessibility of date in real time
- Cost efficiency
- Facilitated documentation of outcome measures
- Improved legibility of the medical record
- Decreased space requirements for storing medical records
- Improved confidentiality of the medical record

of new or rotating staff is made easier and more consistent throughout the organization. Computerized documentation allows for consistent collection of data elements within a patient type, in which the same information can be captured in the same order for all patients. This helps those reading the documentation as they become familiar with the format over time and allows them to locate pertinent information quickly and easily. Automation also can eliminate the use of abbreviations and reduce the need for interpretation when the written documentation is unclear and unknown.

Figure 16-1 illustrates these features in a software program (MediServe Information System, Chandler, Ariz.) with templates designed by a team of rehabilitation professionals (Burke Rehabilitation Hospital, White Plains, NY). In this example, the Impression/Assessment is coded to include key components, such as summarizing and drawing relationships between the patient's impairments, activity limitations, and participation restrictions. All possible options for each of these components are listed as options in a pull-down menu (in this example, Life Role Participation). By using such a format, therapists are prompted

to provide critical information so that it is always included in their documentation. Furthermore, the design of the template is structured so that the terminology is consistent with current practice and, importantly, the *Guide to Physical Therapist Practice* (American Physical Therapy Association, 2001).

ELIMINATION OF REDUNDANCY AND REDUCTION OF ERRORS

Most hospitals and facilities already have computerized registration, financial services, and/or scheduling systems where basic patient demographic information is entered and stored. Through the use of interfaces and connectivity, patient demographic and clinical data can be directly fed into a computerized documentation system by simply selecting the patient name and verifying an account or medical record number. This practice of sharing information between systems will significantly reduce the documentation time normally required to rewrite such necessary information onto a paper form. It also reduces the human error that is associated with such transcription practices.

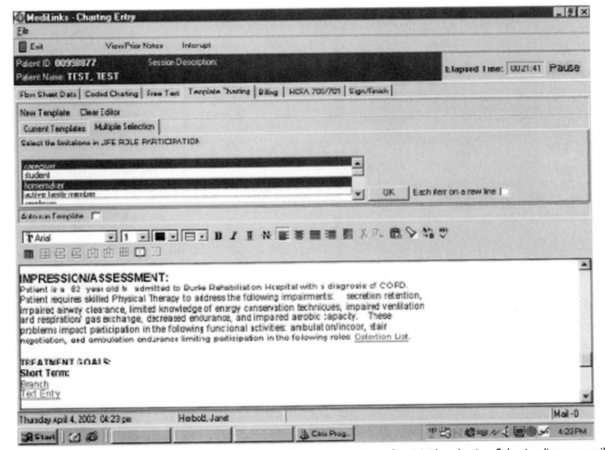

FIGURE 16-1   Computerized documentation template for the Assessment section of an initial evaluation. Selection lists are available at various points throughout the documentation. This figure illustrates the output of selection lists of impairments and functional (activity) limitations.

Just as information can be received *into* an electronic documentation system, it can also be forwarded *out* to another system. This is the case with the interface into a billing or data collection system. Such an interface allows billing/charging elements to be forwarded or interfaced into the financial system, again reducing potential billing error and billing/charting discrepancies by eliminating an extra step in the documentation and billing practices. Payment policy regulations require a perfect match between items billed and treatment rendered. Inconsistencies in documentation and billing could result in reimbursement denials. The practice of "marrying" documentation with billing helps to alleviate those issues, thereby reducing potential denials.

ACCESSIBILITY OF DATA IN "REAL TIME"

In many facilities there is an inherent time delay between when and where the notes are documented and when they are accessible in the medical record. Therapy notes are frequently written and maintained in a working file in the clinic and later transferred into the medical record. Lack of access to clinical data can greatly reduce a clinic or hospital's efficiency and facilitation of the continuum of care by reducing communication and transfer of knowledge. Use of an automated clinical documentation system allows easy accessibility of clinical information at remote locations some distance from where services have been provided, as well as immediately after the documentation of the encounter. Access to therapy notes by physicians, nursing staff, social workers, and case managers allows the rehabilitation process to be continued and reported over a full 24-hour period. Physicians can discuss a patient's present functional status with their patients, family members, and/or caregivers at any time during the patient's stay. The availability of clinical data can help the physician make medical choices and discuss discharge planning options with confidence in a timely manner. The nursing staff can promote and carry through the rehabilitation process 24 hours a day, 7 days per week by having the patient's most recent physical status available. Social workers and case managers can easily access and send updated functional status reports to insurance companies, external case managers, and other necessary medical continuum levels to facilitate communication regarding patient status, transfer, and the discharge process. The benefits of an automated environment help to instill confidence and improve communication in the medical facility, resulting in greater efficiency in the care of the patient.

In addition to sending and receiving information within a facility, connectivity across other hospitals or sites will promote a clinically integrated delivery system. Allowing access to clinical care data across the continuum of patient services—such as from an acute care hospital to a rehabilitation center or to an outpatient environment—facilitates continued medical and rehabilitation care without interruption. Availability of clinical data throughout the rehabilitation continuum will ultimately lead to improved functional outcome, better patient satisfaction, and greater respect among caregivers and personnel. As patients make transitions from one site or facility to another, the evaluation process of getting to know the patient can be reduced through availability of the most recent functional status and rehabilitation report. In addition, the communication of patient information from one therapist to another will help to facilitate professional interaction and development of best practice.

COST EFFICIENCY

The current health care environment mandates demonstration of treatment effectiveness and efficiency of services. For this reason and the need to do so without added cost to the system, it becomes necessary to incorporate monitoring of clinical data as a component of documentation and charting. The availability of data in a computerized form can allow the analysis of clinical outcomes and cost of services. The use of computer analysis will make it easier to demonstrate efficiency and effectiveness to patients, third-party payers, accrediting bodies, and PTs.

USE OF OUTCOME MEASURES

With computerized documentation, outcome data collection elements can be charted during routine documentation and simultaneously entered into its own system. Without computerized documentation, outcomes measures such as the Functional Independence Measure (FIM) and the MDS-RUGS items need to be documented separately in both the physical therapy evaluation and the standardized forms. Automated documentation systems allow for the information to be imbedded in a documentation template and transferred to a freestanding electronic documentation such as an MDS or FIM report. This direct routing of clinical information into regulatory reporting systems for outcome analysis is another example of a more efficient system in which redundancies and errors are reduced.

Figure 16-2 shows an example of a computerized documentation template that incorporates outcome measures. As shown, standardized outcome measures, such as FIM scores and Timed Up and Go, can easily be incorporated into a template. With computerized

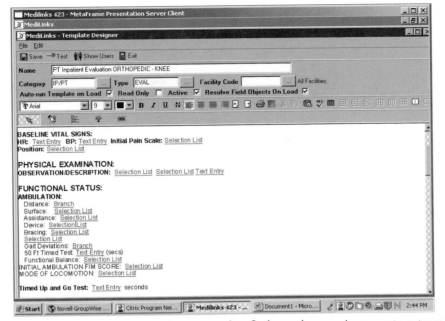

FIGURE 16-2   Computerized printout from an initial evaluation template. Such templates can incorporate outcome measures, such as FIM scores and Timed Up and Go, as shown.

systems, patient's functional or activity status can be assessed and can incorporate standardized assessment tools that capture a picture of the patient at different intervals during rehabilitation (Figure 16-3). Such assessments can be used to determine progress and eventually the outcome of a patient's total rehabilitation encounter.

OTHER BENEFITS

Documentation templates designed for computerized documentation can contain those standard elements needed to comply with a facility's outcome or reimbursement tools, such as FIMware (property of University of Buffalo Foundation Activities, Inc.) and Inpatient Rehabilitation Facility-Patient Assessment Instrument (IRF-PAI) documents. These standard elements can be interfaced directly in the unique system to maintain efficiency and reduce redundancy and potential error. Figure 16-4 shows how a computerized software program can generate an IRF-PAI document.

Other general benefits of computer documentation include improved legibility of the medical record, decreased space requirements for storing medical records, and improved confidentiality of the medical record.

Drawbacks of Computerized Documentation

The primary drawbacks to the use of an automated documentation system include the initial financial investment, the development time, and the need for staff training. An automated electronic rehabilitation system can cost as much as $1 million. Additional expenses include the time for staff development of the software. Some software systems provide "canned" documentation tools with the ability to modify them, whereas others allow the flexibility for total customization but require additional time and resources for development. (The author suggests allowing up to a year to fully develop charting templates or modify canned templates for facility use.) Finally, time and resources must be allocated for staff training for both basic computer literacy and specific application training. Application training should incorporate a thorough understanding of the functionality of the software, practice with actual charting templates that the specific user may use, as well as knowledge of how to view other notes, print, and access clinically relevant patient demographic information.

Uses of Patient Data From Computerized Medical Records

Once clinical data about a patient are available in an automated clinical record, they can provide many benefits to a practice or facility. The following section identifies specific uses for patient information.

INDIVIDUALIZED PATIENT REPORTS

In many hospital settings, team conferences or rounds are used as an opportunity to bring multiple

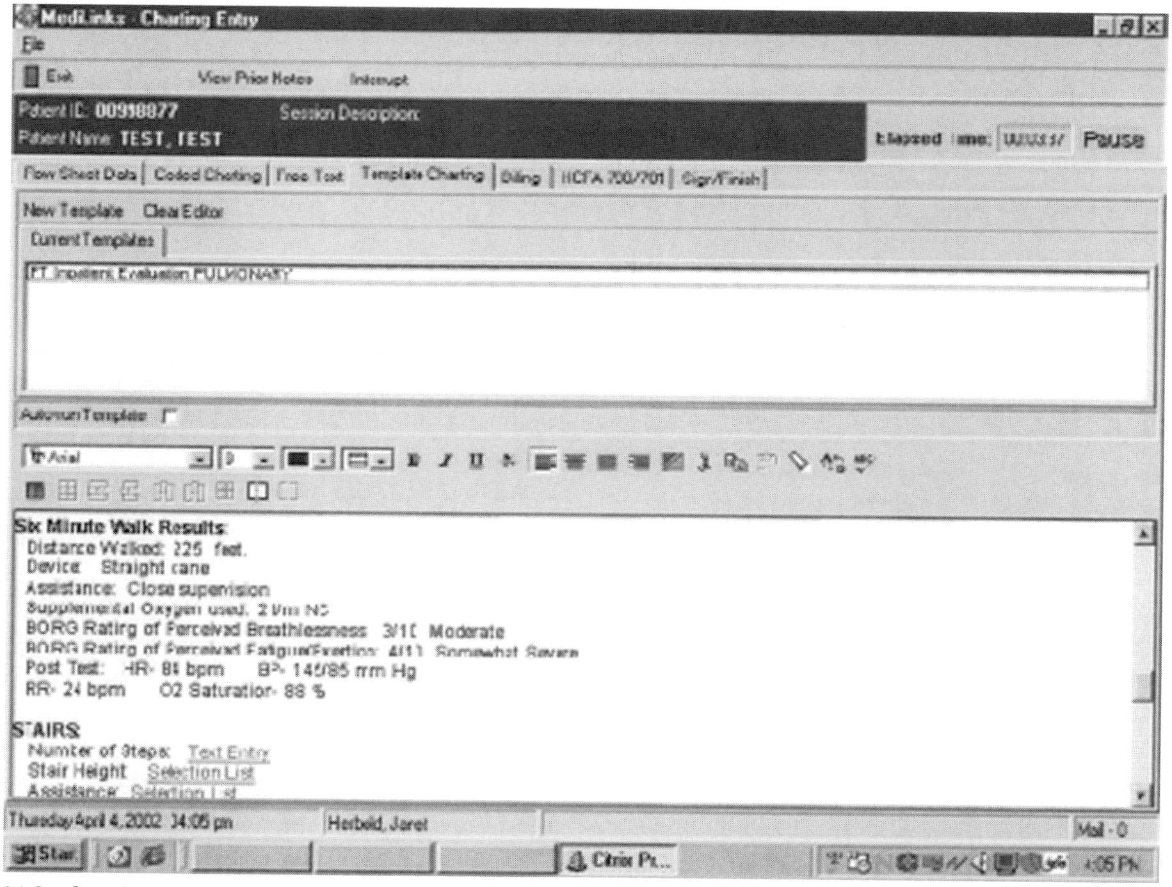

FIGURE 16-3 Sample illustration of how computerized documentation can use standardized assessment tools (e.g., 6-minute walk) in the body of a charting template. This capability provides a means of quickly and easily documenting standard information for a specific patient population.

disciplines together to discuss a patient's condition. In addition to oral communication, a written report is typically generated. Computerized documentation can easily provide data that can be used to create an individualized patient rounds report or profile. In addition, such a summary report can be used to provide an update to a third-party payer. Figure 16-5 is an example of a rounds report that provides a summary of a patient's current status.

AGGREGATED PATIENT DATA

Patient data can also be aggregated for a particular patient population. This is commonly used for performance improvement activities. Information from aggregated data can be summarized for time intervals and viewed periodically to determine whether consistent outcomes of a clinical practice are being maintained. Such data also can be used to identify areas in need of process improvement where action plans can be implemented and reassessed at a later time. Figure 16-6 provides an example of a graph that shows improvement in 6-minute walking for a group of patients with cardiac conditions.

CASE MIX INDEXING

At a facility level, case mix indexing and other management-level information can provide information regarding patient acuity, which may translate to reimbursement measures in a prospective environment such as a skilled nursing facility, home care, or inpatient rehabilitation setting. The *case mix index* (CMI) is an economic indicator that describes the average patient's morbidity in a hospital. It is calculated by determining the total cost of all inpatients for a specified period divided by the number of admissions (Kuster et al., 2008). Figure 16-7 shows a CMI chart generated from computerized documentation records.

CLINICAL RESEARCH

Clinical research efforts can be simplified when data are collected and retrieved from an electronic medical record. During this important time of promoting and using evidence-based practice, documentation of clinical research at all levels—whether a case study, descriptive analysis, or randomized control trial—is an important role of the physical therapy community (Figure 16-8).

Identification Information

1. Facility Information
   A. Facility Name
   Burke Rehabilitation Hospital

   B. Facility Medicare Provider Number

2. Patient Medicare Number

3. Patient Medicaid Number

4. Patient First Name

5. Patient Last Name

6. Birth Date   07/07/1929
                                                MM/DD/YYYY

7. Social Security Number   000000001

8. Gender (1- Male; 2- Female)   1

9. Race/Ethnicity (Check all that apply)
   American Indian or Alaska Native   A
                              Asian   B
         Black or African American   C
              Hispanic or Latino   D
   Native Hawaiian or Other Pacific Islander   E
                              White   F

10. Marital Status   02
    1 - Never Married; 2- Married; 3 - Widowed;
    4 - Separated; 5 - Divorced

11. Zip Code of Patient's Pre-Hospital Residence: 10605

Admission Information*

12. Admission Date   09/12/2002
                                          (MM/DD/YYYY)

13. Assessment Reference Date   09/14/2002
                                          (MM/DD/YYYY)

14. Admission Class   01
    (1- Initial Rehab; 2 - Evaluation; 3 - Readmission; 4 - Unplanned
    Discharge; 5 - Continuing Rehabilitation

15. Admit From   07
    (01 - Home; 02 - Board & Care; 03 - Transitional Living; 04 -
    Intermediate Care; 05 - Skilled Nursing Facility; 06 - Acute Unit of
    Own Facility; 07 - Acute Unit of Another Facility; 08 - Chronic
    Hospital; 09 - Rehabilitation Facility; 10 - Other; 12 - Alternate Level
    of Care Unit; 13 - Subacute Setting; 14 - Assisted Living Residence)

16. Pre Hospital Living Setting   01
    (Use codes from item 15 above)

17. Pre-Hospital Living With   02
    (Code only if item 16 is 01 - Home; Score using 1 - Alone; 2
    - Family/Relatives; 3 - Friends; 4 - Attendant; 5 - Other)

18. Pre-Hospital Vocational Category   06
    (1 - Employed; 2 - Sheltered; 3 - Student; 4 -
    Homemaker; 5 - Not Working; 6 - Retired for Age; 7 -
    Retired for Disability

19. Pre-Hospital Vocational Effort
    (Code only if item 18 is coded 1 - 4; Score using 1 - Full
    time; 2 - Part time; 3 - Adjusted Workload)

Payer Information

20. Payment Source
    A. Primary Source

    B. Secondary Source

    (Score using 01 - Blue Cross; 02 - Medicare non-MCO; 03 - Medicaid
    non-MCO; 04 - Commercial Insurance; 05 - MCO HMO; 06 - Workers
    Compensation; 07 - Crippled Children's Service; 08 - Developmental
    Disabilities Service; 09 - State Vocational Rehabilitation; 10 - Private
    Pay; 11 - Employee Courtesy; 12 - Unreimbursed; 13 - CHAMPUS; 14 -
    Other; 15 - None; 16 - No Fault auto insurance; 51 - Medicare MCO; 52
    - Medicaid MCO)

Medical Information*

21. Impairment Group   0008.51
                           Admission   Discharge
    Condition requiring admission to rehabilitation; code according to
    Appendix A, attached

22. Etiologic Diagnosis: OSTEOAR
    (Use ICD-9 codes to indicate the etiologic problem that led to the
    condition for which the patient is receiving rehabilitation)

23. Date of Onset of Etiologic Diagnosis   09/01/2002
                                            (MM/DD/YYYY)

24. Comorbid Conditions; Use ICD-9 Codes to enter up to ten medical
    conditions existing prior to this rehabilitation admission

    A. _____   B. _____

    C. _____   D. _____

    E. _____   F. _____

    G. _____   H. _____

    I. _____   J. _____

Medical Needs

25. Is patient comatose at admission?
                                        0 - No, 1 - Yes

26. Is patient delirious at admission?
                                        0 - No, 1 - Yes

                                  Admission   Discharge

27. Swallowing Status:

    3 - *Regular Diet:* solids and liquids swallowed safely without
    supervision or modified diet

    2 - *Modified Diet/Supervision*: Subject required Modified diet and/or
    needs supervision for safety

    1 - *Tube/Parenteral Feeding*: tube / parenteral feeding used wholly or
    partially as a means of sustenance
                                  Admission   Discharge

28. Clinical signs of dehydration

    (Evidence of oliguria, dru skin, orthostatic hypotension, somnolence,
    agitation; Score 0 -No; 1 - Yes)

FIGURE 16-4 Standardized assessment tools, such as the Inpatient Rehabilitation Facility–Patient Assessment Instrument (IRF-PAI) shown here, can be incorporated into computerized documentation to maximize efficiency and reduce redundancy in note writing.

Function Modifiers*

Complete the following specific functional items prior to scoring the FIM Instrument:

	ADMISSION	DISCHARGE
29. Bladder Level of Assistance	07	07

Score using FIM Levels 1 - 7; 8 in unable to assess)

	ADMISSION	DISCHARGE
30. Bladder Freq. of Accidents (Score using below)	07	07

7 - Continent
6 - Continent; uses device such as catheter
5 - Incontinent every 8 days or more
4 - Incontinent every 4 - 7 days
3 - Incontinent every 2 - 3 days; not daily
2 - Incontinent daily; some control
1 - Incontinent with every void
8 - Does not void (e.g., due to dialysis)

Score Item 39G (Bladder) as the lowest (most dependent) score from Items 29 and 30 above.

	ADMISSION	DISCHARGE
31. Bowel Level of Assistance (Score using FIM Levels 1 - 7; 8 if unable to assess)	06	06
32. Bowel Freq. of Accidents (Score as below)	06	06

7 - Continent
6 - Continent; uses device such as ostomy
5 - Incontinent every 8 days or more
4 - Incontinent every 4 - 7 days
3 - Incontinent every 2 - 3 days; not daily
1 - Incontinent daily
8 - Could not assess, no bowel movement in 8 days

Score Item 39H (Bowel) as the lowest (most dependent) score of Items 31 and 32

	ADMISSION	DISCHARGE
33. Tub transfer	04	06
34. Shower Transfer	0	☐

(Score using FIM Levels 1 - 7 ; 8 if unable to assess)
Score Item 39K (Tub/Shower Transfer) as the lowest (most dependent) score of Items 33 and 34

	ADMISSION	DISCHARGE
35. Distance Walked (feet)	02	03
36. Distance Traveled Wheelchair (feet)	03	03

Score Items 35 and 36 using the following scale: 3 - 150 feet; 2 - 50 to 149 feet; 1 - Less than 50 feet or unable; 8 - Not applicable)

	ADMISSION	DISCHARGE
37. Walk	02	06
38. Wheelchair	03	03

(Score using FIM Levels 1 - 7; 8 if not applicable)
Score Item 39L (Walk,Wheelchair) as the lowest (most dependent) score of Items 37 and 38

39. FIM™ Instrument*

SELF CARE	ADMISSION	DISCHARGE	GOAL
A. Eating	07	07	☐
B. Grooming	06	06	☐
C. Bathing	03	06	☐
D. Dressing - Upper	04	07	☐
E. Dressing - Lower	04	07	☐
F. Toileting	04	06	☐
SPHINCTER CONTROL			
G. Bladder	07	07	☐
H. Bowel	06	06	☐
TRANSFERS			
I. Bed, Chair, Whlchair	05	06	☐
J. Toilet	05	06	☐
K. Tub, Shower	04	00	☐

W - Walk
C-Wheelchair
B- - Both

LOCOMOTION			
L. Walk/Wheelchair	02 W	06 W	☐
M. Stairs	02	05	☐

A - Auditory
V - Visual
B - Both

COMMUNICATION			
N. Comprehension	04 A	07 A	☐
O. Expression	07 V	07 V	☐

V - Vocal
N - Nonvocal
B - Both

SPINAL COGNITION			
P. Social Interaction	07	07	☐
Q. Problem Solving	05	05	☐
R. Memory	07	07	☐

FIM LEVELS

No Helper
7 Complete Independence (Timely, Safely)
6 Modified Independence (Device)

Helper - Complete Dependence
5 Supervision (Subject = 100%)
4 Minimal Assistance (Subject = 75% or more)
3 Moderate Assistance (Subject = 50% or more)

Helper - Complete Dependence
2 Maximal Assistance (Subject = 25% or more)
1 Total Assistance (Subject less than 25%)

8 Activity does not occur; Use this code only at admission

FIGURE 16-4—cont'd

The Burke Rehabilitation Hosp

ADMIT DATE:
05/12/2004

SEX: F AGE :   DOB: **MR#**

ADMITTING
PHYSICIAN: MITHILESH, SHUBH

AC#: **W00001058053**

FC: MC   WORK AREA : 1E

TEAM CONFERENCE

Date of Rounds: _____   NY

<u>**Admit Diagnosis:**</u> S/P RT TKR

NURSING	
Coumadin Use	No
Pain Scale	4/10
Safety	Red Level
Wound/Surgical Site Status	Clean and dry with staples

SOCIAL WORK/CASE MANAGEMENT	
Insurance/Case management:	Patient is not case managed.
Number of Steps to Bed/Bathroom	4
Number of steps to enter house	4
Prehospital Living Setting	Home
Prehospital Living With	Alone

PHYSICAL THERAPY	
Ambulation/Device	Bent handled/Off-set cane
Ambulation/Distance	320
Ambulation/Level of Assistance	Independent
AROM/(R) Knee Extension	0
AROM/(R) Knee Flexion	100
PROM/(R) Knee Extension	0
PROM/(R) Knee Flexion	102
Stair Negotiation/Device	Bent Handle Cane
Stair Negotiation/Height	7 inch
Stair Negotiation/Level of Assistance	Independent
Stair Negotiation/Number	16
Stair Negotiation/Rail Use	1 Rail

OCCUPATIONAL THERAPY	
DME Used during Toilet Transfer	RTS with arms
DME Used during Tub/Shower Transfer	Tub Safety Rail
Homemaking	With increased time and effort
Initial Bed Mobility / Sit to Supine	Modified Independenct
Initial Bed Mobility / Supine to Sit	Modified Independence
Initial FIM/Dressing - Lower Body	2 Maximal Assistance
Initial FIM/Dressing - Upper Body	5 Supervision
Initial FIM/Transfer - Bed,Chair,WC	5 Supervision
Initial FIM/Transfer - Toilet	4 Minimal Assistance
Initial FIM/Tub Transfer	4 Minimal Assistance
Ongoing Bed Mobility / All position	Minimal Assistance
Ongoing FIM/Dressing-Lower Body	Minimal Assistance
Ongoing FIM/Dressing-Upper Body	Independent
Ongoing FIM/Transfer - Car	Contact Guard
Ongoing FIM/Transfer-Bed, Chair W/C	Modified Independent
Ongoing FIM/Transfer-Toilet	Supervision
Ongoing FIM/Transfer-Tub, Shower	Minimal Assistance

BARRIERS TO DISCHARGE

Print Date: 5/19/2004

GELLER. SHARON   Page 1 of 2

FIGURE 16-5   Example of a rounds report, which can be used to provide summary information of a patient's progress.

Cardiac Six Minute Walk - Study
January 01, 2005 To   March 31, 2005

SIX MINUTE WALK
Initial vs. D/C for Patients with Cardiac Conditions

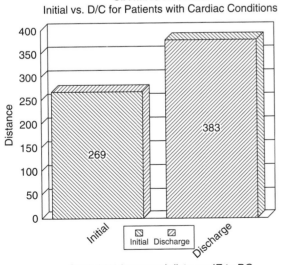

Goal: 25% increased distance IE to DC

FIGURE 16-6   Graph generated from computerized documentation software. The graph provides aggregate data for a 6-minute walk for patients with cardiac conditions at initial evaluation and at discharge, demonstrating a 25% increase in distance walked.

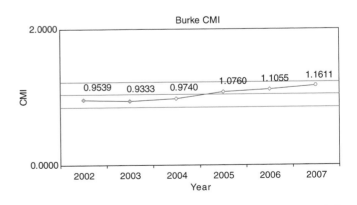

FIGURE 16-7   Graph showing case-mix indexing over a period of 6 years at one hospital. This graph was readily produced with information previously entered into a computerized documentation system.

Rehabilitation following TKR or THR:IRF vs. SNF
Mary Beth Walsh, MD & Janet Herbold, PT
The Burke Rehabilitation Hospital, White Plains, New York 10605

Objective
The purpose of this study was to determine whether outcomes differed between patients following single knee or hip replacement surgery who received rehabilitation in an inpatient rehabilitation facility (IRF) verses Skilled Nursing Facility (SNF).

Characteristics	SNF	IRF
Age:	74.0 ± 9.8	74.0 ± 9.8
Females:	66 (75.9%)	66 (75.9)
Locomotion FIM:	1.63 ± 1.06	1.62 ± 1.04
Comorbidity:	$1.94 \pm .033$	1.93 ± 0.31

Design
87 matched pairs treated in either SNF or IRF

Conclusion
When patients were matched for age, gender, operative procedure and admission FIM scores, those who received rehabilitation in the IRF had, on average, a shorter length of stay and superior functional outcomes with a higher rate of return to community than those treated in SNF's.

Results/Outcomes	SNF	IRF
LOS	20.0 ± 10.8	10.3 ± 3.3
Locomotion FIM at DC	4.90 ± 1.92	5.71 ± 0.91
Ambulation Distance at DC	289 ± 212	380 ± 168
Required Walker (n=81)	65 (80.2%)	31 (38.3%)
Discharge Home	68 (79.1%)	77 (89.5%)
Transfer to Acute Care	6 (6.9%)	3 (3.4%)
Required Home Care post DC	51 (75%)	28 (41.2%)

FIGURE 16-8   Summary of a poster presentation describing results of a research project analyzing outcomes of patients who have undergone total knee replacements and total hip replacements. Computerized documentation readily allows analysis of outcomes data—in this instance, comparing outcomes from two different types of facilities.

Design and Implementation of a New Computerized System

If a facility is considering implementing a computerized documentation system for the first time, managing this process entails several important considerations. Table 16-1 outlines the key components of this process and includes important considerations for ensuring maximum success of such a project.

Summary

The benefits of an automated documentation system used in a physical therapy setting—either freestanding or as a part of an integrated delivery system—are numerous. Automation allows for legible, consistent, standardized documentation that can be completed at the point of care or while the patient is present. Additional benefits include accessibility of clinical information by all members of the medical team, data retrieval for outcomes management, and clinically defined best practice (clinical decision making) in an environment that reduces redundancy and error.

TABLE 16-1	PROCESS OF DEVELOPING AND IMPLEMENTING A COMPUTERIZED DOCUMENTATION SYSTEM
Step	**Responsibilities**
Development of a request for proposal (RFP)	Create a list of all the functionality needed or required. Each item or functional aspect needs to be written and included in a document that is submitted to and answered by each prospective vendor. This document, called an RFP, will become the essence of the vendor/site contract. During vendor selection, the RFP should be used as a check-off document to ensure complete functionality of a proposed system based on the identified needs of the site or institution.
Vendor selection	Choosing a vendor is a critical decision because the institution and the vendor will become partners in a long-term relationship. Institutions should choose a vendor whose system best matches the long-term plans and needs of the institution. It is not necessary to purchase a fully comprehensive electronic medical record-keeping system if the institution does not plan to use all of its functionality. Consider small niche vendors that specialize in your unique area of expertise in rehabilitation, as well as systems with total functionality and the ability to integrate throughout a hospital network.
Creating a timeline	Plan and identify all of the critical elements in your project and the parties responsible for implementing the project/system. This can be done via a timeline and a responsibility list. The maintenance of this document can be time consuming, but it is important to ensure that critical events in the project are identified and completed in a proper sequence. Like building a house, the process begins with the vendor selection (contractor selection) and the contract phase (RFP) and ends with an implementation and final acceptance (final inspection and moving in). As with any building project, realistic timeframes should be proposed with extra time incorporated for unexpected delays.
Design/validation team	The design/validation team will develop the charting or note-writing templates to be used in the system. The staff selected for this role should be experienced and well versed in the reimbursement and financial constraints of the institution. The goal of this team is to develop a standard and consistent format and data elements with corresponding outcome monitoring tools. Templates can differ between diagnostic categories to capture unique clinically significant assessment data, but a standard format should be observed among all charting types. This will assist both those completing and reading the templates to maintain a consistent and predictable flow and order. Whenever possible, selection lists and discrete text data elements should be used for data collection to allow retrieval of data for later analysis. Narrative or text answers cannot be analyzed and used for comparative analysis. Standardized assessment tools should be incorporated into the templates. This facilitates research and outcome studies as a byproduct of treatment note writing. In addition, templates should contain the standard elements needed to comply with the facility's outcome or reimbursement tools such as the FIM, MDS, or IRF-PAI documents. These standard elements should be interfaced directly into that unique system to maintain efficiency and reduce redundancy and potential error.

References

*Items noted with an asterisk (*) are important resources for further information pertinent to functional outcomes and documentation.

Adams MA, Mannion AF, Dolan P: Personal risk factors for first-time low back pain, *Spine* 23:2497–2505, 1999.

Adams J: The purpose of outcome measurement in rheumatology, *Br J Occup Ther* 65(4):172–174, 2002.

*American Physical Therapy Association: *The guide to physical therapist practice*, ed 2, Alexandria, VA, 2001, American Physical Therapy Association.

American Physical Therapy Association: *Guide for professional conduct*, Alexandria, VA, 2004, American Physical Therapy Association.

American Physical Therapy Association: *ICD-9-CM coding: codes for billing diagnosis*, Alexandria, VA, 2007, American Physical Therapy Association. Available at http://www.apta.org/AM/Template.cfm?Section=Future_National_Meetings&TEMPLATE=/CM/ContentDisplay.cfm&CONTENTID=44092.

*American Physical Therapy Association: *Guidelines: physical therapy documentation of patient/client management*, Alexandria, VA, 2008, American Physical Therapy Association. Available at http://www.apta.org/AM/Template.cfm?Section=Home&TEMPLATE=/CM/ContentDisplay.cfm&CONTENTID=31688.

American Physical Therapy Association House of Delegates: *Designation "PT," "PTA," "SPT," and "SPTA,"* HOD 06-99-23-29 [Program 32], 1999.

American Physical Therapy Association House of Delegates: *Diagnosis by physical therapists*, HOD P06-08-06-07 [Program 32], 2007.

Barber-Westin SD, Noyes FR, McCloskey JW: Rigorous statistical reliability, validity, and responsiveness testing of the Cincinnati knee rating system in 350 subjects with uninjured, injured, or anterior cruciate ligament-reconstructed knees, *Am J Sports Med* 27(4):402–416, 1999.

Berg KO, Wood-Dauphinee SL, Williams JI, Maki B: Measuring balance in the elderly: validation of an instrument, *Can J Public Health* 83(Suppl 2):S7–S11, 1992.

Bergner M, Bobbitt RA, Carter, WB, et al: The sickness impact profile: development and final revision of a health status measure, *Med Care* 19:787–805, 1981.

Bickley LS, Hoekelman RA: *JG Bates' guide to physical examination & history taking*, ed 7, Philadelphia, 1999, Lippincott Williams & Wilkins.

Bohannon RW: Manual muscle testing: does it meet the standards of an adequate screening test? *Clin Rehabil* 19:662–667, 2005.

Booher LD, Hench KM, Worrell TW, et al: Reliability of three single leg hop tests, *J Sports Rehabil* 2:165–170, 1993.

Borg G, Linderholm H: Exercise performance and perceived exertion in patients with coronary insufficiency, arterial hypertension and vasoregulatory asthenia, *Acta Med Scand* 187:17–26, 1970.

Bruininks RH, Bruininks BD: *Bruininks-Oseretsky test of motor proficiency (BOT-2)*, ed 2, Circle Pines, MN, American Guidance Center, 2005.

Campbell SK, Wright BD, Linacre JM: Development of a functional movement scale for infants, *J Appl Meas* 3:190–204, 2002.

Carr JH, Shepherd R: *Neurologic rehabilitation: optimizing motor performance*, Sidney, Australia, 1998, Butterworth Heinemann.

Centers for Medicare & Medicaid Services: *HIPAA 101 for health care providers' offices, HIPAA information series 1:1-4*, 2003. Available at http://www.cms.hhs.gov/EducationMaterials/Downloads/HIPAA101-1.pdf

Centers for Medicare & Medicaid Services: *Therapy personnel qualifications and policies effective January 1, 2008*. Available at http://www.cms.hhs.gov/transmittals/downloads/r88bp.pdf.

Centers for Medicare & Medicaid Services: *Program integrity manual*. Available at http://www.cms.hhs.gov/manuals/downloads/pim83c03.pdf.

Centers for Medicare & Medicaid Services: *11 Part B billing scenarios for PTs and OTs, 2009*. Available at http://www.cms.hhs.gov/TherapyServices/02_billing_scenarios.asp#TopOfPage.

Centers for Medicare & Medicaid Services: *Outpatient therapy—additional DRA mandated service edits, 2006*. Available at http://www.cms.hhs.gov/transmittals/downloads/R1019CP.pdf.

Centers for Medicare & Medicaid Services: *2007 PQRI reporting experience*. Available at http://www.cms.hhs.gov/PQRI.

Centers for Medicare & Medicaid Services: *Medicare claims processing manual, Medicare benefit policy manual*. Available at http://www.cms.hhs.gov/manuals/iom/List.asp.

Cole AB: *Physical rehabilitation outcomes measures,* Toronto, 1995, Canadian Physiotherapy Association.

Constant CR, Murley AH: A clinical method of functional assessment of the shoulder, *Clin Orthop Relat Res* 214:160–164, 1987.

Coster WJ, Deeney T, Haltiwanter J, et al: *School function assessment,* San Antonio, TX, 1998, The Psychological Corporation.

Csuka M, McCarty DJ: Simple method for measurement of lower extremity muscle strength, *Am J Med* 78:77–81, 1985.

Curtis KA, Black K: Shoulder pain in female wheelchair basketball players, *J Orthop Sports Phys Ther* 29(4):225–231, 1999.

Davies GJ, Wilk A, Ellenbecker TS: Assessment of strength. In Malone TR, McPoil TG, Nitz AJ, editors: *Orthopedic and sports physical therapy,* ed 2, St Louis, 1996, Mosby.

Davis P: *The American Heritage Dictionary of the English Language,* ed 4, New York, 2000, Houghton Mifflin.

Davis NM: *Medical abbreviations: 30,000 conveniences at the expense of communications and safety,* Huntington Valley, PA, 2009, Neil M Davis Associates.

*Delitto A, Snyder-Mackler L: The diagnostic process: examples in orthopedic physical therapy, *Phys Ther* 75:203–211, 1995.

Dittmar SS, Gresham GE: *Functional assessment and outcome measures for the rehabilitation health professional,* Gaithersburg, MD, 1997, Aspen Publishers.

El-Kareh R, Gandhi TK, Poon EG, et al: Trends in primary care clinician perceptions of a new electronic health record, *J Gen Intern Med* 24:464–468, 2009.

Enderby P, John A, Petheram B: *Therapy outcome measures for rehabilitation professionals,* ed 2, New York, 2006, John Wiley.

Escolar DM, Henricson EK, Mayhew J, et al: Clinical evaluator reliability for quantitative and manual muscle testing measures of strength in children, *Muscle Nerv* 24(6):787–793, 2001.

Fairbank JCT, Couper J, Davies JB, et al: The Oswestry low back pain disability questionnaire, *Physiotherapy* 66:271–273, 1980.

Farrell A, O'Sullivan C, Quinn L: Parent perspectives on early childhood assessment: a focus group inquiry, *Early Childhood Services* 3(1):61–76, 2009.

*Fawcett AJL: *Principles of assessment and outcome measurement for occupational therapists and physiotherapists: theory, skills and application,* Chichester, UK, 2007, John Wiley & Sons.

Fearon H, Levine SM, Lee GR: APTA audio conference presentation, March 26, 2009.

Feuerstein M, Berkowitz SM, Huang GD: Predictors of occupational low back disability: implications for secondary prevention, *J Occup Environ Med* 41(12):1024–1031, 1999.

Folio MR, Fewell RR: *Peabody developmental motor scales (PDMS-2),* ed 2, New York, 2000, Riverside Publishing.

Folstein MF, Robins LN, Helzer JE: The mini-mental state examination, *J Psychiatr Res* 12:189–198, 1975.

Frese E, Brown M, Norton BJ: Clinical reliability of manual muscle testing: middle trapezius and gluteus medius muscles, *Physiotherapy* 67(7):1072–1076, 1987.

Fritz JM, Brennan GP: Preliminary examination of a proposed treatment-based classification system for patients receiving physical therapy interventions for neck pain, *Phys Ther* 87(5):513–524, 2007.

Fugl-Meyer A, Jaasko L, Leyman I, et al: The post-stroke hemiplegic patient: a method for evaluation of physical performance, *Scand J Rehabil Med* 6:13–31, 1975.

Gandek B, Sinclair SJ, Jette AM, et al: Development and initial psychometric evaluation of the participation measure for post-acute care (PM-PAC), *Am J Phys Med Rehabil* 86:57–71, 2007.

Gans BM, Haley SM, Hallenborg SC, et al: Description and inter-observer reliability of the Tufts assessment of motor performance, *Am J Phys Med Rehabil* 67:202–210, 1988.

Gentile AM: Skill acquisition: action, movement, and neuromotor processes. In Shepherd R, Carr J, editors: *Movement science: foundations for physical therapy in rehabilitation,* ed 2, Gaithersburg, MD, 2000, Aspen Publishers.

George SZ, Delitto A: Clinical examination variables discriminate among treatment-based classification groups: a study of construct validity in patients with acute low back pain, *Phys Ther* 85:306–314, 2005.

Goldstein LB, Bertels C, Davis JN: Interrater reliability of the NIH stroke scale, *Arch Neurol* 46:660–662, 1989.

Gordon J, Quinn L: Guide to physical therapist practice: a critical appraisal, *Neurol Report* 23(3):122–128, 1999.

Green SD, Thomas JD: Interdisciplinary collaboration and the electronic medical record, *Pediatr Nurs* 34:225–229, 2008.

Guralnik JM, Simonsick EM, Ferrucci L, et al: A short physical performance battery assessing lower extremity function: association with self-reported disability and prediction of mortality and nursing home admission, *J Gerontol* 49:M85–M94, 1994.

Guccione A: Physical therapy diagnosis and the relationship between impairment and function, *Phys Ther* (71):499–504, 1991.

Guccione AA, Mielenz TJ, DeVellis RF, et al: Development and testing of a self-report instrument to measure actions: outpatient physical therapy improvement in movement assessment log (OPTIMAL), *Phys Ther* 85(6):515–530, 2005.

Guyatt GH, Sullivan MJ, Thompson PJ, et al: The 6-minute walk: a new measure of exercise capacity in patients with chronic heart failure, *Can Med Assoc J* 132:919–923, 1985.

Hakes B, Whittington J: Assessing the impact of an electronic medical record on nurse documentation time, *Comput Inform Nurs* 26:234–241, 2008.

Haley S, Faas R, Coster W, et al: *Pediatric evaluation of disability inventory,* Boston, 1992, New England Medical Center.

Harwood RH, Rogers A, Dickinson E, et al: Measuring handicap: the London handicap scale, a new outcome measure for chronic disease, *Qual Health Care* 3:11–16, 1994.

Hunt SM, McKenna SP, McEwen J, et al: A quantitative approach to perceived health status: a validation study, *J Epidemiol Community Health* 34:281–286, 1980.

Incalzi AR, Capparella O, Gemma A, et al: A simple method of recognizing geriatric patients at risk for death and disability, *J Am Geriatr Soc* 40(1):34–38, 1992.

Jebsen RH, Taylor N, Trieschmann RB, et al: An objective and standardized test of hand function, *Arch Phys Med Rehabil* 50:311–319, 1969.

Jelles F, Van Bennekom CA, Lankhorst GJ, et al: Inter- and intra-rater agreement of the rehabilitation activities profile, *J Clin Epidemiol* 48:407–416, 1995.

Jennett B, Teasdale G: Aspects of coma after severe head injury, *Lancet* 23(1):878–881, 1977.

Jette AM: Diagnosis and classification by physical therapists: a special communication, *Phys Ther* 69(11):967–969, 1989.

*Jette AM: Physical disablement concepts for physical therapy research and practice, *Phys Ther* 74(5):380–386, 1994.

Jette AM, Tao W, Haley SM: Blending activity and participation sub-domains of the ICF, *Disabil Rehabil* 29:1742–1750, 2007.

Jette DU, Halbert J, Iverson C, et al: Use of standardized outcome measures in physical therapist practice: perceptions and applications, *Phys Ther* 89(2):125–135, 2009.

Kaiser Family Foundation: *Health care spending in the United States and OECD countries, 2007.* Available at http://www.kff.org/insurance/snapshot/chcm010307oth.cfm.

Keith RA, Granger CV, Hamilton BB, et al: The functional independence measure: a new tool for rehabilitation, *Adv Clin Rehabil* 1:6–18, 1987.

Kettenbach G: *Writing SOAP notes,* ed 3, Philadelphia, 2003, FA Davis.

Kolobe TH, Bulanda M, Susman L: Predicting motor outcome at preschool age for infants tested at 7, 30, 60, and 90 days after term age using the Test of Infant Motor Performance, *Phys Ther* 84(12):1144–1156, 2004.

Kopec JA, Esdaile JM, Abrahamowicz M, et al: The Quebec Back Pain Disability Scale. Measurement properties, *Spine* 20(3):341–352, 1995.

Kuster SP, Ruef C, Bollinger AK, et al: Correlation between case mix index and antibiotic use in hospitals, *J Antimicrob Chemother* 62:837–842, 2008.

Lamb SE, Guralnik JM, Buchner DM, et al: Factors that modify the association between knee pain and mobility limitation in older women: The Women's Health and Aging Study, *Ann Rheum Dis* 59(5):331–337, 2000.

Law M: Appendix 2: outcome measures rating form guidelines. In Law M, Baum C, Dunn W: *Measuring occupational performance: supporting best practice in occupational therapy,* Thorofare, NJ, 2001, Slack.

Lawton MP, Brody EM: Assessment of older people: self-maintaining and instrumental activities of daily living, *Gerontologist* 9:179–186, 1969.

Lewis C, McNerney T: *Functional Toolbox I,* McLean, VA, 1994, Learn Publications.

Lewis C, McNerney T: *Functional Toolbox II,* McLean, VA, 1997, Learn Publications.

*Lewis K: Do the write thing: document everything!, *PT Magazine* 19(7):30–33, 2002.

Long T, Toscano K: *Handbook of pediatric physical therapy,* ed 2, Philadelphia, 2002, Lippincott Williams & Wilkins.

Mahoney F, Barthel D: Functional evaluation: the Barthel index, *Maryland State Med J* 14:61–65, 1965.

Malone TR, McPoil TG, Nitz AJ, editors: *Orthopedic and sports physical therapy,* ed 2, St Louis, 1996, Mosby.

Martin S: Language shapes thought, *PT Magazine* 7:44–46, 1999.

Mayerson NH, Milano RA: Goniometric measurement reliability in physical medicine, *Arch Phys Med Rehabil* 65(2):92–94, 1984.

McConlogue A, Quinn L: Analysis of physical therapy goals in a school-based setting: a pilot study, *Phys Occup Ther Pediatr* 29:156–171, 2009.

McEwen I: *Providing physical therapy services under parts B & C of the individuals with disabilities education act (IDEA),* Alexandria, VA, 2000, American Physical Therapy Association.

Nagi S: Some conceptual issues in disability and rehabilitation. In Sussman M, editor: *Sociology and rehabilitation,* Washington, DC, 1965, American Sociological Association.

Nagi S: Disability concepts revisited: implication for prevention. In Pope A, Tarlov A, editors: *Disability in America: toward a national agenda for prevention,* Washington, DC, 1991, National Academy Press.

National Advisory Board on Medical Rehabilitation Research: *Report and plan for medical rehabilitation research,* Bethesda, MD, 1991, National Institutes of Health.

National Center for Health Statistics: *International Classifications of Disease, Ninth Revision, Clinical Modification (ICD-9-CM),* Hyattsville, MD, 2007, US Department of Health and Human Services.

Norton BJ: "Harnessing our collective professional power": diagnosis dialog, *Phys Ther* 87(6):635–638, 2007.

O'Sullivan SB, Schmitz TJ: *Physical rehabilitation,* ed 5, Philadelphia, 2006, FA Davis.

Perenboom RJ, Chorus AM: Measuring participation according to the International Classification of Functioning, Disability and Health (ICF), *Disabil Rehabil* 25:577–587, 2003.

Piper MC, Darrah J: *Motor assessment of the developing infant,* Philadelphia, 1994, Saunders.

Podsiadlo D, Richardson S: The timed "up & go": a test of basic functional mobility for frail elderly persons, *J Am Geriatr Soc* 39:142–148, 1991.

*Randall KE, McEwen IR: Writing patient-centered functional goals, *Phys Ther* 80:1197–1203, 2000.

Reese NB, Bandy WD: *Joint range of motion and muscle length testing,* Philadelphia, 2002, Saunders.

Roland M, Jenner J: A revised Oswestry disability questionnaire. In Hudson-Cook N, Tomes-Nicholson K, Breen A, editors: *Back pain: new approaches to rehabilitation and education,* Manchester, UK, 1989, Manchester University Press.

Roland M, Morris R: A study of the natural history of back pain. Part I: development of a reliable and sensitive measure of disability in low-back pain, *Spine* 8(2):141–144, 1983.

Russell DJ, Rosenbaum PL, Cadman DT, et al: The gross motor function measure: a means to evaluate the effects of physical therapy, *Dev Med Child Neurol* 31(3):341–352, 1989.

Research and Training Center on Independent Living: *Guidelines for reporting and writing about people with disabilities,* Lawrence, KS, 2008, RTCIL Publications.

Sackett DL, Haynes RB: The architecture of diagnostic research, *BMJ* 324(7336):539–541, 2002.

Scheets PK, Sahrmann SA, Norton BJ: Diagnosis for physical therapy for patients with neuromuscular conditions, *Neurol Report* 23(4):158–169, 1999.

Scheets PK, Sahrmann SA, Norton BJ: Use of movement system diagnoses in the management of patients with neuromuscular conditions: a multiple-patient case report, *Phys Ther* 87:654–669, 2007.

*Scott RW: *Legal aspects of documenting patient care for rehabilitation professionals*, ed 3, Boston, 2006, Jones and Bartlett.

Skalko T: *Medical abbreviations for the health professions*, Ravensdale, WA, 1998, Idyll Harbor.

Stamer MH: *Functional documentation: a process for the physical therapist*, Tucson, AZ, 1995, Therapy Skill Builders.

*Stewart AL, Hays RD, Ware JE Jr: The MOS short-form general health survey: reliability and validity in a patient population, *Med Care*, 26: 724–735, 1988.

*Stewart DL, Abeln SH: *Documenting functional outcomes in physical therapy*, St. Louis, 1993, Mosby.

Stuck AE, Walthert JM, Nikolaus T, et al: Risk factors for functional status decline in community-living elderly people: a systematic literature review, *Soc Sci Med* 48:445–469, 1999.

Tinetti ME: Performance-oriented assessment of mobility problems in elderly patients, *J Am Geriatr Soc* 34:119–126, 1986.

US Department of Health & Human Services: *Summary of the HIPAA privacy rule*, Washington, DC, 2003, Office of Civil Rights.

Van Dillen LR, Roach KE: Reliability and validity of the acute care index of function for patients with neurologic impairment, *Phys Ther* 68(7):1098–1101, 1988.

Van Dillen LR, Sahrmann SA, Norton BJ, et al: Reliability of physical examination items used for classification of patients with low back pain, *Phys Ther* 78(9):979–988, 1998.

van Straten A, de Haan RJ, Limburg M, et al: A stroke-adapted 30-item version of the sickness impact profile to assess quality of life (SA-SIP30), *Stroke* 28:2155–2161, 1997.

Westhoff G, Listing J, Zink A: Loss of physical independence in rheumatoid arthritis: interview data from a representative sample of patients in rheumatologic care, *Arthr Care Res* 13:11–22, 2000.

Whiteneck GG, Charlifue SW, Gerhart KA, et al: Quantifying handicap: a new measure of long-term rehabilitation outcomes, *Arch Phys Med Rehabil* 73:519–526, 1992.

WHOQOL Group: Development of the WHOQOL-BREF quality of life assessment, *Psychol Med* 28:551–558, 1998.

Wolf SL, Catlin PA, Gage K, et al: Establishing the reliability and validity of measurements of walking time using the Emory functional ambulation profile, *Phys Ther* 79:1122–1133, 1999.

Wong DL, Baker CM: Pain in children: comparison of assessment scales, *Okla Nurse* 33:8, 1988.

Wood-Dauphinee SL, Opzoomer MA, Williams JI, et al: Assessment of global function: the reintegration to normal living index, *Arch Phys Med Rehabil* 69:583–590, 1988.

World Confederation of Physical Therapy: *Declaration of principle—informed consent*, London, 2007, World Confederation of Physical Therapy. Available at http://www.wcpt.org/node/29593

World Health Organization: *International classification of functioning, disability, and health*, Geneva, 1980, World Health Organization.

World Health Organization: *International classification of functioning, disability, and health*, Geneva, 2001, World Health Organization.

World Health Organization: *World Health Organization disability assessment schedule II (WHODAS II)*, Geneva, 2001, World Health Organization.

Wu RC, Straus SE: Evidence for handheld electronic medical records in improving care: a systematic review, *BMC Med Inform Decis Mak* 6:26, 2006.

Guidelines for Physical Therapy Documentation*

GUIDELINES: PHYSICAL THERAPY DOCUMENTA-TION OF PATIENT/CLIENT MANAGEMENT BOD G03-05-16-41 [Amended BOD 02-02-16-20; BOD 11-01-06-10; BOD 03-01-16-51; BOD 03-00-22-54; BOD 03-99-14-41; BOD 11-98-19-69; BOD 03-97-27-69; BOD 03-95-23-61; BOD 11-94-33-107; BOD 06-93-09-13; Initial BOD 03-93-21-55] [Guideline]

Preamble

The American Physical Therapy Association (APTA) is committed to meeting the physical therapy needs of society, to meeting the needs and interests of its members, and to developing and improving the art and science of physical therapy, including practice, education, and research. To help meet these responsibilities, the APTA Board of Directors has approved the following guidelines for physical therapy documentation. It is recognized that these guidelines do not reflect all of the unique documentation requirements associated with the many specialty areas within the physical therapy profession. Applicable for both handwritten and electronic documentation systems, these guidelines are intended to be used as a foundation for the development of more specific documentation guidelines in clinical areas, while at the same time providing guidance for the physical therapy profession across all practice settings. Documentation may also need to address additional regulatory or payer requirements.

Finally, be aware that these guidelines are intended to address documentation of patient/client management, not to describe the provision of physical therapy services. Other APTA documents, including APTA *Standards of Practice for Physical Therapy, Code of Ethics and Guide for Professional Conduct,* and the *Guide to Physical Therapist Practice,* address provision of physical therapy services and patient/client management.

APTA Position on Documentation

DOCUMENTATION AUTHORITY FOR PHYSICAL THERAPY SERVICES

Physical therapy examination, evaluation, diagnosis, prognosis, and intervention shall be documented, dated, and authenticated by the physical therapist who performs the service. Intervention provided by the physical therapist or selected interventions provided by the physical therapist assistant are documented, dated, and authenticated by the physical therapist or, when permissible by law, the physical therapist assistant.

Other notations or flow charts are considered a component of the documented record but do not meet the requirements of documentation in or of themselves.

Students in physical therapist or physical therapist assistant programs may document when the record is additionally authenticated by the physical therapist or, when permissible by law, documentation by physical therapist assistant students may be authenticated by a physical therapist assistant.

Operational Definitions

GUIDELINES

APTA defines a "guideline" as a statement of advice.

AUTHENTICATION

The process used to verify that an entry is complete, accurate and final. Indications of authentication can include original written signatures and computer "signatures" on secured electronic record systems only.

The following describes the main documentation elements of patient/client management: (1) initial examination/evaluation, (2) visit/encounter, (3) reexamination, and (4) discharge or discontinuation summary.

---

*Courtesy American Physical Therapy Association, Alexandria, VA.

INITIAL EXAMINATION/EVALUATION

Documentation of the initial encounter is typically called the *initial examination, initial evaluation,* or *initial examination/evaluation.* The initial examination/evaluation is typically completed in one visit but may occur over more than one visit. Documentation elements for the initial examination/evaluation include the following:

Examination: Includes data obtained from the history, systems review, and tests and measures.

Evaluation: Evaluation is a thought process that may not include formal documentation. It may include documentation of the assessment of the data collected in the examination and identification of problems pertinent to patient/client management.

Diagnosis: Indicates level of impairment and functional limitation determined by the physical therapist.* May be indicated by selecting one or more preferred practice patterns from the *Guide to Physical Therapist Practice.*

Prognosis: Provides documentation of the predicted level of improvement that might be attained through intervention and the amount of time required to reach that level. Prognosis is typically not a separate documentation element, but the components are included as part of the plan of care.

Plan of care: Typically stated in general terms, includes goals, interventions planned, proposed frequency and duration, and discharge plans.

VISIT/ENCOUNTER

Documentation of a visit or encounter, often called a *progress note* or *daily note,* documents sequential implementation of the plan of care established by the physical therapist, including changes in patient/client status and variations and progressions of specific interventions used. Also may include specific plans for the next visit or visits.

REEXAMINATION

Documentation of reexamination includes data from repeated or new examination elements and is provided to evaluate progress and to modify or redirect intervention.

DISCHARGE OR DISCONTINUATION SUMMARY

Documentation is required following conclusion of the current episode in the physical therapy intervention sequence to summarize progression toward goals and discharge plans.

General Guidelines

Documentation is required for every visit/encounter.

All documentation must comply with the applicable jurisdictional/regulatory requirements.

---

*These guidelines use terminology based on the Nagi framework versus the ICF.

All handwritten entries shall be made in ink and will include original signatures. Electronic entries are made with appropriate security and confidentiality provisions.

Charting errors should be corrected by drawing a single line through the error and initialling and dating the chart or through the appropriate mechanism for electronic documentation that clearly indicates that a change was made without deletion of the original record.

All documentation must include adequate identification of the patient/client and the physical therapist or physical therapist assistant.

The patient's/client's full name and identification number, if applicable, must be included on all official documents.

All entries must be dated and authenticated with the provider's full name and appropriate designation.

Documentation of examination, evaluation, diagnosis, prognosis, plan of care, and discharge summary must be authenticated by the physical therapist who provided the service.

Documentation of intervention in visit/encounter notes must be authenticated by the physical therapist or physical therapist assistant who provided the service.

Documentation by physical therapist or physical therapist assistant graduates or other physical therapists and physical therapist assistants pending receipt of an unrestricted license shall be authenticated by a licensed physical therapist or, when permissible by law, documentation by physical therapist assistant graduates may be authenticated by a physical therapist assistant.

Documentation by students (SPT/SPTA) in physical therapist or physical therapist assistant programs must be additionally authenticated by the physical therapist or, when permissible by law, documentation by physical therapist assistant students may be authenticated by a physical therapist assistant.

Documentation should include the referral mechanism by which physical therapy services are initiated; examples include:

• Self-referral/direct access

• Request for consultation from another practitioner

Documentation should include indication of no shows and cancellations.

Initial Examination/Evaluation

EXAMINATION (HISTORY, SYSTEMS REVIEW, AND TESTS AND MEASURES)

History

Documentation of history may include the following:

• General demographics

• Social history

• Employment/work (job/school/play)

• Growth and development

- Living environment
- General health status (self-report, family report, caregiver report)
- Social/health habits (past and current)
- Family history
- Medical/surgical history
- Current condition(s)/chief complaint(s)
- Functional status and activity level
- Medications
- Other clinical tests

Systems Review

Documentation of systems review may include gathering data for the following systems:

- Cardiovascular/pulmonary
  - Blood pressure
  - Edema
  - Heart rate
  - Respiratory rate
- Integumentary
  - Pliability (texture)
  - Presence of scar formation
  - Skin color
  - Skin integrity
- Musculoskeletal
  - Gross range of motion
  - Gross strength
  - Gross symmetry
  - Height
  - Weight
- Neuromuscular
  - Gross coordinated movement (e.g., balance, locomotion, transfers, and transitions)
  - Motor function (motor control, motor learning)

  Documentation of systems review may also address communication ability, affect, cognition, language, and learning style:

- Ability to make needs known
- Consciousness
- Expected emotional/behavioral responses
- Learning preferences (e.g., education needs, learning barriers)
- Orientation (person, place, time)

Tests and Measures

Documentation of tests and measures may include findings for the following categories:

- Aerobic capacity/endurance; examples of examination findings include:
  - Aerobic capacity during functional activities
  - Aerobic capacity during standardized exercise test protocols
  - Cardiovascular signs and symptoms in response to increased oxygen demand with exercise or activity
  - Pulmonary signs and symptoms in response to increased oxygen demand with exercise or activity
- Anthropometric characteristics; examples of examination findings include:
  - Body composition
  - Body dimensions
  - Edema
- Arousal, attention, and cognition; examples of examination findings include:
  - Arousal and attention
  - Cognition
  - Communication
  - Consciousness
  - Motivation
  - Orientation to time, person, place, and situation
  - Recall
- Assistive and adaptive devices; examples of examination findings include:
  - Assistive or adaptive devices and equipment use during functional activities
  - Components, alignment, fit, and ability to care for the assistive or adaptive devices and equipment
  - Remediation of impairments, functional limitations, or disabilities with use of assistive or adaptive devices and equipment
  - Safety during use of assistive or adaptive devices and equipment
- Circulation (arterial, venous, lymphatic); examples of examination findings include:
  - Cardiovascular signs
  - Cardiovascular symptoms
  - Physiological responses to position change
- Cranial and peripheral nerve integrity; examples of examination findings include:
  - Electrophysiological integrity
  - Motor distribution of the cranial nerves
  - Motor distribution of the peripheral nerves
  - Response to neural provocation
  - Response to stimuli, including auditory, gustatory, olfactory, pharyngeal, vestibular, and visual
  - Sensory distribution of the cranial nerves
  - Sensory distribution of the peripheral nerves

- Environmental, home, and work (job/school/play) barriers; examples of examination findings include:
  - Current and potential barriers
  - Physical space and environment
- Ergonomics and body mechanics; examples of examination findings for ergonomics include:
  - Dexterity and coordination during work
  - Functional capacity and performance during work actions, tasks, or activities
  - Safety in work environments
  - Specific work conditions or activities
  - Tools, devices, equipment, and work stations related to work actions, tasks, or activities
- Examples of examination findings for body mechanics include:
  - Body mechanics during self-care, home management, work, community, or leisure actions, tasks, or activities
- Gait, locomotion, and balance; examples of examination findings include:
  - Balance during functional activities with or without the use of assistive, adaptive, orthotic, protection, supportive, or prosthetic devices or equipment
  - Balance (dynamic and static) with or without the use of assistive, adaptive, orthotic, protective, supportive, or prosthetic devices or equipment
  - Gait and locomotion during functional activities with or without the use of assistive, adaptive, orthotic, protective, supportive, or prosthetic devices or equipment
  - Gait and locomotion with or without the use of assistive, adaptive, orthotic, protective, supportive, or prosthetic devices or equipment
  - Safety during gait, locomotion, and balance
- Integumentary integrity; examples of examination findings include:
  - Associated skin:
    - Activities, positioning, and postures that produce or relieve trauma to the skin
    - Assistive, adaptive, orthotic, protective, supportive, or prosthetic devices and equipment that may produce or relieve trauma to the skin
    - Skin characteristics
  - Wound:
    - Activities, positioning, and postures that aggravate the wound or scar or that produce or relieve trauma
    - Burn
    - Signs of infection
    - Wound characteristics
    - Wound scar tissue characteristics

- Joint integrity and mobility; examples of examination findings include:
  - Joint integrity and mobility
  - Joint play movements
  - Specific body parts
- Motor function; examples of examination findings include:
  - Dexterity, coordination, and agility
  - Electrophysiological integrity
  - Hand function
  - Initiation, modification, and control of movement patterns and voluntary postures
- Muscle performance; examples of examination findings include:
  - Electrophysiological integrity
  - Muscle strength, power, and endurance
  - Muscle strength, power, and endurance during functional activities
  - Muscle tension
- Neuromotor development and sensory integration; examples of examination findings include:
  - Acquisition and evolution of motor skills
  - Oral motor function, phonation, and speech production
  - Sensorimotor integration
- Orthotic, protective, and supportive devices; examples of examination findings include:
  - Components, alignment, fit, and ability to care for the orthotic, protective, and supportive devices and equipment
  - Orthotic, protective, and supportive devices and equipment use during functional activities
  - Remediation of impairments, functional limitations, or disabilities with use of orthotic, protective, and supportive devices and equipment
  - Safety during use of orthotic, protective, and supportive devices and equipment
- Pain; examples of examination findings include:
  - Pain, soreness, and nociception
  - Pain in specific body parts
- Posture; examples of examination findings include:
  - Postural alignment and position (dynamic)
  - Postural alignment and position (static)
  - Specific body parts
- Prosthetic requirements; examples of examination findings include:
  - Components, alignment, fit, and ability to care for prosthetic device
  - Prosthetic device use during functional activities

- Remediation of impairments, functional limitations, or disabilities with use of the prosthetic device
  - Residual limb or adjacent segment
  - Safety during use of the prosthetic device
- Range of motion (including muscle length); examples of examination findings include:
  - Functional range of motion
  - Joint active and passive movement
  - Muscle length, soft tissue extensibility, and flexibility
- Reflex integrity; examples of examination findings include:
  - Deep reflexes
  - Electrophysiological integrity
  - Postural reflexes and reactions, including righting, equilibrium, and protective reactions
  - Primitive reflexes and reactions
  - Resistance to passive stretch
  - Superficial reflexes and reactions
- Self-care and home management (including activities of daily living and instrumental activities of daily living); examples of examination findings include:
  - Ability to gain access to home environments
  - Ability to perform self-care and home management activities with or without assistive, adaptive, orthotic, protective, supportive, or prosthetic devices and equipment
  - Safety in self-care and home management activities and environments
- Sensory integrity; examples of examination findings include:
  - Combined/cortical sensations
  - Deep sensations
  - Electrophysiological integrity
- Ventilation and respiration; examples of examination findings include:
  - Pulmonary signs of respiration/gas exchange
  - Pulmonary signs of ventilatory function
  - Pulmonary symptoms
- Work (job/school/play), community, and leisure integration or reintegration (including instrumental activities of daily living); examples of examination findings include:
  - Ability to assume or resume work (job/school/play), community, and leisure activities with or without assistive, adaptive, orthotic, protective, supportive, or prosthetic devices and equipment
  - Ability to gain access to work (job/school/play), community, and leisure environments
  - Safety in work (job/school/play), community, and leisure activities and environments

EVALUATION

Evaluation is a thought process that may not include formal documentation. However, the evaluation process may lead to documentation of impairments, functional limitations, and disabilities using formats such as:

- A problem list
- A statement of assessment of key factors (e.g., cognitive factors, comorbidities, social support) influencing the patient/client status

DIAGNOSIS

Documentation of a diagnosis determined by the physical therapist may include impairment and functional limitations. Examples include:

- Impaired joint mobility, motor function, muscle performance, and range of motion associated with localized inflammation (4E)
- Impaired motor function and sensory integrity associated with progressive disorders of the central nervous system (5E)
- Impaired aerobic capacity/endurance associated with cardiovascular pump dysfunction or failure (6D)
- Impaired integumentary integrity associated with partial-thickness skin involvement and scar formation (7C)

PROGNOSIS

Documentation of the prognosis is typically included in the plan of care. See below.

PLAN OF CARE

Documentation of the plan of care includes the following:

- Overall goals stated in measurable terms that indicate the predicted level of improvement in function
- A general statement of interventions to be used
- Proposed duration and frequency of service required to reach the goals
- Anticipated discharge plans

Visit/Encounter

Documentation of each visit/encounter shall include the following elements:

- Patient/client self-report (as appropriate)
- Identification of specific interventions provided, including frequency, intensity, and duration as appropriate. Examples include:
  - Knee extension, three sets, 10 repetitions, 10# weight

- Transfer training bed to chair with sliding board
- Equipment provided
- Changes in patient/client impairment, functional limitation, and disability status as they relate to the plan of care
- Response to interventions, including adverse reactions, if any
- Factors that modify frequency or intensity of intervention and progression of goals, including patient/client adherence to patient/client-related instructions
- Communication/consultation with providers/patient/client/family/significant other

Documentation to plan for ongoing provision of services for the next visit(s), which is suggested to include, but not be limited to:

- The interventions with objectives
- Progression parameters
- Precautions, if indicated

Reexamination

Documentation of reexamination shall include the following elements:

- Documentation of selected components of examination to update patient's/client's impairment, function, and/or disability status

- Interpretation of findings and, when indicated, revision of goals
- When indicated, revision of plan of care, as directly correlated with goals as documented

Discharge/Discontinuation Summary

Documentation of discharge or discontinuation shall include the following elements:

- Current physical/functional status
- Degree of goals achieved and reasons for goals not being achieved
- Discharge/discontinuation plan related to the patient/client's continuing care. Examples include:
  - Home program
  - Referrals for additional services
  - Recommendations for follow-up physical therapy care
  - Family and caregiver training
  - Equipment provided

Relationship to Vision 2020: Professionalism (Practice Department, ext. 3176)
[Last updated: 12/22/08; Contact: executivedept@apta.org]

Rehabilitation Abbreviations

This list provides abbreviations most commonly used by rehabilitation professionals. It is divided into the categories of general, professional, medical diagnosis, and symbols. In addition, the entire list is organized alphabetically by name.

General

A or Ⓐ	assistance
A	assessment
AAA	abdominal aortic aneurysm
AAFO	articulating ankle foot orthosis
AAROM	active assistive range of motion
Abd or ABD	abduction
ABG	arterial blood gases
abn	abnormal
AC	alternating current
ACA	anterior cerebral artery
ACL	anterior cruciate ligament
AD	assistive device
Add or ADD	adduction
ADL	activities of daily living
ad lib	at discretion
Afib	atrial fibrillation
AFO	ankle foot orthosis
AG	against gravity
AK	above knee
amb	ambulatory, ambulation
ant	anterior
AP	anteroposterior
approx	approximate, approximately
appt	appointment
A&O	alert and oriented
AROM	active range of motion
ASIA	American Spinal Injury Association
ASIS	anterior superior iliac spine
assist	assistant, assistance
ATNR	assymetrical tonic neck reflex
AV	atrioventricular
B or Ⓑ	bilateral
B&B	bowel and bladder
bal	balance
BE	below elbow
b.i.d.	twice a day
bil	bilateral
b.i.w.	biweekly
BK	below knee
BM	bowel movement
BNL	below normal limits
BOS	base of support
BP	blood pressure
bpm	beats per minute
BS	breath sounds
$\bar{c}$	with
CA	cancer, cardiac arrest
CICU	cardiac intensive care unit
CG	contact guarding
cm	centimeter
CNS	central nervous system
c/o	complained of, complains of
cont'd	continued
CO_2	carbon dioxide
CPAP	continuous positive airway pressure
CPT	chest physical therapy
CS	close supervision
CSF	cerebrospinal fluid
CT	computed tomography
d	day
D or Ⓓ	dependent
DAI	diffuse axonal injury
DBE	deep breathing exercise
D/C	discharge; discontinue

Dep	dependent	H_2O	water
DF	dorsiflexion	I or Ind or Ⓘ	independent
DIP	distal interphalangeal (joint)	I&O	intake and output
dist	distance, distant	ICU	intensive care unit
DME	durable medical equipment	IM	intramuscular
DS	distant supervision	inf	inferior
DTR	deep tendon reflex	int	internal
dx	diagnosis	int rot, IR	internal rotation
ECF	extended care facility	IQ	intelligence quotient
ECG	electrocardiogram	IV	intravenous
EEG	electroencephalogram	jt	joint
EMG	electromyogram	J-tube	jejunostomy tube
ENT	ear, nose, throat	K	potassium
equip	equipment	KAFO	knee-ankle-foot orthosis
ER	emergency room; external rotation	KCAL	kilocalorie
e-stim	electrical stimulation	kg	kilogram(s)
eval	evaluation	L or Ⓛ	left
ex	exercise	L	liter
exam	examination	lat	lateral
ext	external; extension	lb	pound
ext rot, ER	external rotation	LBP	lower back pain
F	fair (muscle grade)	LBQC	large-based quad cane
FES	functional electric stimulation	LE	lower extremity
flex	flexion	LLB	long leg brace
freq	frequently, frequency	LLE	left lower extremity
FT	full time	LLL	left lower lobe
F/U	follow-up	LLQ	left lower quadrant
FWB	full weight bearing	lig(s)	ligament(s)
Fx	function, fracture	LOA	level of assistance
G	good (muscle grade)	LOB	loss of balance
GCS	Glasgow Coma Scale	LOC	loss of consciousness
GE	gravity eliminated	L/min	liters per minute
GI	gastrointestinal	LTG	long-term goal(s)
G-tube	gastrostomy tube	LTC	long-term care
h	hour	LTM	long-term memory
HA	headache	LUE	left upper extremity
HEP	home exercise program	LUL	left upper lobe
HHA	home health aide	LUQ	left upper quadrant
H/O	history of	LVH	left ventricular hypertrophy
HOH	hard of hearing	m	meters
HR	heart rate	max	maximal, maximum
HS	heel strike	MCA	middle cerebral artery
HTN	hypertension	MCP	metacarpophalangeal joint
hx	history	med	medical

MH	moist heat	P&V	percussion and vibration
min	minute(s), minimal	PWB	partial weight-bearing
MMT	manual muscle test	q	every
mod	moderate	q.d.*	every day, daily
mo	month	quads	quadriceps
MRI	magnetic resonance imaging	R or Ⓡ	right
MVA	motor vehicle accident	re	concerning, regarding
mvt	movement	rehab	rehabilitation
N	normal (muscle grade)	rep(s)	repetition(s)
N/A	not applicable, not available	RLE	right lower extremity
NBQC	narrow-based quad cane	RLL	right lower lobe
NC	nasal canula	RLQ	right lower quadrant
Neg	negative	RML	right middle lobe
NG	nasogastric	R/O	reports of, rule out, ruled out
NICU	neonatal intensive care unit	ROM	range of motion
NPO	nothing by mouth	RR	respiratory rate
N/T	not tested	RROM	resisted range of motion
NWB	non–weight-bearing	R/T	related to
OOB	out of bed	RUE	right upper extremity
OR	operating room	RUL	right upper lobe
ORIF	open reduction internal fixation	RUQ	right upper quadrant
O_2	oxygen	RW	rolling walker
$\bar{p}$	after	Rx	prescription; treatment; orders
P	poor (muscle grade)	S or Ⓢ	supervision
PA	posteroanterior	$\bar{s}$	without
PCA	posterior cerebral artery	SAQ	short arc quads
PET	positron emission tomography	SB	sliding board
PF	plantar flexion	SBA	standby assistance
PIP	proximal interphalangeal (joint)	SBQC	small-based quad cane
PLS	posterior leaf splint	SBT	sliding board transfers
PMH	past medical history	SCM	sternocleidomastoid muscle
PO	by mouth	sec	second(s)
post	posterior	sig	significant
post op	postoperative	SLR	straight-leg raise
PRE	progressive resistive exercise(s)	SNF	skilled nursing facility
prn	as needed	S/O	standing order
PROM	passive range of motion	SOB	shortness of breath
prox	proximal	SOS	step-over-step (stair climbing)
PRW	platform rolling walker	s/p	status post
PSH	past surgical history	SPT	stand pivot transfers
PSIS	posterior superior iliac spine	staph	*Staphylococcus*
PT	part time		
PTA	prior to admission		
pt	patient		

*q.i.d. and q.o.d. (every other day) are on the Joint Commission's "do not use" list and should be avoided. Write "daily" instead. (See www.jointcommission.org.)

stat	immediately, at once
STG	short-term goal(s)
STM	short-term memory
STNR	symmetrical tonic neck reflex
str cane	straight cane
strep	*Streptococcus*
STS	sit to stand; step-to-step (stair climbing)
supp	supported
surg	surgical, surgery
sx	symptoms
symm	symmetrical, symmetry
T	trace (muscle grade)
TBA	to be assessed
TBE	to be evaluated
TDWB	touch-down weight bearing
temp	temperature
TENS	transcutaneous electrical nerve stimulation
ther ex	therapeutic exercise
t.i.w.	three times per week
TMJ	temporomandibular joint
TO	toe off
T/O	throughout
TOL	tolerate(s)
trach	tracheostomy
trans	transverse, transferred
trng	training
TTWB	toe-touch weight bearing
Tx	treatment
UE	upper extremity
U/L	unilateral
unsupp	unsupported
URI	upper respiratory infection
US	ultrasound
UTI	urinary tract infection
VAS	visual analog scale
VC	verbal cues, vital capacity, vocal cord
V/O	verbal order
VS	vital signs
Vtach	ventricular tachycardia
WB	weight bearing
WBAT	weight bearing as tolerated
WBQC	wide-based quad cane

W/C	wheelchair
WFL	within functional limits
WNL	within normal limits
WS	weight shift
wk	week(s)
x	times (e.g., 6×d = six times daily); for (e.g., ×5 yr = for 5 years); of (e.g., 3 sets × 10 reps)
$\bar{x}$	except
y/o or y.o.	years old

Professional

ATC	Athletic Trainer Certified
CCC-A	Certificate of Clinical Competence–Audiology
CCC-SLP	Certificate of Clinical Competence–Speech-Language Pathology
CDN	Certified Dietitian
CFY-SLP	Clinical Fellowship Year–Speech-Language Pathology
CNA	Certified Nursing Assistant
CNS	Clinical Nurse Specialist
COTA	Certified Occupational Therapy Assistant
CSW	Certified Social Worker
CTRS	Certified Therapeutic Recreation Specialist
CRTT	Certified Respiratory Therapy Technician
DC	Doctor of Chiropractic
DO	Doctor of Osteopathic Medicine
DPM	Doctor of Podiatric Medicine
DTR	Registered Dietetic Technician
GYN	Gynecologic, gynecology
HHA	Home Health Aide
LPN	Licensed Practical Nurse
MD	Medical Doctor
MSW	Master of Social Work
NP	Nurse Practitioner
OB	Obstetrics
OT	Occupational Therapy
OTOL	Otolaryngology
OTR	Occupational Therapist Registered
OTR/L	Occupational Therapist Registered/Licensed
PED	Pediatrics, pediatrician

PA	Physician's Assistant
PT	Physical Therapist, physical therapy
PTA	Physical Therapist Assistant
RD	Registered Dietitian
RN	Registered Nurse
RRT	Registered Respiratory Therapist
SLP	Speech-Language Pathologist
ST	Speech Therapist
TR	Therapeutic Recreation

Medical Diagnosis

ADD	attention deficit disorder without hyperactivity
ADHD	attention deficit–hyperactivity disorder
AIDS	acquired immunodeficiency syndrome
AKA	above-knee amputation
ALS	amyotrophic lateral sclerosis
ASD	arterioseptal defect
ASHD	arteriosclerotic heart disease
AVM	arteriovenous malformation
BKA	below-knee amputation
CA	carcinoma
CABG	coronary artery bypass graft
CAD	coronary artery disease
CFS	chronic fatigue syndrome
CHF	congestive heart failure
CHI	closed head injury
COPD	chronic obstructive pulmonary disease
CVA	cerebrovascular accident
DVT	deep vein thrombosis
DJD	degenerative joint disease
GBS	Guillain-Barré syndrome
GSW	gunshot wound
HD	Huntington's disease
HIV	human immunodeficiency virus
IDDM	insulin-dependent diabetes mellitus (type 1)
MI	myocardial infarction
MS	multiple sclerosis
NIDDM	non–insulin-dependent diabetes mellitus (type 2)
OA	osteoarthritis

OBS	organic brain syndrome
PD	Parkinson's disease
PSP	progressive supranuclear palsy
PVD	peripheral vascular disease
RA	rheumatoid arthritis
SAH	subarachnoid hemorrhage
SCI	spinal cord injury
TB	tuberculosis
TBI	traumatic brain injury
THI	traumatic head injury
THR	total hip replacement
TIA	transient ischemic attack
TKR	total knee replacement
TSR	total shoulder replacement

Symbols

1°	initial, primary, first degree
2°	secondary, second degree
3°	tertiary, third degree
=	equal
≠	not equal
−	negative, minus, inhibitory
+	positive, plus, facilitory
>	greater than
<	less than
/	extension, extensor
✓	flexion, flexor
♀	female
♂	male
‖	parallel
@	at
Δ	change
↑	increase, up, improve
↓	decrease, down, decline
↔	to and from
#	pound, number

Abbreviations by Word

abdominal aortic aneurysm	AAA
abduction	Abd or ABD
abnormal	abn
above the knee	AK
above-knee amputation	AKA

acquired immunodeficiency syndrome	AIDS	below the elbow	BE
		below the knee	BK
active assistive range of motion	AAROM	below-knee amputation	BKA
active range of motion	AROM	below normal limits	BNL
activities of daily living	ADL	bilateral	bil, B, or Ⓑ
adduction	Add or ADD	biweekly	b.i.w.
after	p̄	blood pressure	BP
against gravity	AG	bowel and bladder	B&B
alert and oriented	A&O	bowel movement	BM
alternating current	AC	breath sounds	BS
ambulatory, ambulation	amb	by mouth	PO
American Spinal Injury Association	ASIA	cancer	CA
		carbon dioxide	CO_2
amyotrophic lateral sclerosis	ALS	carcinoma	CA
ankle-foot orthosis	AFO	cardiac arrest	CA
anterior	ant	cardiac intensive care unit	CICU
anterior cerebral artery	ACA	centimeter	cm
anterior cruciate ligament	ACL	central nervous system	CNS
anterior superior iliac spine	ASIS	cerebrovascular accident	CVA
anteroposterior	AP	cerebrospinal fluid	CSF
appointment	appt	Certificate of Clinical Competence–Audiology	CCC-A
approximate, approximately	approx		
arterial blood gases	ABG	Certificate of Clinical Competence–Speech-Language Pathology	CCC-SLP
atrial septal defect	ASD		
arteriosclerotic heart disease	ASHD		
arteriovenous malformation	AVM	Certified Dietitian	CDN
articulating ankle-foot orthosis	AAFO	Certified Nursing Assistant	CNA
as needed	prn	Certified Occupational Therapy Assistant	COTA
assessment	A		
assistance	A or Ⓐ	Certified Respiratory Therapy Technician	CRTT
assistant, assistance	assist		
assistive device	AD	Certified Social Worker	CSW
asymmetrical tonic neck reflex	ATNR	Certified Therapeutic Recreation Specialist	CTRS
at	@		
at discretion	ad lib	change	Δ
Athletic Trainer Certified	ATC	chest physical therapy	CPT
atrial fibrillation	Afib	chronic fatigue syndrome	CFS
atrioventricular	AV	chronic obstructive pulmonary disease	COPD
attention deficit disorder without hyperactivity	ADD		
		Clinical Fellowship Year–Speech-Language Pathology	CFY-SLP
attention deficit–hyperactivity disorder	ADHD		
		Clinical Nurse Specialist	CNS
balance	bal	close supervision	CS
base of support	BOS	closed head injury	CHI
beats per minute	bpm	complained of, complains of	c/o
		computed tomography	CT

congestive heart failure	CHF	fair (muscle grade)	F
contact guarding	CG	female	♀
continued	cont'd	first degree	1°
continuous positive airway pressure	CPAP	flexion, flex	✓
coronary artery bypass graft	CABG	flexor	✓
coronary artery disease	CAD	follow-up	F/U
day	d	for (e.g., ×5 yr = for 5 years)	×
decrease, down, decline	↓	fracture	Fx
deep breathing exercise	DBE	frequently, frequency	freq
deep tendon reflex	DTR	full time	FT
deep vein thrombosis	DVT	full weight bearing	FWB
degenerative joint disease	DJD	function	Fx
dependent	D, dep	functional electric stimulation	FES
diagnosis	dx	gastrointestinal	GI
diffuse axonal injury	DAI	gastrostomy tube	G-tube
discharge	D/C	Glasgow Coma Scale	GCS
discontinue	D/C	good (muscle grade)	G
distal interphalangeal (joint)	DIP	gravity eliminated	GE
distance, distant	dist	greater than	>
distant supervision	DS	Guillain-Barré syndrome	GBS
Doctor of Chiropractic	DC	gunshot wound	GSW
Doctor of Osteopathic Medicine	DO	gynecology	GYN
Doctor of Podiatric Medicine	DPO	hard of hearing	HOH
dorsiflexion	DF	headache	HA
durable medical equipment	DME	heart rate	HR
ear, nose, throat	ENT	heel strike	HS
electrical stimulation	e-stim	history	hx
electrocardiogram	ECG	history of	H/O
electroencephalogram	EEG	home exercise program	HEP
electromyogram	EMG	home health aide	HHA
emergency room	ER	hour	h
equal	=	human immunodeficiency virus	HIV
equipment	equip	Huntington's disease	HD
evaluation	eval	hypertension	HTN
every	q	immediately, at once	stat
examination	exam	increase, up, improve	↑
except	x̄	independent	I or Ind or ①
exercise	ex	inferior	inf
extended care facility	ECF	inhibitory	–
extension	ext, /	initial	1°
extensor	/	insulin-dependent diabetes mellitus (type 1)	IDDM
external	ext		
external rotation	ext rot, ER	intake and output	I&O
facilitory	+		

intelligence quotient	IQ	meters	m
intensive care unit	ICU	middle cerebral artery	MCA
internal	int	minus	–
internal rotation	int rot, IR	minute(s), minimal	min
intramuscular	IM	moderate	mod
intravenous	IV	moist heat	MH
improve	≠	month	mo
jejunostomy tube	J tube	motor vehicle accident	MVA
joint	jt	movement	mvt
kilocalorie	kcal	multiple sclerosis	MS
kilogram(s)	kg	myocardial infarction	MI
knee-ankle-foot orthosis	KAFO	narrow-based quad cane	NBQC
large-based quad cane	LBQC	nasal canula	NC
lateral	lat	nasogastric	NG
left	L or Ⓛ	negative	–, neg
left lower extremity	LLE	neonatal intensive care unit	NICU
left lower lobe	LLL	non–insulin-dependent diabetes mellitus (type 2)	NIDDM
left lower quadrant	LLQ	non–weight-bearing	NWB
left upper extremity	LUE	normal (muscle grade)	N
left upper lobe	LUL	not applicable, not available	N/A
left upper quadrant	LUQ	not equal	≠
left ventricular hypertrophy	LVH	not tested	N/T
level of assistance	LOA	nothing by mouth	NPO
less than	<	number	#
Licensed Practical Nurse	LPN	Nurse Practitioner	NP
ligament(s)	lig(s)	obstetrics	OB
liters	L	Occupational Therapy	OT
liters per minute	L/min	Occupational Therapist Registered	OTR
long leg brace	LLB	Occupational Therapist Registered/Licensed	OTR/L
long-term goal(s)	LTG		
long-term care	LTC	of (e.g., 3 sets × 10 reps)	×
long-term memory	LTM	open reduction internal fixation	ORIF
loss of balance	LOB	operating room	OR
loss of consciousness	LOC	orders	Rx
lower back pain	LBP	organic brain syndrome	OBS
lower extremity	LE	osteoarthritis	OA
magnetic resonance imaging	MRI	otolaryngology	OTOL
male	♂	out of bed	OOB
manual muscle test	MMT	oxygen	O₂
Master of Social Work	MSW	parallel	‖
maximal, maximum	max	Parkinson's disease	PD
medical	med	part time	PT
medical doctor	MD	partial weight bearing	PWB
metacarpophalangeal joint	MCP		

passive range of motion	PROM	rheumatoid arthritis	RA
past medical history	PMH	right	R or Ⓡ
past surgical history	PSH	right lower extremity	RLE
patient	pt	right lower lobe	RLL
pediatrics	PED	right lower quadrant	RLQ
percussion and vibration	P&V	right middle lobe	RML
peripheral vascular disease	PVD	right upper extremity	RUE
Physician's Assistant	PA	right upper lobe	RUL
Physical Therapist, physical therapy	PT	right upper quadrant	RUQ
		rolling walker	RW
Physical Therapist Assistant	PTA	rule out, ruled out	R/O
plantar flexion	PF	second(s)	sec
platform rolling walker	PRW	secondary, second degree	2°
poor (muscle grade)	P	short arc quads	SAQ
positive, plus	+	shortness of breath	SOB
posterior	post	short-term goal(s)	STG
posteroanterior	PA	short-term memory	STM
posterior cerebral artery	PCA	significant	sig
positron emission tomography	PET	sit to stand	STS
posterior leaf splint	PLS	skilled nursing facility	SNF
posterior superior iliac spine	PSIS	sliding board	SB
postoperative	post op	sliding board transfers	SBT
potassium	K	small-based quad cane	SBQC
pound	lb, #	Speech-Language Pathologist	SLP
prescription	Rx	Speech Therapist	ST
primary	1°	spinal cord injury	SCI
prior to admission	PTA	standby assistance	SBA
progressive resistive exercise(s)	PRE	stand pivot transfers	SPT
progressive supranuclear palsy	PSP	standing order	S/O
proximal	prox	*Staphylococcus*	staph
proximal interphalangeal (joint)	PIP	status post	s/p
quadriceps	quads	step-over-step (stair climbing)	SOS
range of motion	ROM	step-to-step (stair climbing)	STS
regarding, concerning	re	sternocleidomastoid muscle	SCM
Registered Dietitian	RD	straight cane	str cane
Registered Nurse	RN	straight-leg raise	SLR
Registered Respiratory Therapist	RRT	*Streptococcus*	strep
Registered Dietetic Technician	DTR	subarachnoid hemorrhage	SAH
rehabilitation	rehab	supervision	S or Ⓢ
related to	R/T	supported	supp
repetition(s)	rep(s)	surgical, surgery	surg
reports of	R/O	symmetrical, symmetry	symm
resisted range of motion	RROM	symmetrical tonic neck relfex	STNR
respiratory rate	RR	symptoms	sx

temperature	temp	treatment	Tx, Rx
temporomandibular joint	TMJ	tuberculosis	TB
tertiary	3°	twice a day	b.i.d.
therapeutic exercise	ther ex	ultrasound	US
therapeutic recreation	TR	unilateral	U/L
third degree	3°	unsupported	unsupp
three times per week	t.i.w.	upper extremity	UE
throughout	T/O	upper respiratory infection	URI
times (e.g., 6×d = six times daily)	×	urinary tract infection	UTI
		ventricular tachycardia	Vtach
to and from	⟷	verbal cues	VC
to be assessed	TBA	verbal order	V/O
to be evaluated	TBE	visual analog scale	VAS
toe off	TO	vital capacity	VC
toe-touch weight bearing	TTWB	vital signs	VS
total hip replacement	THR	vocal cord	VC
total knee replacement	TKR	water	H_2O
total shoulder replacement	TSR	week(s)	wk
touch-down weight bearing	TDWB	weight bearing	WB
trace (muscle grade)	T	weight bearing as tolerated	WBAT
tracheostomy	trach	weight shift	WS
training	trng	wheelchair	W/C
transcutaneous electrical nerve stimulation	TENS	wide-based quad cane	WBQC
		with	c̄
transient ischemic attack	TIA	within functional limits	WFL
transverse, transferred	trans	within normal limits	WNL
traumatic brain injury	TBI	without	s̄
traumatic head injury	THI	years old	y/o or y.o.

Answers to Exercises

Chapter 1

EXERCISE 1-1

1. **I**—Range of motion is an impairment at the level of body structures and function. Musculoskeletal flexibility is measured in units of joint rotation.

2. **A**—A person's ability to walk is generally measured at the activity level.

3. **HC**—A tear of the anterior cruciate ligament is a medical diagnosis specifying location and type of tissue damage.

4. **P**—The ability to fulfill occupational role is at the level of participation.

5. **I**—Strength measures at the level of body structures and function.

6. **A**—Dressing is a functional activity.

7. **HC**—This is a medical diagnosis that specifies the location and nature of tissue damage.

8. **I or A**—The observation focus is on the patient's cardiopulmonary function, a description of the function of a body function. However, this is described within the context of an activity (walking), so for documentation purposes it could be justified being included in either Impairments or Activities.

9. **HC**—Multiple sclerosis describes a type of disease. This is a medical diagnosis.

10. **A**—Eating is a functional activity. Here the word *independently* is used, specifying how the performance is achieved.

11. **I**—Lateral pinch strength represents a body function of the musculoskeletal system.

12. **A**—Transfers are functional activities, described here in terms of goal attainment and with use of adaptive equipment (sliding board).

13. **I**—Passive range of motion represents a body function of the musculoskeletal system.

14. **A**—Crawling is an activity of locomotion for a child.

15. **A**—Reaching and grasping a cup is an activity.

16. **A**—Standing at a kitchen sink is an important functional activity.

17. **I**—A straight-leg raise reflects performance of a body system (musculoskeletal). This is a way of specifying active range of motion.

18. **I**—Pain is considered an impairment. A functional activity is not mentioned.

19. **P**—Daily household chores describe a range of activities that encompass a person's participation related to his or her personal roles in life.

20. **A**—Cooking and preparing dinner are specific functional activities.

21. **A**—Getting in and out of a wheelchair is an important functional activity for a person who uses a wheelchair for mobility.

22. **HC**—A spinal cord injury is a specific pathologic condition; the motor vehicle accident specifies the mechanism of injury.

23. **P**—Accessibility to a person's community encompasses that person's participation in society. It is a global measure rather than specifically identifying his or her functional skill in wheelchair mobility, for example.

24. **HC**—A rotator cuff tear is a pathologic condition of the shoulder.

25. **P**—Work represents a component of a person's participation (occupational role).

Chapter 2

EXERCISE 2-1

1. Manual muscle test 3/5 right quadriceps.

2. Patient can stand without assistance for 30 seconds without loss of balance.

3. Patient can transfer from bed to wheelchair with moderate assistance using sliding board.

4. Patient instructed in performing right short arc quads, 3 sets of 10 repetitions.

5. Passive range of motion of right ankle dorsiflexion is 5 degrees.

6. Received order from (or prescription from) medical doctor for weight bearing as tolerated on left lower extremity.

7. Patient instructed to perform home exercise program twice a day, 10 repetitions each exercise.

8. Patient admitted to emergency department on 10/12/09 with Glasgow Coma Scale score of 4.

9. Medical diagnosis: right hip fracture with open reduction, internal fixation.

10. Active range of motion bilateral lower extremities within normal limits.

11. Patient instructed in use of transcutaneous electrical nerve stimulator unit as needed.

12. Chest physical therapy for 20 minutes, percussion and vibration to right lower lobe.

13. Patient was discharged from the neonatal intensive care unit on 3/3/09.

14. Past medical history: insulin-dependent diabetes mellitus for 5 years, high blood pressure for 10 years.

15. Magnetic resonance imaging revealed moderate left middle cerebral artery cerebral vascular accident.

EXERCISE 2-2

1. Pt. underwent CABG 3/17/08; or pt. s/p CABG 3/17/08.

2. PT to coordinate ADL trng c̄ OT and RN staff.

3. Pt.'s HR Δ'd from 90 → 120 bpm p̄ 3 min of amb. at comfortable speed.

4. Pt.'s OB/GYN reported pt. had LBP t/o pregnancy.

5. Pt.'s daughter reports pt. has had recent ↓ in fx abilities and h/o falls.

6. BS ↓ B. Pt. instructed in DBE b.i.d.

7. Pt.'s wife reports pt. has h/o chronic LBP × 15 yr.

8. Pt.'s LTG is to walk using only str. cane. Or, Pt.'s LTG is to amb. using only str. cane.

9. DTR R biceps 2+.

10. Pt. can ↑↓ 1 flight of stairs Ⓘ, 1 hand on railing.

11. Rx received for PT: ther ex and gait trng.

12. 82 y.o. c̄ 1° med dx of CHF.

13. ECG revealed v-tach.

14. Pt. s/p CVA c̄ hemiplegia R UE & LE.

15. HHA instructed to assist pt. in AAROM exer: SLR and hip abd in supine.

EXERCISE 2-3*

1. *A person with quadriplegia will often require help with transfers.*
   Quadriplegic is a label that reduces an individual to a disability or physical condition. Terms such as *quad* or

para (or *paraplegic*) should never be used to refer to a person.

2. *The patient was diagnosed with multiple sclerosis when she was in her 20s.*
   Expressions such as *afflicted with, suffers from,* or *is a victim of* sensationalize a person's health status and may be considered patronizing. Simply say the patient was first diagnosed with multiple sclerosis in her 20s or that the condition developed in the patient.

3. *Many PTs are involved in foot clinics for people with diabetes.*
   Here again, the problem is a label.

4. *Have you finished the documentation for Mrs. Jones, who had a shoulder injury?*
   Unbelievable as it may seem, some health care providers still can be heard referring to patients as body parts. This question could easily be reworded as "Have you finished the documentation for the patient with shoulder pain in room 316?"

5. *The patient reported pain in the right upper extremity.*
   Complaining of may suggest that the patient is overreacting to his or her symptoms or is difficult to work with.

6. *OK*

7. *Although this computer program was designed for users with disabilities, users without disabilities will also find it helpful.*
   In this sentence, the term *disabled* has the effect of grouping individuals into a distinct "disability class." Again, focus on the person and not on the disability.

8. *Because of a spinal cord injury, the patient used a wheelchair for mobility.*
   To a person who lives an active, full life with the use of a wheelchair, *confined to* can have a patronizing tone.

9. *OK*

10. *The patient stated he was not doing his home exercises because they were not helping "at all."*
    This has a negative connotation and is derogatory. Statements should be kept to objective facts (e.g., stating what the patient's behavior was, rather than interpreting it).

11. *Which therapist is treating Mr. Smith in room 216, who has a brain injury?*
    People-first language should be used.

12. *A person who has had a stroke can often return to work.*
    Patients are not victims.

13. *After a discussion of heel height, the patient reported that she believed it wasn't necessary to modify her heel height choice.*
    Refused may be too strong a word.

*Some answers are adapted with permission from Martin (1999).

14. *Mr. Johnson will first go on the bike for 10 minutes; then I will sent up Ms. Glaser with moist heat.*
    Patients have names and it is important to use them or at least refer to patients as people.

15. *The patient has a diagnosis of Parkinson's disease.*
    The original wording implies that people with Parkinson's disease (or any other disease) suffer in some way, which is not always the case.

Chapter 4

EXERCISE 4-1

1. **G**—This sentence states that the child "will" be able to do something; this reflects a goal and thus belongs in the expected outcomes section.
2. **I**—Limitation in range of motion is a common impairment.
3. **I**—Blood pressure and heart rate also are impairments; they represent the "organ" level of impairments.
4. **R**—A seizure represents a pathologic condition (damage to the cellular process or homeostasis); thus it belongs in Reason for Referral, where health condition information is listed.
5. **PC**—Patient education is an important component of the Plan of Care.
6. **R**—Describing a patient's work status or occupation information is a component of his or her participation and is listed in Reason for Referral.
7. **Ac**—Stair climbing is a functional activity.
8. **As**—This statement links impairments (poor expiratory ability) with activity (ineffective cough and lowered endurance for daily care activities). The link provides the foundation for a diagnosis and is stated in the Assessment section of a report.

9. **R**—Describing a patient's profession or occupation is listed in Reason for Referral.
10. **G**—This sentence states that the patient "will" be able to stand at the bathroom sink; this reflects a goal and thus belongs in the Goals section.
11. **PC**—Therapeutic exercise is a commonly used intervention by physical therapists, which is described in the Plan of Care.
12. **I**—Muscle strength is a measure of impairments.
13. **As**—This statement links impairments (ineffective right toe clearance; weak R hip musculature) with function (slow and unsafe ambulation indoors). The link is related to a PT diagnosis and is stated in the Assessment section of a report.
14. **Ac**—Lifting a box is an activity.
15. **PC**—Coordinating intervention with other professionals (OT and nursing staff) is documented in the Plan of Care.

Chapter 5

EXERCISE 5-1

1. PMH
2. N/A
3. CC
4. MED
5. N/A
6. OTHER
7. CC
8. CC
9. PMH
10. N/A
11. PI
12. CC

EXERCISE 5-2

Example	What Is Wrong?	Rewrite Statement (Examples)
1. Pt. had heart surgery yesterday.	DP—Type of surgery not described. Also best to indicate date of surgery rather than "yesterday."	Pt. underwent L total hip replacement (posterior approach) 7/2/07.
2. Pt. reports pain starting 5/10/09.	L—Location of pain is not described in detail; does not provide meaningful information about the health condition.	Pt. reports pain in central low back, radiating into left buttock, starting 5/10/09 after a slip near her pool.
3. Pt. had a right-sided stroke.	L—Location of stroke not specified. TC—Date stroke occurred.	Pt. s/p R MCA stroke on 12/5/08.

(Continued)

Example	What Is Wrong?	Rewrite Statement (Examples)
4. Pt. is an amputee.	L—Location and type of amputation are not included. TC—Date of amputation not indicated; avoid use of "amputee"; statement is labeling; person-first terminology is not used.	Pt. is an 18 y.o. male s/p R transtibial amputation 5/12/08.
5. Pt. has typical problems related to aging.	DP—Describe specific problems the patient is experiencing. TC—How long has problem existed?	Pt. reports general forgetfulness of short-term events over past 2 mo but does not report any problems with long-term memory.
6. Pt. complains of fatigue.	DP—Type of fatigue not specified. TC—Time course not specified. "Complains of" has a negative connotation and should be avoided.	Pt.'s primary problem is general fatigue, which has been constant for the past 3 wk, and does not change based on activity level or time of day.
7. Pt. has a broken leg.	DP—Type of fracture not specified. L—Specific bone needs to be documented. TC—Date fracture occurred needs to be included.	Pt. fractured his R femur (comminuted) on 1/23/09 after skiing accident.
8. Pt. diagnosed with cancer 11/07.	L—Location of cancer not specified. More specifics of cancer could be included (e.g., stage of cancer, primary or secondary site).	Pt. was diagnosed c̄ stage II colon cancer on 8/2/05.

EXERCISE 5-3

Statement	Rewrite Statement (Examples)
PAST MEDICAL HISTORY	
1. Pt. has h/o cardiac problems.	Pt. has h/o coronary artery disease with stable angina, dx on 10/04.
2. Pt. has h/o several surgeries.	Pt. had C-section 6/6/04 and appendectomy 12/2/08.
3. Pt. is a diabetic.	H/o IDDM ×10 yr.
MEDICATIONS	
4. Pt. is taking multiple medications for various medical conditions.	Pt. is currently taking 2.0 mg Haldol daily to minimize involuntary movements; 20 mg Paxil for depression.
5. Pt. is taking antispasticity meds.	Pt. is currently taking Baclofen 20 mg t.i.d. to reduce upper extremity spasticity.

Chapter 6

EXERCISE 6-1

Statement	Discussion	Rewrite Statement
1. Pt. is confined to a wheelchair.	This statement could be more descriptive about the type of wheelchair and what the patient uses the wheelchair for. Also, *confined to* has a negative connotation.	Pt. uses a lightweight W/C with gel seat cushion for primary means of indoor and outdoor mobility.
2. Has poor motivation to return to work.	*Poor motivation* has a negative connotation and reflects your opinion rather than an objective finding. Stick to objective findings about a patient's participation in rehabilitation program.	Pt. reports that he is "not interested in returning to work."
3. Works on a loading dock.	Not enough detail. Pt.'s general responsibilities and level of physical activity required on the job need to be included.	Pt. works on a loading dock lifting boxes as heavy as 50 lbs, up to 8 hr/day.

Statement	Discussion	Rewrite Statement
4. Client enjoys sports.	Not enough detail provided about specific sports and level of participation.	Client enjoys hiking 1-2×/month and skiing 10-12× during winter months.
5. Pt. cannot return to work 2° to architectural barriers.	Description of the architectural barriers is needed.	Pt. reports that 8 stairs in front entrance of office building limit her ability to enter the building with her wheelchair and thus return to work.
6. Pt. was very active before her injury.	*Very active* does not provide enough detail. Specify the type of activity the patient was involved in.	Pt. led a very active lifestyle prior to her injury – she bicycled 15 miles 3×/wk and played tennis 1 hr, 2×/wk.
7. Pt. is in poor shape.	This statement has a negative connotation. There is not enough specific detail about the person's lifestyle or activity level that would be relevant to the rehabilitation program.	Pt. reports he has led a relatively inactive lifestyle and has not participated in a regular exercise routine for the past 5 yr.
8. Pt. lives in an apartment.	It is important to include whether there are stairs to enter, or stairs within the house, and with whom the patient lives.	Pt. lives alone on 4th floor of an apt. building, with elevator. No steps to enter building.
9. Pt. has a history of bad health habits.	Describing a patient's health habits as *bad* is making a judgment and does not provide useful information that is pertinent to physical therapy.	Pt. has hx of smoking 1 pack of cigarettes/day for past 10 yr.
10. Pt. uses adaptive equipment.	The type of equipment used by the patient should be listed or described.	Pt. uses a raised toilet seat and a shower chair with handheld shower.

EXERCISE 6-2

1. **S**
2. **S**
3. **NP**
4. **P**
5. **S**
6. **NP**
7. **P**
8. **NP**
9. **P**
10. **S**

EXERCISE 6-3

Case Report A

Setting: Outpatient
   Name: Terry O'Connor **D.O.B.:** 3/23/43 **Date of Eval.:** 7/2/09

Reason for Referral

Current Condition: Right hip bursitis, onset around 5/10/99. Pt. is a 66 y.o. female who had a gradual onset of pain approximately 2 mo ago in her R thigh, which progressed to a continuous "throbbing pain." Pain radiates from the R hip to the R knee. Pt. does not attribute it to any particular incident.

Social History: Pt. lives with husband in a 2-story house, 5 steps to enter, with bedroom on 2nd floor.

Participation: Pt. is retired secretary. Volunteers 1 day/wk at the local hospital but has not volunteered since late May 2° to pain. Pt. reports that husband has recently been assisting with laundry and household cleaning, which patient previously performed independently. Sleep is frequently disturbed 1-2×/night, especially after rolling onto R side, and she has difficulty falling asleep due to the pain.

Pt. enjoys cooking and golfing. Doctor advised her to discontinue playing golf until pain subsides. Pt. enjoys playing bridge with her friends once/wk. She is still able to do this but has to modify her position (change from sitting to standing approximately every 10 min). Goes out to lunch or dinner 2-3×/week with husband or friends; quality of this activity reduced due to constant position changes.

EXERCISE 6-3

Case Report B

Setting: Inpatient Rehabilitation
Name: Tommy Jones **D.O.B.:** 5/12/89 **Date of Eval.:** 7/2/09 **Admission date:** 7/2/09

Reason for Referral

Current Condition: C7 incomplete SCI 2° to MVA on 6/15/09. Pt. was transferred this morning from County Acute Care Hospital, where he has been since his accident. Medical records reveal one episode of orthostatic hypotension upon coming to sitting and two episodes of autonomic dysreflexia. Pt. underwent surgery on 6/16/99 for anterior cervical fusion. Currently cleared for all rehabilitation activities per Dr. Johnston (per phone conversation this morning).

Social History: Before hospital admission, pt. lived at home with his parents while attending college full-time. His parents are very supportive, and his mother is able to stay home to assist with pt.'s care if needed.

Participation: Pt was full-time engineering student on a large campus. He drove to school and walked long distances (10-15 minutes) between classes. Worked part-time at a local pub as a bartender 2 nights per week. Before injury, household responsibilities included laundry, cleaning room, and mowing lawn weekly. Pt. enjoyed running (completed several marathons), biking, and hiking. Very busy social life in college and with family. Enjoyed going out to dinner and to pubs and to friends' homes. Described health as "good" before injury.

Chapter 7

EXERCISE 7-1

Statement	Discussion	Rewrite Statement
1. Able to walk 50 ft.	Context not specified; not enough detail. Describe where pt. can walk, such as surface conditions or specific environment. Also should indicate level of assistance and assistive devices, if applicable.	Pt. can walk a maximum of 50 ft I'ly, using str cane in hospital corridor; limited due to fatigue (HR ↑ from 78 to 115).
2. Able to eat with a spoon with occasional assistance.	*Occasional assistance* is not measurable.	Able to eat c̄ a spoon c̄ A required 25% of time to prevent spilling.
3. Pt. is confined to using a wheelchair for long-distance mobility.	*Confined* has a negative connotation; long-distance mobility is not measurable.	Pt. reports propelling W/C I'ly for distances up to 1000 ft outside home.
4. Able to climb a few stairs.	Not enough detail. Provide more details on capability. *A few* is not measurable. Indicate # of stairs, pattern of stair climbing, or speed.	Pt. can ↑↓ 10 steps, step-over-step, c̄ 1 hand on R ↑ railing.
5. Can throw a ball but cannot catch one.	Not enough detail; not measurable. Describe size of ball, distance thrown.	Can throw an 8-inch ball 5 ft 3/4 trials; unable to catch from 3 ft distance 0/4 trials.
6. Can walk on uneven surfaces.	The term *uneven surfaces* is not sufficiently detailed; not measurable.	Pt. can walk outdoors on grass I'ly for distance up to 500 ft before fatigue reported (Borg RPE = 12).
7. Pt. is not motivated to walk.	*Not motivated* has a negative connotation and is an interpretation by the therapist, not an objective statement.	Pt. would not attempt ambulation. Pt. reports he is not yet "ready to try to walk," despite advice by PT and MD that he is medically ready.
8. Dresses upper body with difficulty.	*Difficulty* is not measurable; specify degree of difficulty—which components of dressing are problematic?	Pt. needs min A to get arms through shirts and do most buttons.
9. Walks slowly.	Not enough detail; not measurable; context not specified. Provide speed of ambulation to provide measurable data.	Pt's avg walking speed on indoor level surface is 60 m/min (avg. for an adult her age is 90 m/min).

Statement	Discussion	Rewrite Statement
10. Pt. doesn't drive.	Not enough detail; specify why the patient does not drive.	Pt. does not drive >20 min at a time 2° to pain in neck and R arm.
11. C/o pain during standing.	Focus should be on standing (an activity) not on pain (an Impairment). "Complains of" has a negative connotation. Also not measurable—specify time the patient can stand and where the pain is.	Pt. is able to stand for max. 15 min. After this, pt. reports gradual increase in LBP (rated up to 4/10) and needs to sit after 20-25 min.
12. Transfers with assistance.	Assistance is not measurable; not enough detail; specify how much assistance is required and the type of transfer.	Transfers from bed → W/C c̄ max A using SPT.
13. Pt. can lift various-sized boxes.	Not measurable; provide more information about boxes (e.g., weight) and also to what height boxes can be lifted.	Pt. can lift boxes up to 10 lb from floor to waist-height shelf.
14. Pt. can't get up from a low chair.	Not measurable; quantify amount of assistance needed and height of chair.	Sit → stand c̄ min A from 16-inch height chair.
15. Pt. is having trouble sitting for extended periods at work.	Not measurable; quantify how long pt. can sit for and specify why he cannot sit longer.	Pt. unable to sit at work desk for >20 min at a time 2° to back pain.

EXERCISE 7-2

1. Ambulation
2. Self-care
3. Climbing stairs
4. N/A
5. N/A
6. Transfers
7. Standing ability
8. N/A
9. Travelling to work/school (or community mobility)
10. N/A
11. Dressing
12. Transfers
13. Food preparation

EXERCISE 7-3

Bus Driver

Sitting
Turning wheel
Operating door
Shifting gears
Walking up and down stairs
Walking (approx. 50 ft)
Turning head to look behind both ways

Homemaker

Cooking—carrying pots and pans, standing to cook
Cleaning—mopping, vacuuming, washing dishes
Laundry
Financial management
Shopping (walking, pushing cart, reaching to shelves, carrying groceries)

College Student

Sitting
Reading/turning pages
Traveling to and from classes
Traveling up and down stairs

Administrative Assistant

Typing
Filing
Computer skills
Sitting
Walking

Professional Basketball Player

Dribbling
Free throw
Running
Blocking
Jumping
Passing
Shooting
Walking backwards and sideways

Chapter 8

EXERCISE 8-1

Impairment Statement	Impairment Category
1. R elbow flexion PROM 0-60°.	Range of motion
2. Walks with uneven step lengths and ↑ weight-bearing time on R side.	Gait, locomotion, and balance
3. Sensation intact B LEs below knee, 10/10 correct responses.	Sensory integrity
4. Mini-Mental State Examination score 19/30 (cognitive assessment).	Arousal, attention, and cognition
5. AROM B UEs—no limitations noted.	Range of motion
6. Right facial nerve intact.	Cranial and peripheral nerve integrity
7. Circumference midpatella L knee: 10″; R knee: 9.25″.	Anthropometric characteristics
8. Rates pain in low back as 5/10 sitting for 10 min; pain described as aching/throbbing.	Pain
9. Skin intact B LE and trunk.	Integumentary integrity
10. Berg Balance Scale score = 31/56 indicating high risk for falls.	Gait, locomotion, and balance
11. Demonstrates antalgic gait pattern.	Gait, locomotion, and balance
12. B patellar tendon reflexes 2+.	Reflex integrity
13. B lung fields clear to auscultation.	Aerobic capacity/endurance ventilation AND respiration/gas exchange
14. Incentive spirometry in sitting c̄ maximal volume = 1750 mL.	Aerobic capacity/endurance ventilation AND respiration/gas exchange
15. Pt. has forward head and flattened lumbar lordosis.	Posture
16. Pt. is alert and oriented to ×2 (person and place).	Arousal, attention, and cognition
17. HR ↑'d to 110 beats/min p̄ 5 min walking at 1.0 m/sec.	Aerobic capacity/endurance
18. Proprioception sensation impaired L ankle 2/8 correct responses.	Sensory integrity
19. R hand grip strength 15 kg as measured by handheld dynamometer, avg. 3 trials.	Muscle performance
20. Eye movements, smooth pursuit, and visual fields intact (cranial nerves II, III, IV, and VI).	Cranial and peripheral nerve integrity

EXERCISE 8-2

Statement	Discussion	Rewrite Statement
1. Sensation is impaired.	Impaired is not measurable. Not enough detail; describe where sensation is impaired; quantify extent of impairment.	Sensation impaired dorsal aspect R foot, 2/5 correct responses.
2. ROM is moderately limited.	Moderately limited is not measurable; ROM can be measured in degrees. Not enough detail; specify ROM of a specific joint and motion.	ROM R knee flexion 0-85°.

Statement	Discussion	Rewrite Statement
3. Pt. c/o excruciating pain.	Excruciating is not measurable; describe location, quality, severity, timing, intensity, what makes pain better/worse.	Pt. reports pain in L shoulder at glenohumeral joint ("stabbing"), onset 3 days ago. Rates pain as 4/10 in AM, 8/10 in PM. Pain is relieved by lying down (2/10).
4. Pt. has L leg edema.	Not enough detail; specify where the edema is (ankle, calf, knee, etc.). Not measurable; quantify degree of edema.	2+ pitting edema L ankle; circumference L ankle at malleoli 26 cm, R ankle 22 cm.
5. Pt. demonstrates a significant ↑ in HR c̄ stair climbing.	*Significant* is not measurable; HR can be measured quantitatively.	HR increases from 80 to 120 bpm p̄ pt. ↑≠ 24 steps.
6. Pt's. reflexes are hyperactive.	Not enough detail; specific reflex not identified. *Hyperactive* is not measurable; reflexes can be quantified.	Patellar tendon reflex: L 2+; R 3+.
7. Pt. doesn't know what's going on.	Not appropriate; if pt.'s cognitive status is being documented, not enough detail is provided.	Pt. is alert and oriented ×3 (person, place, and time).
8. Pt. has abnormal gait pattern.	*Abnormal* is not measurable; should identify what specifically is not normal.	Pt. walks c̄ L Trendelenburg gait, indicative of gluteus medius weakness.
9. Pt. has poor endurance.	*Poor* is not measurable; not specific to an activity, which is important for endurance. Endurance can be measured on a perceived exertion scale.	Pt. reports SOB (11/15 on Borg RPE) and has HR ↑ to 140 bpm p̄ amb 200 ft.
10. Pt. walks c̄ L knee pain.	Not measurable; not enough detail. Focus is on walking and not on pain. For this statement to belong in the Impairment section, it should focus on the pain specifically. Describe location, quality, severity, timing, and what makes pain better/worse.	Pt. reports L knee pain began approx. 2 mo ago. Pain described as "sharp," located on medial aspect of L knee. Pt. rates pain as 3/10 at rest (sitting or lying down), ↑ to 7/10 p̄ walking 5 min.

Chapter 9

EXERCISE 9-1

Case 1: Outpatient

Case Information	Assessment
59 y.o. man, s/p R THR 2° to osteoarthritis, 3 wk previous. Pt. past acute stage—no significant pain or swelling; incision well healed. **Participation:** Sales representative, travels by car, unable to work since surgery. **Activity Limitations:** Needs assist for transfers into car, walks slowly with walker, up to 100 ft at a time, needs assist on steps. **Impairments:** Weakness in R hip flexors, abductors, and extensors; habitual gait deviations from preop antalgic gait. R hip √ and abduction ROM limited.	Pt. is a 59 y.o. male, 3 wks s/p R THR 2° to osteoarthritis. Incision is healing well, and pt. experiences no significant pain or swelling. Weakness in hip musculature, hip ROM limitations, and preop gait deviations have resulted in limited speed and distance for walking. Weakness also makes transfer in and out of car impossible without assistance. Limitations in walking and car transfers are currently preventing pt. from returning to work as a sales rep. Pt. requires PT intervention to improve strength, ROM, and walking ability, facilitating pt.'s return to work.

Case 2: Outpatient

Case Information	Assessment
43 y.o. female with MS diagnosed 3 yr previous; recovering from recent exacerbation. **Participation:** Clerical worker in major downtown office building; rides train and bus to work; resists using cane. Pt. is fearful of falling during commute and needs extra time to commute. **Activity Limitations:** Requires assist to go up and down steps; walks slowly; walking difficulties exacerbated in crowded places. **Impairments:** Only mild weakness; standing balance easily disturbed, esp. when pt. is distracted.	Pt. is a 43 y.o. female diagnosed c̄ MS 3 yr ago. Pt. presents c̄ significantly impaired standing balance, resulting in slowed walking speed and difficulties walking in crowded places and negotiating stairs. These problems are limiting pt.'s ability to safely and efficiently commute to work. Pt. requires PT intervention to address balance and ambulation difficulties and improve ability to commute to work.

Case 3: Inpatient

Case Information	Assessment
48 y.o. woman admitted to an acute care hospital with complaints of severe abdominal pain, diminished appetite with nausea and diarrhea for 4 days. PMH, end-stage live disease; liver transplant 4 yr ago, end-stage renal disease with hemodialysis 2×/wk hypertension and a DVT with onset 4 mo ago; sacral onset ×4 mo. **Activity Limitations:** Mobility limited to wheelchair. Mod. to maximal assistance for all bed mobility and transfers. **Impairments:** Posture: the supine position most frequently observed was with the head of bed elevated >6°. Muscle strength: 2+/5 gross lower extremity strength, 3-/5 gross upper extremity strength. Wound: 3.7 × 3.4 cm with 2-3 cm of undermining); 85% yellow rubbery eschar; 15% red granulation.	Pt. is a 48 y.o. female diagnosed c̄ end-stage liver disease. Pt. admitted to hospital for current episode of care for abdominal pain, diminished appetite, nausea, and diarrhea. Pt. presents with upper and lower extremity weakness 2° to current medical conditions, which have led to significant mobility limitations including dependence in all forms of mobility and transfers. This lack of independent mobility has led to further complications, including a sacral pressure sore. Pt. requires PT intervention to address strength deficits and deconditioning, treatment to facilitate healing of pressure sore, and functional training to minimize caregiver burden for mobility and transfers.

Case 4: Outpatient

Case Information	Assessment
39 y.o. female c̄ diagnosis of cervical strain. Onset of symptoms occurred 6 wk ago. **Participation:** CPA at local firm, currently unable to tolerate typical 8-10 hr workday 2° to symptoms. Majority of time typically spent on phone and computer. **Activity Limitations:** Occasionally requires pain medication to assist with sleeping at night. Unable to talk on phone 2° to pain with phone cradling position. Unable to tolerate computer work >2 hr 2° to increased pain. **Impairments:** Static sitting posture presents with a decrease in cervical lordosis and an increase in thoracic kyphosis. Limited AROM with right-side flexion and rotation at C-spine. Flexed, rotated, and sidebent left at C5 and C6. Weakness in bilateral lower trapezius: 3/5, bilateral middle trapezius/rhomboids: 4/5, and cervical extensors: 3+/5. Pain rated as 3/10 at rest and 6/10 after working 2 hr; described as throbbing and occasionally shooting.	Pt. is a 39 y.o. female with recent diagnosis of cervical strain; onset of symptoms 6 weeks ago. Pt. presents with poor cervical and thoracic postures, moderate ROM and strength deficits in the cervical and thoracic spine regions, cervical facet dysfunction, and increased pain that results in limited tolerance with computer and phone duties, as well as sleep disturbance. These issues are restricting the pt.'s work endurance and performance. Pt. requires PT to address postural dysfunction, ROM, and strength deficits as well as facet dysfunction. Postural education, proper body mechanics, ergonomic assessment, and pain management would be addressed as well.

Case 5: Inpatient Rehabilitation—Burn Center

Case Information	Assessment
23 y.o. female college student, sustained 11% TBSA full-thickness scald burn to right anterior thigh, anterior lower leg, and dorsal foot. s/p skin grafting surgery to excise burn eschar and skin graft the wound 5 days ago. **Participation:** Previously active in playing tennis weekly. Full-time graduate student; lives in apartment with 2 roommates; elevator to enter, all living on one floor. **Activity Limitations:** Able to amb. independently 20 ft in 19.5 sec; step to gait; Tinetti Gait assessment 7/12. Stands independently without support; independent and safe with transfers. **Impairments:** 11% TBSA, full-thickness burns to right anterior thigh, anterior lower leg, dorsal foot; potential for scarring after healing/surgery. Pain in right lower extremity 4/10 at rest, with movement 6/10. ROM: R knee ext/flex 0-90°; right ankle dorsiflexion 5°, plantar flexion 20°. Edema noted right lower extremity.	Pt. is a 25 y.o. female s/p 11% full-thickness scald burn to right leg and foot and is 5 days s/p skin graft surgery. Pt. presents with wounds and grafts 2° to burn injury, which have resulted in significant pain and ROM limitations in R LE in addition to edema postsurgery. These impairments have led to limitations in ambulation speed and balance, which will limit pt.'s ability to function independently at home and return to previous active lifestyle and attend full-time graduate school. Pt. requires impatient PT to address ROM limitations and edema, facilitate graft healing, and address ambulation and balance deficits, facilitating pt.'s return to independent and full participation in previous lifestyle.

Chapter 10

EXERCISE 10-1

1. Independent in transfers in 2 wk. Patient (A) will transfer (B) independently (D) bed → W/C (C) 100% of time (D) within 2 wk (E).	Type: Activity *Problem:* A, B, C
2. Patient will be functional in ADL within 3 wk. Patient (A) will perform (B) all ADLs (C) independently (D) within 3 wk (E).	Type: Participation *Problem:* B, C, D
3. Return to work in 3 mo. Patient (A) will return (B) to work as kindergarten teacher (C) and be able to participate (B) in all required activities (C) within 3 months (E).	Type: Participation *Problem:* A, C, D
4. Increased strength in quadriceps to 5/5 bilaterally. Strength B quadriceps (C) will ↑ (B) to 5/5 (D) within 3 wk (E). NOTE: Actor is typically not specified for Impairment goal.	Type: Impairment *Problem:* B, E
5. Pt. will ↑↓ 1 flight of stairs in 1 min. Pt. (A) will ↑↓ (B) 1 flight/12 steps (C) at 7″ height (C) c̄ 1 rail (C) step-over-step pattern (D) in 1 min (D) I'ly (D) within 3 wk (E).	Type: Activity *Problem:* C, E
6. Pt. will demonstrate increased R hip ROM. AROM R hip flexion (C) will ↑ (B) to 110° (D) in 2 wk (E).	Type: Impairment *Problem:* C, D, E
7. Pt. will return to school. Pt. (A) will return (B) to college (C) taking 2 classes (D) within 1 mo (E).	Type: Participation *Problem:* C, D, E
8. Pt. will get from his room to therapy. Pt. (A) will propel his W/C (B) from his room to therapy gym (approx. 250 ft) (C) in less than 3 min (D) within 2 weeks (E).	Type: Activity *Problem:* B, D, E

EXERCISE 10-2

Statement	Discussion	Rewrite Statement
1. Pt. will experience less pain.	Reports of pain are related to impairment goals. Focus should be on task or function. Less pain is not measurable. Where is the pain? During what activity?	Pt. will walk >500 ft distance c̄ pain <4/10 4/5 days, within 2 wk.
2. Pt. will progress from a walker to a cane within 3 wk.	Not enough detail regarding distance/speed or context. Progress will be obvious when all notes are reviewed. Reflects the process rather than the goal.	Pt. will walk 100 m at speed ≤0.80 m/sec in clinic hallway using a cane in 3 wk.

(Continued)

Statement	Discussion	Rewrite Statement
3. Educate pt. on hip precautions within 2 sessions.	Educating the pt. is part of the intervention, not a goal. Reflects the process rather than the goal.	Pt. will verbally demonstrate knowledge of total hip precautions when asked by therapist 100% of the time.
4. Pt. will walk with a normal gait pattern within 4 wk.	Not measurable. Normal is a relative term and depends on status prior to recent injury.	Pt. will amb. 500 ft s̄ an assistive device, in the hospital hallways, c̄ CG in 3 wk.
5. ①ADLS in 2 wk.	Not enough detail; "all activities" is too vague.	Pt. will transfer I'ly W/C → toilet c̄ SB in <1 min in 2 wk.
6. Pt. will ascend and descend stairs within 3 days.	Not concrete; not enough detail. Height of stairs, time to complete, use of railing can all be used to clarify goal.	Pt. will ↑↓ 12 8" height steps, using step-over-step pattern in 30 sec, within 5 days.
7. Pt. will not have pain when reaching.	Emphasis is on pain, which relates to impairments; not enough detail describing functional skill of reaching; no time course.	Pt. will put away dishes from dishwasher to all shelves without report of pain (0/10), within 1 wk.
8. Pt. will sit for 5 min.	Sitting can occur in many different locations. Describe chair or surface and other conditions. No time course specified.	Pt. will be able to sit on office chair for up to 30 min s̄ pain.
9. Pt. will improve standing balance.	Actor is not specified; need to be more specific about surface and task; time course not specified.	Pt. will stand I'ly at kitchen counter for 5 min c̄ 2-hand support.
10. Pt. will transfer from sit → stand in 2 wk.	Describe conditions more specifically (e.g., level of assistance) and degree (e.g., success rate)	Pt. will transfer from sit → stand and c̄ min A 4/5 trials within 2 wk.

Chapter 11

EXERCISE 11-1

1. **PI**—Pt. will be instructed in self-stretching of right wrist and elbow.

2. **NP**—Past medical hx is significant for HTN. (Belongs in Reason for Referral/Past Medical History.)

3. **CC**—Referral to orthotist to evaluate for specific AFO.

4. **I**—Functional training to address balance and coordination during morning bathroom routine.

5. **I**—RLE strengthening exercises such as squats, stair stepping, and obstacle negotiation to improve standing and walking ability.

6. **NP**—Pt. will be able to negotiate walking over 6-inch high obstacles (this is a goal).

7. **CC**—Discuss with pt. options for long-distance mobility, including use of wheelchair.

8. **NP**—Strength of right hip abductors will increase to 4/5 (this is a goal).

9. **I**—Trng with appropriate assistive device (straight cane or quad cane) during ambulation indoors and outdoors, and transfers to improve safety, speed, and distance.

10. **PI**—Pt. will view video modeling strategies for improved UE function in patients who have had a stroke.

11. **PI**—Pt. will be instructed in home walking program to improve speed and endurance; walking daily beginning with 10 min and progressing to 20 min over 4 wk.

12. **PI**—Instruct pt.'s wife in soft tissue massage for right upper extremity and guarding techniques for outdoor ambulation.

EXERCISE 11-2

Statement	Discussion	Rewrite Statement
1. Practice walking.	Practice of a task does not mean the need for skilled services. Describe circumstances, type of walking, type of training.	Gait training within home from bedroom to bathroom, living room, and kitchen to address safety and teach compensatory strategies for visual field deficits and L spatial neglect.
2. Apply hot packs.	Rationale not provided; not enough detail. Why is a hot pack needed? Specify to address pain, relax tissues, etc. Area of body needs to be stated. No indication of skilled services required.	Moist heat to cervical spine to promote relaxation and improve cervical spine flexibility.

Statement	Discussion	Rewrite Statement
3. Pt. will be able to walk 10 ft to the bathroom.	Not appropriate for this section. This is a goal, not an intervention. Need to state it in terms of what the pt. or therapist will do.	Gait training for short distances to bathroom using manual guidance as needed to improve foot clearance.
4. Pt. will be given strengthening exercises.	Not enough detail. Describe what type of strengthening exercises. Be specific to muscle group. "Instructed" is a better term than "given."	Pt. will be instructed in home program to include isometric strengthening for left quadriceps.
5. Coordinate care with all nursing personnel.	Not enough detail. What care will be coordinated? Clarify the PT-related activities you will coordinate with nurses on—transfers, bed mobility, etc.	Will review transfers and bed mobility strategies with nursing staff, to facilitate pt.'s use of right side of body.
6. Assess work environment.	Not enough detail. This could involve many different things; try to clarify which areas of the work environment will be addressed. What is the purpose of assessing work environment?	Work environment to be assessed within 2 wk to make modification recommendations before returning to work.
7. Pt. will increase right hamstring strength.	Not appropriate for this section. This is a goal, not an intervention. Need to state this as what the patient or therapist will do.	Progressive resistive strengthening exercises for R hamstrings.
8. Balance training.	Not enough detail. Need to identify what specifically will be addressed with this training.	Training of sitting balance including proactive (reaching, ball play activities) and reactive (response to perturbations in sitting, activities on therapeutic ball) to improve overall sitting ability.
9. Pt. will receive ultrasound at 1.0 W/cm^2, 1 MHz to R quadriceps (VMO), in a 10-cm area just proximal and slightly medial to R knee, moving ultrasound head slowly in circular fashion for 10 min, each session.	Too much detail is provided. It would be sufficient to eliminate some of the details; parameters could be specified in treatment notes. Rationale for the intervention is not stated.	Pt. will receive ultrasound to R quadriceps (VMO) to improve mobility and promote tissue healing.
10. Pt. will take pain relief medication as needed.	Prescribing or recommending medication is not within the scope of physical therapy practice. Therapists can discuss and coordinate with other health care personnel regarding a patient's medication management as it pertains to physical therapy.	Pt.'s pain medication regimen will be coordinated with MD and nursing staff to be administered 1-2 hours before PT treatment for optimal exercise tolerance.
11. Home evaluation.	Not enough detail; rationale for doing a home evaluation not provided.	Home evaluation will be conducted prior to D/C to evaluate pt.'s home environment and accessibility.
12. Reduce R ankle edema.	Not appropriate for this section. This is a general goal, not an intervention. The method used to reduce the edema would be appropriate to document in the intervention section.	Ice to be applied to R ankle to ↓ swelling and pain.
13. Teach family to care for pt.	Not enough detail; document specific skills being taught.	Educate pt.'s family members on safe techniques for W/C transfers → car and bed.
14. Practice pressure-relief techniques.	Not enough detail; not specific as to type of pressure relief.	Educate pt. in effective pressure-relief techniques while sitting in W/C to prevent skin breakdown.
15. E-stim to anterior tibialis.	Rationale not provided.	E-stim to anterior tibialis for muscle re-education.

Chapter 12

EXERCISE 12-1

Statement	Section	Discussion	Rewrite
1. Pt. states he hates using his walker.	S	Not enough detail. It would be helpful to know why he dislikes using his walker.	Pt. states that he "prefers to use a cane rather than a walker" because it is too difficult to carry things while using the walker.
2. Pt. has an awkward gait.	O	Not enough detail; *awkward* is not measurable.	Pt. walks on indoor level surfaces $\bar{s}$ assistive device $\bar{c}$ decreased stance time on R 2° to pain in R foot on weight bearing.
3. PROM at the knee is getting better.	O	Not enough detail; not measurable.	PROM of R knee √ is 0-95°.
4. Pt. is very confused.	O	Not enough detail. What is pt. confused about? If performing a mental status assessment, report findings in an objective manner.	Pt. is alert & oriented × 1 (person). Mini-Mental State examination score: 16/30.
5. Pt. reports that his son is concerned.	S	Not enough detail. Need to document son's specific concerns.	Pt. reports that his son is concerned about his ability to care for his father when he returns home. Son has a full-time job and 2 small children of his own.
6. Pt. c/o fatigue after walking for 5 min.	S	*Complains of* has a negative connotation; fatigue could be quantified.	Pt. reports feeling fatigued (Borg RPE 14) $\bar{p}$ amb 5 min outdoors.
7. Pt. complains of pain in left shoulder.	S	*Complains of* has a negative connotation. Not enough detail about pain (location, quality, severity, timing, etc.).	Pt. continues to report pain in her L shoulder that radiates down to her elbow, 6/10. It aches all of the time except when she is lying down.
8. Pt. performed 10 reps of knee exercises.	O	Not enough detail; specific exercises should be documented.	Pt. performed 10 reps of isometric quad sets.

EXERCISE 12-2

SOAP Statement	SOAP Section G, S, O, A, P
1. Performed 10 reps SLR B.	O
2. Pt. reports she was able to walk with her daughter out to get the mail yesterday and did not experience any dizziness.	S
3. Treatment next session will include progression to stationary bike × 10 min.	P
4. Pt. walked 15 ft from bed to bathroom without SOB in 30 sec.	O
5. Pt. states that she "felt sore" after last treatment session.	S
6. Pt. is progressing well with increasing repetitions of LE strengthening exercises and has achieved goal 1.	A
7. Pitting edema noted in R ankle.	O

SOAP Statement	SOAP Section G, S, O, A, P
8. Pt. was instructed to continue to maintain R leg in elevated position while sitting at desk during the day.	O
9. Pt. will transfer from bed to wheelchair independently, 4/5 trials within 2 wk.	G
10. Pt. states she is anxious to return to work.	S
11. Pt. will continue with daily walking program at home during off-therapy days, progressing to 20 min each day by next wk.	P
12. Pt. will stand s̄ A for up to 1 min within 1 wk.	G
13. Pt. reports pain in low back while walking as 5/10 and 8/10 while sitting at desk at work.	S
14. Pt.'s fear of falling is limiting his progress in improving his ability to ambulate in crowded environments and outdoors.	A
15. Pt. reports that she is going back to work on a trial basis next week.	S

Chapter 14

EXERCISE 14-1

Statement	Discussion	Rewrite Statement
1. The child was uncooperative.	Describing a child as uncooperative has a negative connotation and is subjective. Instead, describe the child's behavior objectively.	Child refused to attempt several tasks on the evaluation, including hopping on one foot and skipping, preferring to play with the puzzles.
2. John has poor strength.	While "poor" is a muscle grade used in manual muscle testing, in this sentence it is used as a vague descriptor of strength. Rather, describe the child's ability to perform a task that is related to a particular muscle action.	John seems to have weakness of bilateral hip musculature: he could squat with only approx. 10° of knee flexion, and demonstrated a + Gower's sign upon coming from floor to stand.
3. Lucy has spasticity of B hamstrings and gastrocs.	Spasticity is a term that should be defined if the report is to be read by the parent (which in all likelihood it is). Hamstrings and gastrocs may also be unfamiliar terms to a layperson.	Lucy demonstrates spasticity (increased muscle tone and reflexes leading to stiffness and involuntary muscle contraction) in both her hamstrings (muscle group in the back of the leg) and her gastrocsoleus (muscles of the calf)
4. Kelly cannot walk and is currently wheelchair bound.	This sentence has a very negative tone. It should include more information about Kelly's abilities, and not just her disabilities.	Kelly is able to stand for short periods (up to 30 sec) but has not yet demonstrated the ability to take steps. She uses a manual W/C as a primary means of mobility within the home, which she can independently maneuver. For community distance Kelly is pushed in her W/C by a family member.
5. Tommy can climb stairs but can only do so with one hand held by his mother.	A child's abilities should not always be followed by a "but…" statement. This type of statement focuses the reader on what the child can't do rather than on what he can do.	Tommy is able to climb stairs with one hand held by his mother.
6. ROM R knee √ 100°.	This statement uses abbreviations that will likely be unfamiliar to a parent or school personnel reading the report.	Amelia demonstrates some limitation in range of motion (ability to move a joint) in her right knee (100°; typical range for a child her age is 160°)

(Continued)

Statement	Discussion	Rewrite Statement
7. Samantha sits in W-sitting with excessive kyphotic posture.	W-sitting and kyphotic posture are likely to be unfamiliar terms. They should be defined, and the tone of this sentence should be softened.	Samantha prefers sitting in a W-sitting position (sitting on her bottom with her knees bent and feet out to either side of her hips) when playing on the floor. In this position, she tends to have an increase in normal thoracic kyphosis (outward curvature of the upper part of the spine), so that she appears very hunched over.
8. Timmy performed very poorly on the PEDI with a standard score of 20.	Report scores on standardized tests objectively without drawing judgment. Avoid abbreviations for tests or spell out the name.	Timmy received a standard score of 20 on the Pediatric Evaluation of Disability Inventory (PEDI). This test has a mean of 50 and a standard deviation of 10, which means Timmy's score falls 3 standard deviations below the mean.

EXERCISE 14-2

Examples of possible goals:

1. Tim will walk in school hallway with Loftstrand crutches and use a backpack to carry books from classroom to lunchroom with avg. speed of 1.0 m/sec within 3 mo.
2. Tim will use the stairs (ascending) to get to art/music class 3x/wk.
3. Tim will amb. 200 ft from bus to school building with Pictorial Children's Effort Rating Table (PCERT) of <6/10.

Sample Forms

Following are examples of forms that can be used in PT documentation.

Documentation Review Sample Checklist

APTA
American Physical Therapy Association
The Science of Healing. The Art of Caring. •

REVIEW FOR MEDICAL RECORDS DOCUMENTATION
Physical Therapy

Note: This is meant to be a sample documentation review checklist only. Please check payer, state law, and specific accreditation organization (i.e., Joint Commission, CARF, etc) requirements for compliance.

Therapist reviewed: Privileged and Confidential

PT Initial Visit Elements for Documentation Date:	N/A	Yes	No
Examination:			
1. Date/time 2. Legibility			
3. Referral mechanism by which physical therapy services are initiated			
4. History – medical history, social history, current condition(s)/chief complaint(s), onset, previous functional status and activity level, medications, allergies			
5. Patient/client's rating of health status, current complaints			
6. Systems Review – Cardiovascular/pulmonary, Integumentary, Musculoskeletal, Neuromuscular, communication ability, affect, cognition, language, and learning style			
7. Tests and Measures – Identifies the specific tests and measures and documents associated findings or outcomes, includes standardized tests and measures, e.g., OPTIMAL, Oswestry, etc.			
Evaluation:			
1. Synthesis of the data and findings gathered from the examination: A problem list, a statement of assessment of key factors (e.g., cognitive factors, co-morbidities, social support, additional services) influencing the patient/client status.			
Diagnosis:			
1. Documentation of a diagnosis - include impairment and functional limitations which may be practice patterns according to the Guide to Physical Therapists Practice, ICD9-CM, or other descriptions.			
Prognosis:			
1. Documentation of the predicted functional outcome and duration to achieve the desired functional outcome			
Plan of Care:			
1. Goals stated in measurable terms that indicate the predicted level of improvement in function			
2. Statement of interventions to be used; whether a PTA will provide some interventions			
3. Proposed duration and frequency of service required to reach the goals (number of visits per week, number of weeks, etc)			
4. Anticipated discharge plans			
Authentication:			
1. Signature, title, and license number (if required by state law)			

FORM A   Develop a documentation review checklist. (Courtesy American Physical Therapy Association, Alexandria, Va.)

PT Daily Visit Note Elements for Documentation Date:	N/A	Yes	No
1. Date			
2. Cancellations and no-shows			
3. Patient/client self-report (as appropriate) and subjective response to previous treatment			
4. Identification of specific interventions provided, including frequency, intensity, and duration as appropriate			
5. Changes in patient/client impairment, activity, and participation status as they relate to the plan of care.			
6. Response to interventions, including adverse reactions, if any.			
7. Factors that modify frequency or intensity of intervention and progression toward anticipated goals, including patient/client adherence to patient/client-related instructions.			
8. Communication/consultation with providers/patient/client/family/ significant other. Patient/caregiver education.			

9. Documentation to plan for ongoing provision of services for the next visit(s), which is suggested to include, but not be limited to:
          The interventions with objectives
          Progression parameters
          Precautions, if indicated			

10. Continuation of or modifications in plan of care			
11. Signature, title, and license number (if required by state law)			

PT Progress Report Elements for Documentation ** Date:	N/A	Yes	No
1. Labeled as a Progress Report/Note or Summary of Progress 2. Date			
3. Cancellations and no-shows			
4. Treatment information regarding the current status of the patient/client			
5. Update of the baseline information provided at the initial evaluation and any needed reevaluation(s)			
6. Documentation of the extent of progress (or lack thereof) between the patient/client's current functioning/disability and that of the previous progress report or at the initial evaluation			
7. Factors that modify frequency or intensity of intervention and progression toward anticipated goals, including patient/client adherence to patient/client-related instructions.			
8. Communication/consultation with providers/patient/client/family/significant other. Patient/caregiver education.			
9. Documentation of any modifications in the plan of care (i.e., goals, interventions, prognosis)			
10. Signature, title, and license number (if required by state law)			

** The physical therapist may be required by state law or by a payer, such as Medicare, to write a progress report. The daily note is not sufficient for this purpose unless it includes the elements listed above.

FORM A—cont'd

PT Re-examination Elements for Documentation Date:	N/A	Yes	No
1. Date			
2. Documentation of selected components of examination to update patients/client's impairment, function, and/or disability status.			
3. Interpretation of findings and, when indicated, revision of goals.			
4. Changes from previous objective findings			
5. Interpretation of results			
6. When indicated, modification of plan of care, as directly correlated with goals as documented.			
7. Signature, title, and license number (if required by state law)			

PT Discharge/Discontinuation/Final Visit Elements for Documentation Date: Note: discharge summary must be written by the PT and may be combined with the final visit note if seen by the PT on final visit	N/A	Yes	No
1. Date			
2. Criteria for termination of services			
3. Current physical/functional status.			
4. Degree of goals and outcomes achieved and reasons for goals and outcomes not being achieved.			
5. Discharge/discontinuation plan that includes written and verbal communication related to the patient/client's continuing care.			
6. Signature, title, and license number (if required by state law)			

PTA Visit Note Elements for Documentation Date:	N/A	Yes	No
1. Date			
2. Cancellations and no-shows			
3. Patient/client self-report (as appropriate) and subjective response to previous treatment			
4. Identification of specific interventions provided, including frequency, intensity, and duration as appropriate and as established by the PT in the plan of care.			
5. Changes in patient/client impairment, activity, and participation status as they relate to the interventions provided.			
6. Subjective response to interventions, including adverse reactions, if any			
7. Continuation of intervention(s) as established by the PT or change of intervention(s) as authorized by PT. Consultation with PT or other healthcare provider is documented.			
8. Signature, title, and license number (if required by state law)			

FORM A—cont'd

Strength & Range of Motion					
Extremities & Trunk:		Strength		ROM	
		Left	Right	Left	Right
Neck	Flexion				
	Extension				
	Rotation				
Shoulder	Flexion 0-180°				
	Extension 0-45°				
	Abduction 0-180°				
	Int Rot 0-70°				
	Ext Rot 0-90°				
Elbow	Flexion 0-145°				
	Extension 0°				
Wrist	Flexion 0-80°				
	Extension 0-70°				
	Fingers				
Trunk	Flexion				
	Extension				
Hip	Flexion 0-125°				
	Extension 0-10°				
	Abduction 0-45°				
	Adduction 0-10°				
	Int Rot 0-45°				
	Ext Rot 0-45°				
Knee	Flexion 0-140°				
	Extension 0°				
Ankle	Dorsiflex 0-20°				
	Plantarflex 0-45°				
	Inversion 0-40°				
	Eversion 0-20°				

FORM B   A sample form used for an examination of strength and range of motion. Norm values from Randall et al. (1993).

BODY DIAGRAM

Name:_____ Date:_____

Directions: On the body diagram below, please mark the areas of your symptoms as they are at this moment of your evaluation.

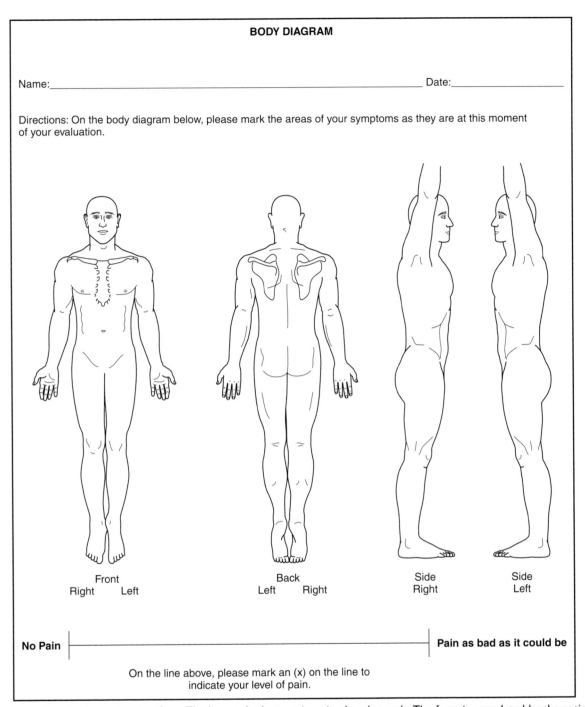

Front	Back	Side	Side
Right Left	Left Right	Right	Left

No Pain |————————————————————————————| **Pain as bad as it could be**

On the line above, please mark an (x) on the line to
indicate your level of pain.

FORM C   A sample pain documentation form. The line at the bottom is a visual analog scale. The form is completed by the patient and should be included as part of the medical record.

Wong-Baker FACES Pain Rating Scale

All patients may experience some pain from cancer or cancer treatment. Only the patient knows how much pain he/she has. Patients need to be able to communicate their pain to members of the health care team as well as to family members.

Communicating the Pain

Using a pain rating scale, like the one below, is helpful for young patients to communicate how much pain they are feeling.

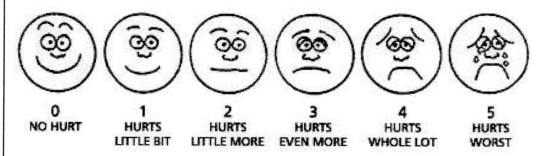

| 0 | 1 | 2 | 3 | 4 | 5 |
| NO HURT | HURTS LITTLE BIT | HURTS LITTLE MORE | HURTS EVEN MORE | HURTS WHOLE LOT | HURTS WORST |

Wong-Baker FACES Pain Rating Scale

Instructions

Explain to the child that each face is for a person who feels happy because he has no pain (hurt) or sad because he has some or a lot of pain.

Face 0 is very happy because he doesn't hurt at all.
Face 1 hurts just a little bit.
Face 2 hurts a little more.
Face 3 hurts even more.
Face 4 hurts a whole lot more.
Face 5 hurts as much as you can imagine, although you do not have to be crying to feel this bad.

Ask the child to choose the face that best describes how he/she is feeling

From Wong, DL, Hockenberry-Eaton M, Wilson D, Winkelstein ML, Schwartz P: *Wong's Essentials of Pediatric Nursing*, ed. 6, St. Louis, 2001, p.1301. Copyrighted by Mosby, Inc. Reprinted by permission.

FORM D   The FACES scale to document pain in younger clients. (From Wong, DL, Hockenberry-Eaton M, Wilson D, et al. *Wong's essentials of pediatric nursing*, ed. 6, St Louis, 2001, Mosby, p 1301.)

PHYSICAL THERAPY HOMECARE INITIAL EVALUATION

Name:_____ D.O.B.:_____ Date of Evaluation visit:_____

Address:_____ Phone:_____

Primary MD:_____ Phone:_____

Admitting Diagnosis/date of onset:_____

Past Medical History:_____

_____

Home living situation:_____

Prior functional status:_____

Employment/Recreation/Social Activities:_____

_____

HOME SAFETY ASSESSMENT:

	Safe	Unsafe	Comments/Action taken
1. Kitchen			
2. Bathroom			
3. Living room			
4. Bedroom			
5. Hallways			
6. Stairs in the home			
7. Stairs outside the home			
8. Equiment in the home Specify:_____			
9. Other Specify:_____			

SITTING/STANDING ABILITY *(indicate time & physical limitations, environmental modification and amount of assistance)*

	STATIC	REACTIVE	PROACTIVE
Sitting	Independent	Able to maintain	Able to reach in all directions
	Needs assist	Unable to maintain	Reaching limited
Comments	_____	_____	_____
	_____	_____	_____
Standing	Independent	Able to maintain	Able to reach in all directions
	Needs assist	Unable to maintain	Reaching limited
Comments	_____	_____	_____
	_____	_____	_____

Standardized tests: ❏ Berg Balance Scale_____ ❏ Activities of Balance Confidence_____ ❏ Other:_____

FORM E   A sample evaluation form used in a home care setting. This form standardizes data collected by therapists while allowing opportunity for narrative descriptions of a patient's functional abilities and impairments.

DAILY LIVING SKILLS

Activity	Assist Code	Comments (strategy, speed, endurance)	Activity	Assist Code	Comments (strategy, speed, endurance)
Bed mobility			Assumes standing position		
Assumes sitting from supine position in bed			Negotiates thresholds		
Lying down in bed from sitting position			Negotiates stairs		
Transfers bed to wheelchair			Bathing		
Transfers to tub			Dressing		
Transfers to toilet			Grooming		
Management of wheelchair			Feeding		
Wheelchair mobility			Housework		
Negotiates doorways			Meal prep		

AMBULATION

Device(s) used:_____

Weight Bearing Status:_____

Assistance needed (see assist code):_____

Distance:_____ time:_____ # steps:_____

Gait:_____
_____

FORM E—cont'd

IMPAIRMENTS

Passive Range of Motion

Upper:_____

Lower:_____

Trunk & Neck:_____

*Strength/AROM:*_____

_____

Posture: Sitting_____

Standing_____

*Skin Integrity*_____

Sensation   Normal   Abnormal   _____

*Pain:*_____

*Neurological Findings:*_____

Babinski: Positive   Negative   Reflexes:_____

Clonus: Present   Absent   Muscle tone:_____

Cardiopulmonary/Vital signs: HR_____   BP_____   RR_____   Comments:_____

*Cognitive/mental status:*_____

Other: (include other systems review or pertinent impairments):_____

_____

===

Patient education/home instructions_____

_____

Patient goals:_____

Patient attitude:_____

Short Range Goals (indicate time frame for each):_____

_____

_____

Long Range Goals (indicate time frame for each):_____

_____

_____

Plan of care:_____

_____

_____

Recommendations:_____

_____

_____   _____
Therapist's name   Therapist's signature

FORM E—cont'd

INPATIENT REHABILITATION FACILITY – PATIENT ASSESSMENT INSTRUMENT

Identification Information*

1. Facility Information
   A. Facility Name
   _____
   _____
   _____

   B. Facility Medicare
      Provider Number _____

2. Patient Medicare Number _____

3. Patient Medicaid Number _____

4. Patient First Name _____

5A. Patient Last Name _____

5B. Patient Identification Number _____

6. Birth Date _____ / _____ / _____
                   MM / DD / YYYY

7. Social Security Number _____

8. Gender (1 - Male; 2 - Female) _____

9. Race/Ethnicity (Check all that apply)
   American Indian or Alaska Native A. _____
   Asian B. _____
   Black or African American C. _____
   Hispanic or Latino D. _____
   Native Hawaiian or Other Pacific Islander E. _____
   White F. _____

10. Marital Status _____
    (1 - Never Married; 2 - Married; 3 - Widowed;
    4 - Separated; 5 - Divorced)

11. Zip Code of Patient's Pre-Hospital Residence _____

Admission Information*

12. Admission Date _____ / _____ / _____
                    MM / DD / YYYY

13. Assessment Reference Date _____ / _____ / _____
                    MM / DD / YYYY

14. Admission Class _____
    (1 - Initial Rehab; 2 - Evaluation; 3 - Readmission;
    4 - Unplanned Discharge; 5 - Continuing Rehabilitation)

15. Admit From _____
    (01 - Home; 02 - Board & Care; 03 - Transitional Living;
    04 - Intermediate Care; 05 - Skilled Nursing Facility;
    06 - Acute Unit of Own Facility; 07 - Acute Unit of Another
    Facility; 08 - Chronic Hospital; 09 - Rehabilitation Facility;
    10 - Other; 12 - Alternate Level of Care Unit; 13 – Subacute
    Setting; 14 - Assisted Living Residence)

16. Pre-Hospital Living Setting _____
    (Use codes from item 15 above)

17. Pre-Hospital Living With _____
    (Code only if item 16 is 01 - Home;
    Code using 1 - Alone; 2 - Family/Relatives;
    3 - Friends; 4 - Attendant; 5 - Other)

18. Pre-Hospital Vocational Category _____
    (1 - Employed; 2 - Sheltered; 3 - Student;
    4 - Homemaker; 5 - Not Working; 6 - Retired for
    Age; 7 - Retired for Disability)

19. Pre-Hospital Vocational Effort _____
    (Code only if item 18 is coded 1 - 4; Code using
    1 - Full-time; 2 - Part-time; 3 - Adjusted Workload)

Payer Information*

20. Payment Source
    A. Primary Source _____

    B. Secondary Source _____

    (01 - Blue Cross; 02 - Medicare non-MCO;
    03 - Medicaid non-MCO; 04 - Commercial Insurance;
    05 - MCO HMO; 06 - Workers' Compensation;
    07 - Crippled Children's Services; 08 – Developmental
    Disabilities Services; 09 - State Vocational Rehabilitation;
    10 - Private Pay; 11 - Employee Courtesy;
    12 - Unreimbursed; 13 - CHAMPUS; 14 - Other;
    15 - None; 16 – No-Fault Auto Insurance;
    51 – Medicare MCO; 52 - Medicaid MCO)

Medical Information*

21. Impairment Group _____ _____
                    Admission Discharge
    Condition requiring admission to rehabilitation; code
    according to Appendix A, attached.

22. Etiologic Diagnosis _____
    (Use an ICD-9-CM code to indicate the etiologic problem
    that led to the condition for which the patient is receiving
    rehabilitation)

23. Date of Onset of Impairment _____ / _____ / _____
                    MM / DD / YYYY

24. Comorbid Conditions; Use ICD-9-CM codes to enter up to
    ten medical conditions

    A. _____   B. _____

    C. _____   D. _____

    E. _____   F. _____

    G. _____   H. _____

    I. _____   J. _____

Medical Needs

25. Is patient comatose at admission? _____
                    0 - No, 1 - Yes

26. Is patient delirious at admission? _____
                    0 - No, 1 - Yes

27. Swallowing Status _____ _____
                    Admission Discharge

    3 - _Regular Food_: solids and liquids swallowed safely
        without supervision or modified food consistency
    2 - _Modified Food Consistency/ Supervision_: subject
        requires modified food consistency and/or needs
        supervision for safety
    1 - _Tube /Parenteral Feeding_: tube / parenteral feeding
        used wholly or partially as a means of sustenance

28. Clinical signs of dehydration _____ _____
                    Admission Discharge

    (Code 0 – No; 1 – Yes) e.g., evidence of oliguria, dry
    skin, orthostatic hypotension, somnolence, agitation

*The FIM data set, measurement scale and impairment
codes incorporated or referenced herein are the property of
U B Foundation Activities, Inc. ©1993, 2001 U B Foundation
Activities. Inc. The FIM mark is owned by UBFA. Inc.

FORM F The Inpatient Rehabilitation Facility–Patient Assessment Instrument (IRF-PAI). Information on the IRF-PAI is collected for all Medicare Part A fee-for-service patients who receive services under Part A from an inpatient rehabilitation facility. (Courtesy Department of Health and Human Services, Centers for Medicare & Medicaid Services.)

INPATIENT REHABILITATION FACILITY – PATIENT ASSESSMENT INSTRUMENT

Function Modifiers*

Complete the following specific functional items prior to scoring the FIM™ Instrument:

	ADMISSION	DISCHARGE
29. Bladder Level of Assistance (Score using FIM Levels 1 - 7)	☐	☐
30. Bladder Frequency of Accidents (Score as below)	☐	☐

7 - No accidents
6 - No accidents; uses device such as a catheter
5 - One accident in the past 7 days
4 - Two accidents in the past 7 days
3 - Three accidents in the past 7 days
2 - Four accidents in the past 7 days
1 - Five or more accidents in the past 7 days

Enter in Item 39G (Bladder) the lower (more dependent) score from Items 29 and 30 above.

	ADMISSION	DISCHARGE
31. Bowel Level of Assistance (Score using FIM Levels 1 - 7)	☐	☐
32. Bowel Frequency of Accidents (Score as below)	☐	☐

7 - No accidents
6 - No accidents; uses device such as an ostomy
5 - One accident in the past 7 days
4 - Two accidents in the past 7 days
3 - Three accidents in the past 7 days
2 - Four accidents in the past 7 days
1 - Five or more accidents in the past 7 days

Enter in Item 39H (Bowel) the lower (more dependent) score of Items 31 and 32 above.

	ADMISSION	DISCHARGE
33. Tub Transfer	☐	☐
34. Shower Transfer	☐	☐

(Score Items 33 and 34 using FIM Levels 1 - 7; use 0 if activity does not occur) See training manual for scoring of Item 39K (Tub/Shower Transfer)

	ADMISSION	DISCHARGE
35. Distance Walked	☐	☐
36. Distance Traveled in Wheelchair	☐	☐

(Code items 35 and 36 using: 3 - 150 feet; 2 - 50 to 149 feet; 1 - Less than 50 feet; 0 – activity does not occur)

	ADMISSION	DISCHARGE
37. Walk	☐	☐
38. Wheelchair	☐	☐

(Score Items 37 and 38 using FIM Levels 1 - 7; 0 if activity does not occur) See training manual for scoring of Item 39L (Walk/Wheelchair)

*The FIM data set, measurement scale and impairment codes incorporated or referenced herein are the property of U B Foundation Activities, Inc. ©1993, 2001 U B Foundation Activities, Inc. The FIM mark is owned by UBFA, Inc.

39. FIM™ Instrument*

	ADMISSION	DISCHARGE	GOAL
SELF-CARE			
A. Eating	☐	☐	☐
B. Grooming	☐	☐	☐
C. Bathing	☐	☐	☐
D. Dressing - Upper	☐	☐	☐
E. Dressing - Lower	☐	☐	☐
F. Toileting	☐	☐	☐
SPHINCTER CONTROL			
G. Bladder	☐	☐	☐
H. Bowel	☐	☐	☐
TRANSFERS			
I. Bed, Chair, Whlchair	☐	☐	☐
J. Toilet	☐	☐	☐
K. Tub, Shower	☐	☐	☐

W - Walk
C - wheelChair
B - Both

LOCOMOTION	ADMISSION	DISCHARGE	GOAL
L. Walk/Wheelchair	☐ ☐	☐ ☐	☐
M. Stairs	☐	☐	☐

A - Auditory
V - Visual
B - Both

COMMUNICATION	ADMISSION	DISCHARGE	GOAL
N. Comprehension	☐ ☐	☐ ☐	☐
O. Expression	☐ ☐	☐ ☐	☐

V - Vocal
N - Nonvocal
B - Both

SOCIAL COGNITION	ADMISSION	DISCHARGE	GOAL
P. Social Interaction	☐	☐	☐
Q. Problem Solving	☐	☐	☐
R. Memory	☐	☐	☐

FIM LEVELS

No Helper
7 Complete Independence (Timely, Safely)

6 Modified Independence (Device)

Helper - Modified Dependence
5 Supervision (Subject = 100%)

4 Minimal Assistance (Subject = 75% or more)

3 Moderate Assistance (Subject = 50% or more)

Helper - Complete Dependence
2 Maximal Assistance (Subject = 25% or more)

1 Total Assistance (Subject less than 25%)

0 Activity does not occur; Use this code only at admission

FORM F—cont'd

INPATIENT REHABILITATION FACILITY – PATIENT ASSESSMENT INSTRUMENT

Discharge Information*

40. Discharge Date

                         __ / __ / ____
                         MM / DD / YYYY

41. Patient discharged against medical advice?

                       (0 - No, 1 -Yes)

42. Program Interruption(s)

                       (0 - No; 1 - Yes)

43. Program Interruption Dates
    (Code only if Item 42 is 1 - Yes)

A. 1st Interruption Date   B. 1st Return Date

    MM / DD / YYYY   MM / DD / YYYY

C. 2nd Interruption Date   D. 2nd Return Date

    MM / DD / YYYY   MM / DD / YYYY

E. 3rd Interruption Date   F. 3rd Return Date

    MM / DD / YYYY   MM / DD / YYYY

44A. Discharge to Living Setting
    (01 - Home; 02 - Board and Care; 03 - Transitional Living; 04 - Intermediate Care; 05 - Skilled Nursing Facility; 06 - Acute Unit of Own Facility; 07 - Acute Unit of Another Facility; 08 - Chronic Hospital; 09 - Rehabilitation Facility; 10 - Other; 11 - Died; 12 - Alternate Level of Care Unit; 13 - Subacute Setting; 14 - Assisted Living Residence)

44B. Was patient discharged with Home Health Services? ____
                               (0 - No; 1 - Yes)
    (Code only if Item 44A is 01 - Home, 02 - Board and Care, 03 - Transitional Living, or 14 - Assisted Living Residence)

45. Discharge to Living With
    (Code only if Item 44A is 01 - Home; Code using 1 - Alone; 2 - Family / Relatives; 3 - Friends; 4 - Attendant; 5 - Other)

46. Diagnosis for Interruption or Death
    (Code using ICD-9-CM code)

47. Complications during rehabilitation stay
    (Use ICD-9-CM codes to specify up to six conditions that began with this rehabilitation stay)

    A. _____   B. _____

    C. _____   D. _____

    E. _____   F. _____

Quality Indicators

RESPIRATORY STATUS
(Score items 48 to 50 as 0 - No; 1 - Yes)

	Admission	Discharge
48. Shortness of breath with exertion		
49. Shortness of breath at rest		
50. Weak cough and difficulty clearing airway secretions		

*The FIM data set, measurement scale and impairment codes incorporated or referenced herein are the property of U B Foundation Activities, Inc. ©1993, 2001 U B Foundation Activities, Inc. The FIM mark is owned by UBFA, Inc.

FORM F—cont'd

Quality Indicators

PAIN

51. Rate the highest level of pain reported by the patient within the assessment period:

    Admission: _____   Discharge: _____

(Score using the scale below; report whole numbers only)

0	1	2	3	4	5	6	7	8	9	10
No Pain					Moderate Pain					Worst Possible Pain

Pressure Ulcers

52A. Highest current pressure ulcer stage
    Admission _____   Discharge _____

    (0 - No pressure ulcer; 1 - Any area of persistent skin redness (Stage 1); 2 - Partial loss of skin layers (Stage 2); 3 - Deep craters in the skin (Stage 3); 4 - Breaks in skin exposing muscle or bone (Stage 4); 5 - Not stageable (necrotic eschar predominant; no prior staging available)

52B. Number of current pressure ulcers
    Admission _____   Discharge _____

PUSH Tool v. 3.0 ©

SELECT THE CURRENT LARGEST PRESSURE ULCER TO CODE THE FOLLOWING. Calculate three components (C through E) and code total score in F.

52C. Length multiplied by width (open wound surface area)
    Admission _____   Discharge _____

    (Score as   0 - 0 cm^2; 1 - < 0.3 cm^2; 2 - 0.3 to 0.6 cm^2; 3 - 0.7 to 1.0 cm^2 ; 4 - 1.1 to 2.0 cm^2; 5 - 2.1 to 3.0 cm^2; 6 - 3.1 to 4.0 cm^2; 7 - 4.1 to 8.0 cm^2; 8 - 8.1 to 12.0 cm^2; 9 - 12.1 to 24.0 cm^2; 10 - > 24 cm^2)

52D. Exudate amount
    Admission _____   Discharge _____
    0 - None;   1 - Light; 2 - Moderate; 3 - Heavy

52E. Tissue type
    Admission _____   Discharge _____
    0 - Closed/resurfaced: The wound is completely covered with epithelium (new skin); 1 - Epithelial tissue: For superficial ulcers, new pink or shiny tissue (skin) that grows in from the edges or as islands on the ulcer surface. 2 - Granulation tissue: Pink or beefy red tissue with a shiny, moist, granular appearance. 3- Slough: Yellow or white tissue that adheres to the ulcer bed in strings or thick clumps or is mucinous. 4 - Necrotic tissue (eschar): Black, brown, or tan tissue that adheres firmly to the wound bed or ulcer edges.

52F. TOTAL PUSH SCORE (Sum of above three items -- C, D and E)
    Admission _____   Discharge _____

SAFETY   Admission   Discharge

53. Balance problem   _____   _____
    (0 - No; 1 - Yes)
    e.g., dizziness, vertigo, or light-headedness

                                       Discharge

54. Total number of falls during the rehabilitation stay   _____

Index